WOMEN'S GROWTH IN DIVERSITY

WOMEN'S GROWTH IN DIVERSITY

More Writings from the Stone Center

Edited by

JUDITH V. JORDAN

THE GUILFORD PRESS
New York   London

Library of Congress Cataloging-in-Publication Data

Women's growth in diversity : more writings from the Stone Center /
    edited by Judith V. Jordan
        p.   cm..
    Includes bibliographical references and index.
    ISBN 1-57230-205-4 (hc : alk. paper).—ISBN 1-57230-206-2 (pbk.
    alk. paper)
        1. Women—Psychology.   2. Minority women—Psychology.   3. Minority
    women—Social conditions.   4. Marginality, Social—Psychological
    aspects.   5. Psychotherapy—Social aspects.   I. Jordan, Judith V.
    II. Stone Center for Developmental Services and Studies.
    HQ1206.W863   1997
    305.4—dc21   96-52883
                                                        CIP

About the Authors

Stephen Bergman, M.D., Ph.D. Co-Director, Gender Relations Project, the Stone Center. Psychiatrist, Harvard Medical School.

Cynthia García Coll, Ph.D. Professor of Education, Psychology, and Pediatrics, Chair of the Education Department, and Associate Director of the Center for the Study of Human Development at Brown University. Former Director of the Stone Center.

Natalie Eldridge, Ph.D. Clinical Coordinator of the Boston University Counseling Center. Member of the Lesbian Theory Group at the Stone Center. Steering committee of the Feminist Therapy Institute. Faculty of the Jean Baker Miller Training Institute.

Judith V. Jordan, Ph.D. Director of Training and Founding Scholar, Jean Baker Miller Institute at the Stone Center. Member, Diversity Theory Group, the Stone Center. Assistant Professor in Psychology at Harvard Medical School. Former Director of Women's Treatment Network and Psychology Training, McLean Hospital. Attending Psychologist, McLean Hospital.

Alexandra Kaplan, Ph.D. Former Director of the Counseling Program at the Stone Center. Lecturer in Psychiatry at the Harvard Medical School. Member Diversity Process Group, the Stone Center.

Julie Mencher, M.S.W. Psychotherapist, Mount Holyoke College Counseling Center. Adjunct Faculty, Smith College for Social Work. Affiliated Scholar, the Stone Center. Faculty, Jean Baker Miller Training Institute.

Jean Baker Miller, M.D. Clinical Professor of Psychiatry, Boston University School of Medicine. Director, Jean Baker Miller Training Institute. Founding scholar and former Director, the Stone Center.

Robin Cook-Nobles, Ed.D. Chief Psychologist and Director of Counseling Services, the Stone Center. Faculty, the Jean Baker Miller Training Institute. Member, Diversity Process Group, the Stone Center.

Wendy Rosen, M.S.W., Ph.D. Attending staff at McLean Hospital. Faculty of the Jean Baker Miller Training Institute. Adjunct faculty of Smith College School for Social Work. Board of Advisors for the Massachusetts Institute for Gay, Lesbian, and Bisexual Studies. Member of the Stone Center Lesbian Theory Group.

Suzanne Slater, M.S.W. Member of the Stone Center Lesbian Theory Group. Faculty of the Jean Baker Miller Training Institute.

Irene Stiver, Ph.D. Founding Scholar, Jean Baker Miller Institute at the Stone Center. Senior Consultant, McLean Hospital. Lecturer, Harvard Medical School. Former Director of the Psychology Department, McLean Hospital.

Janet Surrey, Ph.D. Founding Scholar, Jean Baker Miller Institute at the Stone Center. Co-director of Gender Relations Project, the Stone Center. Member Diversity Theory Group, the Stone Center. Attending Psychologist, McLean Hospital. Instructor, Harvard Medical School.

Beverly Daniel Tatum, Ph.D. Professor of Psychology and Education at Mount Holyoke College. Former Visiting Scholar at the Stone Center.

Clevonne Watkins Turner, M.S.W. Assistant Director of Continuing Education and Adjunct Faculty Instructor at the University of Tennessee College of Social Work, Knoxville. Former Assistant Clinical Director of the Stone Center.

Contents

WOMEN'S GROWTH IN DIVERSITY

Introduction

JUDITH V. JORDAN

Since the publication of *Women's Growth In Connection* those of us working at, and with, the Stone Center at Wellesley College have taken some new directions in our efforts to broaden and deepen our understanding of women's development. We have also sought to address more explicitly the differences that exist among many women from different backgrounds, be they racial, cultural, socioeconomic, or involving sexual orientation. This volume is one part of our ongoing work to extend the relational model, in both societal and clinical applications.

Our initial work, developed in a spirit of trying to better understand women and give voice to women's special paths of development, contained a clear, acknowledged bias: it represented largely white, middle-class, well-educated heterosexual experience. While we struggled not to reproduce the errors that occur when one subgroup speaks as if *its* reality is *the* reality, we inevitably were bound by our own blindspots and biases. We became more and more aware of the dangers of speaking about or for "all women." We were indeed speaking about "some women" or about partial aspects of many women's experience. Our appreciation of diversity needed to be broadened and deepened. Early on we attempted to facilitate the creation of expanded theory and research by bringing together groups of women with differing life experiences. A lesbian theory group was established and members of that group have contributed to the Stone Center theory and colloquia in many ways. Two study groups of women of color and white women have also been meeting to grapple with the complexities of trying to represent the many different experiences of women. Most recently a group of women with disabilities and chronic illness have begun to work on theory building. In addition, invited presenters at the Stone Center have contributed to our knowledge about diverse cultural experiences. While we have begun to appreciate more deeply the powerful learning that occurs across diversity, we have by no means expanded in all the ways we could. We have not yet had representation from Asian American or Native American women. And, very importantly, we have not sufficiently studied or articulated the influence of class for all groups of women.

In this second volume of papers from the Stone Center we wish to invite the reader to accompany us in two directions: to further elaborate selected topics in relational theory such as sexuality, shame, anger, depression, and applications to therapy; and to begin an exploration of some of the richness and complexity that arise from the diverse life experiences of women. While all women suffer in a patriarchal society where our experience is not represented in the dominant discourse, women in various cultural/ethnic groups suffer additional marginalization based on race, sexual orientation, socioeconomic standing, able-bodiedness, and age. Women who are marginalized also develop strengths that may differ from those of white, privileged heterosexual women.

Writers from differing backgrounds, as Kaplan noted, remind us "that those who label themselves the so-called 'mainstream' represent but one small segment of a broad and diverse" range of experience, "and in fact, as privileged women within the world community, constitute a decided minority" (Kaplan, 1991, p. 6). Unfortunately those in a dominant position often "presume the right to determine which aspects of identities are core, and by which aspects others will be known" (Kaplan, p. 6); "people are known only in terms of where they fit in an arbitrary hierarchy of worth as defined by the dominant culture" (Kaplan, p. 6).

Engaging with difference in relationship can be a source of enlargement and growth. But when differences are organized hierarchically by dominant groups, with some characteristics viewed as "normal" or "desirable" and others as deviant or undesirable, diversity can be a source of disempowerment and pain.

Both white people and people of color are affected by "white privilege" (McIntosh, 1988) as well as sexist, classist, and heterosexist privilege. It is crucial that those who enjoy the privilege of being part of the dominant group know and acknowledge that privilege, not to move into a state of guilt, but to take responsibility for the impact of that privilege on themselves and on those who do not enjoy it. And we need to develop a clear and active sense of responsibility and awareness of the impact of this privilege in shaping and limiting our own growth and understanding of the larger world. It is equally important that we all recognize and take responsibility for the biases and assumptions which result from that privilege. These biases contribute to major disconnections at a societal and personal level.

The Stone Center relational model emphasizes the centrality of connection in women's lives. Disconnection is viewed as the source of most human suffering. In particular, we suggest that women grow through growth fostering relationships. Due to our culture's handling of difference, through a system of hierarchy and dismissal, major, chronic, and painful disconnections occur around diversity; racism, sexism, heterosexism, classism, and ageism all become forces in creating disconnection rather than connection. Often these forces interact in complicated ways creating even deeper and confusing sources of isolation. Differences that could be sources of great growth and expansion instead lead to closing down and withdrawal, fear, shame, and chronic disconnection. A tendency to "blame the victim" or project one's own unwanted vulnerability or anxiety onto others also leads to destructive perceptions and behavior towards marginalized groups. "Empathy across difference," however, can be one of the most compelling paths to personal and relational growth. "While some mutual empathy involves an acknowledgment of sameness in the other, an appreciation of the differentness of the other's experience is also vital. The movement towards the other's differentness is actually central to growth in relationship and also can provide a powerful sense of validation for both people. Growth occurs because as I stretch to match or understand your experience, something new is acknowledged or grows in me" (Jordan, 1986).

In a context of highly individualistic values and antirelational biases, bringing awareness to the profound importance of relationship in people's lives could be thought of as revolutionary. Western culture has devalued women's skills in empathy and our capacity and motivation to foster growth in others. We are advocating not just a more accurate understanding of women (important and essential in and of itself) but we are suggesting a major paradigm shift in all of western psychology . . . from a psychology of the separate self to a psychology of relational being. We are suggesting that we need to put connection rather than "the separate self" or power over others at the center of our focus. This is indeed revolutionary and, we hope, ultimately healing. And this is indeed a work in progress, taking small steps here, leaps there, getting bogged down in the complexities of our own misunderstandings, blindspots, and relational shortcomings. The struggle to work with our own perceptions and misperceptions, to rethink the distorting messages we have grown up with, to re-place ourselves in our social context is a process of internal as well as external revolution and transformation. This is a painful, complex but enormously important undertaking. Again, we invite the reader to join us in our journey of exploration and hope.

The book begins with some general review and preliminary updating of the relational approach. The first chapter, "A Relational Perspective for Understanding Women's Development," presents a summary of many of the core ideas of the Stone Center relational model of development. It examines some of the convergences with, and differences from, other psychodynamic theories and suggests the usefulness of moving from a psychology of separate self to a psychology of relational being.

In "Some Misconceptions and Reconceptions of a Relational Approach," the authors individually address several recurring questions that have been posed regarding the Stone Center model of women's development. Jean Baker Miller first discusses the concern, expressed by some, that our model idealizes women and relationships. Judith Jordan looks at the usefulness of the concepts of self and autonomy in understanding women's experience. Alexandra Kaplan examines some of the core ideas (presented elsewhere in this book) which have to do with how the Stone Center model has dealt with diversity and essentialism. Irene Stiver responds to some clinical questions, especially the role of transference in relational therapy, and Janet Surrey continues the exploration of therapy by looking at how we use the concept of mutuality in therapy. Many of these themes are also elaborated in later chapters of the book.

In a continuing emphasis on theory development, Judith Jordan (Chapter 3) first looks at two broad ways of conceptualizing and organizing our ways of being in the world: the power/control mode and the empathy/love mode. She then goes on to point out how boys and girls are socialized differently regarding these two modes and how this may create complications for adolescents as they attempt to relate to one another.

Clevonne Turner's chapter, "Clinical Applications of the Stone Center Theoretical Approach to Minority Women," emphasizes the importance of connection and relatedness in black women's lives. Turner notes that the relational approach validates important parts of black women's maturation process. She further suggests that racial oppression and the requirement to be bicultural in this country increase the possibilities for connectedness of women within the oppressed culture. These experiences often enhance a sense of connection to people of other marginalized groups.

Continuing the themes of relational theory and black women's development, in "Racial Identity Development and Relational Theory: The Case of Black Women in White Communities," Beverly Tatum examines the connection between racial identity development theory and relational theory. The points of intersection between these two theoretical perspectives are used to understand the experiences of young black women growing up in predominantly white communities. Racial identity development theory describes a process of moving from internalized racism to a position of empowerment based on a positively affirmed sense of racial identity. As Tatum notes, racism is "a pervasive system of advantage based on race . . . , which has personal, cultural, and institutional implications for our daily lives. . . . [W]e must acknowledge its daily impact on interpersonal relationships. If mutual empathy requires the interest and motivation to know the other, then everyday racism often, if not always, represents the failure of mutual empathy."

In "The Conundrum of Mutuality: A Lesbian Dialogue," Natalie Eldridge, Julie Mencher, and Suzanne Slater explore different aspects of mutuality in psychotherapy with lesbian clients and lesbian therapists. In the first of these three separate sections, Mencher examines the structural elements in the therapeutic relationship, particularly issues related to the power and role differentials inherent in the therapy relationship, the therapist's uses of herself and the construction of boundaries. Next, Slater looks at the development of intimacy in the therapeutic relationship. Eldridge outlines principles of ethical thinking from a relational orientation and offers practical suggestions for an ethical use of mutuality in psychotherapy.

In "Relational Development: Therapeutic Implications of Empathy and Shame," Jordan suggests that we need to move away from "the self" as the basic unit of study with its corresponding emphasis on independence, security, and separation from others. Instead she suggests we begin to learn more about "relational development." Because the need for connection is basic, experiences of disconnection or isolation become important for us to understand. Shame involves a profound sense of longing for connection and feeling unworthy to be in connection; this is a major force in the lives of most women and other marginalized groups. The action of shaming people also serves as a major weapon by any dominant group to silence nondominant or marginalized people's views of reality. It behooves us, then, to pay careful attention to shame in social, developmental, and therapeutic arenas.

In "Psychosocial Barriers to Black Women's Career Development," Clevonne Turner looks at the burdens of racism, sexism, classism, and ageism in the lives of black women. While emphasizing the particularity of each multifaceted person, often hidden in the words Black, female or "other," Turner presents some common themes and threads that "most Black women share with each other more than with other women." She explores in particular the themes of inclusion–exclusion, "not belonging." She concludes with a review of coping strategies.

In "Building Connection through Diversity," drawing upon personal experience and the Stone Center relational model of connections and disconnections, Coll, Cook-Nobles, and Surrey explore the questions of what interferes with the development of cross-cultural connections and what is needed for the establishment of such connections. This is done from the point of view of three women coming from very different backgrounds: a colonial, culturally and racially mixed Caribbean island society (Puerto Rican), the racially segregated South just before the civil rights movement (African American), and a white, Jewish, middle class community.

In "Revisioning Women's Anger," Miller first points out that anger is a necessary part of the movement of relationships. Anger is a signal that something is wrong, that something "hurts" in a relationship, that something needs to change. Miller then goes on to point out the complications that occur in relationships when anger is not allowed expression. In order for anger to be a resource in relationships, the relationship needs to be safe for each person to express anger. Clearly not all relationships or social contexts create that safety and it is important for women to distinguish between these (e.g., acknowledging anger is not safe for many marginalized groups). Surrey addresses the shared anger and vulnerability that many women feel and suggests that this can be a source of positive action and an important response to injustice.

The final four chapters of the book attempt to extend the model by reframing several clinical concepts. In Stiver and Miller's "From Depression to Sadness in Women's Psychotherapy," the authors examine some of the reasons for the higher incidence of depression in women and they make a distinction between sadness and depression. In fact, Stiver and Miller suggest that a primary task in therapy with depressed women is to help them move into the more effectively clear and intense state of sadness. Movement into sadness involves the capacity to bring feelings such as sadness and anger more authentically into relationship.

Wendy Rosen points out in "On the Integration of Sexuality: Lesbians and their Mothers" that "the bulk of clinical literature on homosexuality is riddled with heterosexist and homophobic assumptions, and thus, inevitably casts lesbianism in a pathological light." Rosen also points out that most of the literature, whether biased or gay-affirmative, is focused on gay men. Lesbians are underrepresented in the literature. Using the relational concepts of mutual empathy, relationship authenticity, and relationship differentiation, Wendy Rosen looks at the process of disclosure/coming-out for lesbians. She gives us a clear picture of a cultural context characterized by sexism and heterosexism in which this disclosure process occurs. By providing us with a clinical case example, Rosen enriches and deepens our understanding of this complex process.

Bergman and Surrey, in "The Woman–Man Relationship: Impasses and Possibilities," describe a format of workshops designed to bring men and women together to explore the impact of gender differences in relationships and to provide a context in which to work towards creating mutuality in woman–man relationships. They identify prototypical impasses between women and men, suggest structures to help relationships move through these impasses and describe different pathways to mutuality.

In "A Relational Approach to Therapeutic Impasses," Stiver explores the inevitability of impasses in the course of therapy and notes that their resolution can lead to growth and change in both therapist and patient. Stiver explains the paradox of connections and disconnections and how to understand the dynamics of these impasses and guides us in our efforts to move the therapy out of impasse and into more authentic relationship.

Julie Mencher's "Intimacy in Lesbian Relationships: A Critical Reexamination of Fusion" explores the relational patterns of lesbian couples from the perspective of the Stone Center model. She suggests that the dynamics that have been called "fusion" do not necessarily create or represent pathology in lesbian relationship and that the intense intimacy in lesbian relationships actually leads to a high degree of expressed satisfaction. Mencher reframes the notion of fusion in lesbian relationships in such a way that the positive, constructive qualities of these relational patterns are seen.

This volume brings together several threads of the relational patterns which remain loosely woven. We hope that we stimulate the reader to search for connections among the various points of view. The similarities and differences among people can be both challenging and reassuring; they can be a source of exhilarating connection and profoundly disturbing disconnection. As we continue to struggle with relating across difference in a culture that has done little to assist us in working creatively with difference, we hope for growth and a greater sense of connection and empowerment. In a process of mutual empowerment between two people, both people are transformed. Potentially, in a broader movement of mutual empowerment, chronic disconnections between groups of people can be transformed. We believe mutual relationships are the source of healing and growth. We are all joined in our primary need for this healing and growth. We hope that this volume will aid in the journey towards growth, understanding, and increasing connection at a personal and societal level. Perhaps the essence of our being as humans is contained in the simple words of E. M. Forster, who wrote in *Howard's End*: "Only connect."

These chapters, "works in progress," are stepping stones in our own continuing search for a more full and accurate portrayal of women's life experiences. We look forward to future volumes in which we can present currently evolving ideas. Simply by listening more carefully to all women's experience and by learning to speak as clearly as we can the many truths we hear, we hope we will contribute to an increasingly accurate representation of women's lives. Ultimately, our goal is to develop an appreciation of the centrality of connection to life itself and thereby, we believe, to increase our understanding of all people's lives.

REFERENCES

Jordan, J. (1986). *The meaning of mutuality*. (Work in Progress No. 23.) Wellesley, MA: Stone Center Working Paper Series.

Kaplan, A. (1991). *How can a group of white, heterosexual women claim to speak of "women's" experience?* (Work in Progress No. 49.) Wellesley, MA: Stone Center Working Paper Series.

McIntosh, P. (1988). *White privilege and male privilege: A personal account of coming to see correspondence through work in women's studies.* (Working Paper No. 189.) Wellesley, MA: Center for Research on Women.

1

A Relational Perspective
for Understanding
Women's Development

JUDITH V. JORDAN

In traditional Western psychological theories of development, the "self" has long been viewed as the primary reality and unit of study. Typically, the self has been seen as separated out from its context, a bounded, contained entity that has both object and subject qualities. Clinical and developmental theories generally have emphasized the growth of an autonomous, individuated self. Increasing self-control, a sense of self as origin of action and intention, an increasing capacity to use abstract logic, and a movement toward self-sufficiency characterize the maturation of the ideal Western self. Although most theorists have struggled with the issue of reification of the self, all have to some degree succumbed to the powerful pull to de-contextualize, abstract, and spatialize this concept. I will examine some of these models in terms of their limited applicability to the psychology of women and suggest an alternative conceptualization of self, a "relational self" or, as Jean Miller has suggested, a model of "being in relation" (Miller, 1984).

ESTABLISHED THEORY

Several biases have prominently shaped clinical-developmental theory about the self. Psychology as a discipline emulated Newtonian physics, seeking thus to be recognized as a bona fide "hard" science rather than as an arm of philosophy, theology, or other humanistic traditions. Newtonian physics posited discrete, separate entities existing in space and acting on each other in predictable and measurable ways. This easily led to a study of the self as a comparably bounded and contained "molecular" entity, a notion most visibly supported by the existence of separate body-identities. It became very seductive to equate self with embodied person. As Helen Lynd notes:

> The assumption that understanding proceeds by means of first seeking the discrete, supposedly unchanging elements into which a phenomenon under study can be analyzed and only later turning attention to the changes going on in the elements and to the relations among them is still very much with us. (Lynd, 1958, p. 67)

> The separation having been initially assumed, the problems of relation and integration are posed. (Lynd, 1958, p. 81).

A further influence on theory building about the self was provided by the social–political context in Western, democratic societies, where the sanctity and freedom of the individual greatly overshadowed the compelling reality of the communal and deeply interdependent nature of human beings. In this societal paradigm, as represented particularly in the American culture, there is an imperative in socializing children to wean the "helpless" and "dependent" infant toward greater self-sufficiency and independence; so engrained is this bias that it is hard for most of us to appreciate that other cultures may in fact perceive the infant as born independent and needing acculturation toward dependency!

Major support for the "separate self" model came from Freudian theory. While Freud did not explicitly theorize about the self, his original "das Ich," later translated as "ego," had much in common with the subjective "I" aspect of self delineated by James (1890/1968). Certainly, many of his ideas have been influential in subsequent concepts of the self. Specifically, his understanding of the psyche grew from a view of pathology in which the ego was seen as coming into being to protect the person from assaults both by internal impulses and external demands. Its relational function was obscured. Freud commented that, "Protection against stimuli is an almost more important function for the living organism than reception of stimuli" (Freud, 1920/1955, p. 27). Derivative psycho-analytic theories view the individual as growing from an undifferentiated, then embedded and symbiotic phase into an ultimately separate, individuated state (Mahler, Pine, & Bergman, 1975). Until quite recently in psychoanalytic theories, healthier, more mature modes of functioning were predicated on greater separation of self and other.

Furthermore, Freudian theory stressed the power of innate instinctual forces and the development of increasing internal structure and freedom from dependence on others for gratification of needs. Relationships were seen as secondary to or deriving from the satisfaction of primary drives (e.g. hunger or sex). Intrapsychic development was seen as the ultimate area of interest; and "self development" (or ego development) was seen as a process of internalization of resources from caretakers and others to create an increasingly unique, separate, self-sufficient structure: the self. Connotations of control, ownership of action, and mastery over both impulses and outer reality abound in this model.

Pivotal to this individualistic picture of human beings is the pleasure principle (Freud, 1920/1955; Jordan, 1987) Attainment of satisfaction, motivated by desire or need, is framed as the primary goal of behavior and therefore shapes the self. In this tradition (both psychoanalytic and behaviorist) "the self" is the personal history of gratifications and frustrations of desire and the projection of these into the future in the form of intention (Jordan, 1987).

Although disagreements with Freudian theory occurred as quickly as the theory was put forth, the dissenters never gained a hold on the cultural vision of "Man" or on the imagination of clinical practitioners in the way that Freud's original ideas did. Sullivan (1953), in this country, took a major step away from the instinct–drive model, as did Horney (1926/1967) and Thompson (1941). In addition, Sullivan placed the development of the self directly within the interpersonal realm: "A personality can never be isolated from the complex of interpersonal relations in which the person lives and has his being" (1953, p. 10). While this was an enormous contribution and gave impetus to the movement away from construction of the self as separate being, the basic inactivity of the self and the unidirectional quality of development survived in his model. The self was seen as being constructed of "reflected appraisals" (1953).

Erikson's ego identity (1963), comparable in many ways to what others call a sense of self, is importantly constructed as an outcome of a psychosocial line of development; this represents a definite and important move beyond the earlier Freudian psychosexual model. But in Erikson's schema, identity is early predicated on establishment of autonomy. Intimacy is established later, only after identity is consolidated. As such, the basic relationality of development is lost in much of this model.

The object relations theorists in Britain advanced our understanding of the centrality of relationships in human development. But they, unfortunately, were unable to free themselves of many of the core premises of Freudian psychology and continued to view the other person as "object" to the subject; that is, defined by drive factors in the subject. The language and naming of this theory perpetuate the biological approach these theorists struggled against. The bias of an instinctually driven and basically selfish and aggressive being is also carried forward in this theory. Melanie Klein (1953) thus traces the development of a capacity for love to the infant's wish to make reparations to the mother for harm inflicted.

Fairbairn (1946/1952) and Guntrip (1973) distance themselves most clearly from the Freudian model of the developing organism. Fairbairn stated, "It is impossible to gain any adequate conception of the nature of an individual organism if it is considered apart from its relationship to its natural objects, for it is only in its relationship to these objects that its true nature is displayed" (1946/1952, p. 39)

Most recently in the clinical realm, Kohut (1984) has emphasized the ongoing need for relationships throughout life. His concept of the "selfobject" pertains to the importance of others in shaping our self image and maintaining self esteem. But this theory, too, is built on a model of drives, with others used as objects to perform some function for a self that still remains intrinsically and ideally separate, if at best empathically connected.

In a study both psychoanalytic and developmental, Daniel Stern has creatively delineated modes of "being with the other." Early patterns of differentiation and relatedness, in which mother and infant participate in a mutually regulated relationship, are traced in his work (Stern, 1986). Trevarthan (1979) has pointed to a "primary intersubjectivity" in human development, which is innate and unfolding. Earlier, George Klein posited the existence of "we" identities in the development of a concept of self, an "aspect of one's self construed as a necessary part of a unit transcending one's autonomous actions." (G. Klein, 1976, p. 178).

A contextual-relation view of self also has much in common with the earlier work of the symbolic interactionists (Baldwin, 1897/1968; Cooley, 1902/1968; Mead 1925/1968), typified by Mead's idea that "selves exist only in relation to other selves" (Mead, 1925/1968). Cooley addressed the relation of the self to context in noting: "It [the self] might also, and perhaps more justly, be compared to the nucleus of a living cell, not altogether separate from the surrounding matter, out of which indeed it is formed, but more active and definitely organized" (Cooley, 1902/1968, p. 89). A relational model also resembles the existential approach in which the "being-with-others" (Milsein) is stressed as fully as the concrete existence (Dasein) (Tiryakian, 1968).

The change in emphasis involved in a relational point of view is comparable to what other theorists have described as a movement to dialectical schemata. Basseches (1980), writing about dialectical thinking, captures the quality of the shift in perspective:

> Conceptualizing entities as forms of existence rather than as elements of existence emphasizes the sense of coherence, organization, and wholeness implicit in the notion of form over against the sense of separateness implicit in the notion of elements. Secondly since these entities are viewed as temporary rather than immutable, the entities themselves are deemphasized relative to that process of existence as a whole, which is viewed as characterized by continual differentation and integration. (Basseches, 1980, p. 404)

Existence ceases to be seen as being "composed of independent monads" (Basseches, 1980).

Piaget's (1952) model of adaptation, with accommodation and assimilation in an ever shifting process of equilibration, is helpful in conceptualizing the changing, active, ongoing, and interactive quality of a relational model of development.

RELATIONAL BEING

In the past decade, an important impetus for shifting to a different paradigm of "the self" in developmental-clinical theory has come from feminist psychologists who have been increasingly vocal and articulate about their dissatisfaction with existing models of female development and the "female self." Although not always explicitly stated, the adequacy of old models for describing male development is also questioned.

> Feminist thought [has been described as] different in every respect: as a practical, particular, contexted, open, and nonsystematic knowledge of the social circumstances in which one has one's being, concerned with achieving a heterarchy of times and places for a plurality of otherwise conflicting voices. (Shotter & Logan, 1988, pp. 75–76)

Miller (1976), Chodorow (1978), and Gilligan (1982) are the most notable of the new wave of women challenging existing conceptualizations of women's development and personal organization. All note the male (phallocentric) bias in clinical-developmental theory.

Miller's work takes a broad psychological-cultural approach to the problem; she explicitly notes, "As we have inherited it, the notion of 'a self' does not appear to fit women's experience" (Miller, 1984, p. 1). More recently, she has been drawing on clinical work to broaden and deepen her alternative perspective of "being in relation."

Gilligan's ideas about the nature of female development derived from her awareness that prevailing theories of moral development (Kohlberg, 1984) were not applicable to women but were being used in such a way that women consistently appeared as defective or deficient moral selves. As Gilligan notes: "The disparity between women's experience and the representation of human development, noted throughout the psychological literature, has generally been seen to signify a problem in women's development. Instead, the failure of women to fit existing models of human growth may point to a problem in the representation, a limitation in the conception of human condition, an omission of certain truths about life" (Gilligan, 1982, pp. 1–2). An important truth being omitted was the power of the ethic of caretaking and relationship in women's lives.

Chodorow (1978) re-examined object relations theory and found that traditional theory failed to acknowledge the importance of the early and longer lasting bond between the girl and her mother. This bond leads to a different experience of boundaries and identity than what the boy, as objectified other, experiences with mother.

What all of these theorists allude to, and seek to begin to correct, in psychological theory reflects an old tradition, captured in Aristotle's statement that: "the female is a female by virtue of a certain lack of qualities; we should regard the female nature as afflicted with a natural defectiveness" (Sanday, 1988, p. 58). When men are studied, when men do the studying, and when male values hold sway in the culture, one cannot expect any other outcome; the "other" will always be defined in the terms of the subject, and differences will be interpreted as deficiencies, especially in a hierarchical system. (Broverman, Broverman, Clarkson, Rosenkrantz, & Vogel, 1970). Very specifically, all of these theorists note the failure of previous theories of "human development" to appreciate the relational nature of women's sense of themselves. Miller (1976) and Gilligan (1982) also explicitly or implicitly posit a more contextual, relational paradigm for the study of all self experience.

One perspective of the "interacting sense of self," sometimes called "self-in-relation" (Jordan & Surrey, 1986; Surrey, 1985), "relational-self" (Jordan, 1985), or "being in relation" (Miller, 1984), is currently being developed by Miller (1984), Jordan (1984, 1985, 1987), Kaplan (1984) Stiver (1984), and Surrey (1985) at the Stone Center at

Wellesley College New relational theory of self, perhaps like the "new physics" of quantum theory and uncertainty, emphasizes the contextual, approximate, responsive and process factors in experience. In short, it emphasizes relationship and connection. Rather than a primary perspective based on the formed and contained self, this model stresses the importance of the intersubjective, relationally emergent nature of human experience. While there is still a "felt sense of self," which is acknowledged by this point of view it is a "self inseparable from a dynamic interaction" (Miller, 1984, p. 4) an "interacting sense of self," (Miller, 1984). From this intersubjective perspective, the movement of relating, of mutual initiative and responsiveness, are the ongoing central organizing dynamics in women's (but probably all people's) lives (Jordan, 1989). This goes beyond saying that women value relationships; we are suggesting that the deepest sense of one's being is continuously formed in connection with others and is inextricably tied to relational movement. The primary feature, rather than structure marked by separateness and autonomy, is increasing empathic responsiveness in the context of interpersonal mutuality.

Empathy, the dynamic cognitive–affective process of joining with and understanding another's subjective experience, is central to this perspective (Jordan, 1984). Mutual empathy, characterized by the flow of empathic attunement between people, alters the traditional boundaries between subject and object and experientially alters the sense of separate self in a profound way. In true empathic exchange, each is both object and subject, mutually engaged in affecting and being affected, knowing and being known. In interpersonal language, in a mutually empathic relationship, each individual allows and assists the other in coming more fully into clarity, reality, and relatedness; each shapes the other (Jordan, 1987)

Thus, in mutual empathic understanding, the inner conviction of the "separate self" is challenged. Descriptions of the empathic process refer to the "sharing in and comprehending the momentary psychological state of another person" (Schafer, 1959, p. 345) or "trial identification" (Fliess, 1942), which occur during empathy. The boundaries as well as functional differences between subject and object, knower and known, cognitive and affective are altered in the process of empathy. As two people join in empathic subjectivity, the distinctions between "subject" and "object" blur; knower and known connect and join in mutual empathy. The other's subjective experience becomes as one's own; this is at the heart of "relational being." Action, creativity, and intentionality occur within this context.

Empirical work on empathy demonstrates that in addition to cognitive awareness of another's inner subjective state, in empathic attunement people resonate emotionally and physically with the other's experience (this mirroring physiological arousal is sometimes called vicarious affective arousal). Women typically demonstrate more emotional-physical resonance with others' affective arousal than do men (Hoffman, 1977). Also of note, is that 1- to 2-day-old infants demonstrate distress cries to other infants' wails of distress; sex differences exist at that time as well, with girls showing more resonant distress. (Sagi & Hoffman, 1976; Simmer, 1971). The sex differences at this age are not easily explained, and the greater import of this study is to suggest that intrinsic empathic responsiveness exists in all human beings. This is a simple, yet dramatic example of the deep interconnectedness between people that "separate self" theory overlooks. Not just at the level of goals, values, and beliefs do women experience a sense of connected self but at the very concrete and compelling level of feelings and body experience. The study of the development of empathy, then, may provide a route to the delineation of relational development and intersubjective processes, slighted for so long in Western psychology.

THE QUESTION OF BOUNDARIES

In moving from a theory of separate self to a perspective of relational being, the question of how we experience and depict boundaries becomes very important. Our metaphors for "being" are heavily spatialized. Thus, the self typically is portrayed as existing in space, characterized by the "possession" of various unique attributes (a particular organization of physical, cognitive, psychological, and spiritual attributes), demarcated or bounded in some way (typified either by "open boundaries" or "closed boundaries") and interacting from a place of separation or containment with "the world out there." This is a profoundly de-contextualized self. The emphasis on boundary functions as protecting and defining, rather than as meeting or communicating, reinforces especially the self as "separate" entity rather than "being" as a contextual, interactional process.

The way one conceptualizes one's "place" in the world broadly affects interpretive, meaning-making, value-generating activity. The nature of relatedness, the nature of the boundary concept shapes the openness to new experience and the quality of revelations about inner experience that occur between people. If "self" is conceived of as separate, alone, "in control," personally achieving and mastering nature, others may tend to be perceived as potential competitors, dangerous intruders, or objects to be used for the self's enhancement. A system that defines the self as separate and hierarchically measurable is usually marked in Western cultures by power-based dominance patterns. In such systems, the self-boundary serves as protection from the impinging surround and the need for connection with, relatedness to, and contact with others is subjugated to the need to protect the separate self. Abstract logic is viewed as superior to more "connected knowing" (Belenky, Clinchy, Goldberger, & Tarule 1986). Safety in a power-based society seems to demand solid boundaries; self-disclosure is carefully monitored, lest knowledge about the inner experience be used against one. As caricatured in this way, this actually prescribes much of the socialization of Western males.

If, on the other hand, self is conceived of as contextual and relational, with the capacity to form gratifying connections, with creative action becoming possible through connection, and a greater sense of clarity and confidence arising within relationship, others will be perceived as participating in relational growth in a particular way that contributes to the connected sense of self. In empathic resonance, the person experiences, at a cognitive and physical level, the powerful sense of connection. Further, if mutuality prevails, not only will I be influenced, moved, changed by context, and most importantly by my relational context, but I will also be shaping and participating in the development of others' "selves." This growth and movement is participatory and synergistic. This view of "self with other" typifies much of the socialization toward care-taking and empowerment of others that occurs for females in Western cultures.

Hence, it should be no surprise to find important differences between men's and women's experiences of boundaries, contributing to vastly different experiences of "self with other" or the "interacting sense of self." As Carol Gilligan notes, women "define themselves in the context of human relationship" (1982, p. 17). For men, what is crucial is "separation as it defines and empowers the self" (Gilligan, 1982, p. 156). Women feel most themselves, most safe, most alive in connection, men . . . in separation (Gilligan and Pollack, 1982).

Chodorow (1978) gives one explanation for gender differences in the sense of identity vis-à-vis boundaries. She suggests that Western cultures allow a much longer pre-oedipal period for the girl, in which the immediate and close attachment and consequent identification with mother is uninterrupted for an extended time. The boy's experience is marked, on the other hand, by an abrupt interruption of the earliest identification with the mother and a shift of the identification to father when he discovers the "defective," penis-less state of the mother and the superior power of the father. He is further treated as an object rather than as an identified-with subject by the mother. This difference in intrapsychic development, in Chodorow's opinion, leads to more "permeable boundaries" in girls and a greater premium on separation and protection from other in boys. Lynn (1962) hypothesized that the nature of the identification process is quite different in boys and girls by virtue of the very different roles mothers and fathers traditionally play in raising children; that is, mothers are present in an ongoing way while fathers are typically more absent. Thus, it is suggested, boys are left having to identify with an "abstract role" rather than a specific, particular, interacting person. This dynamic, alone, would shed light on the greater contextuality of girls and the greater tendency toward abstracted and separate functioning of boys. I would also like to suggest that boys are actively socialized toward a power–dominance experience of selfhood, while girls are socialized towards a love–empathy mode of being in the world (Jordan, 1987). The former stresses discontinuity between self and other, decreased empathic resonance; the latter enhances the movement of mutual impact and growth. These two very different approaches to organizing "self with other" experience also have far-reaching effects on every aspect of our lives, including the theories of self and science that we construct. Psychological theories of self, especially value-laden notions of the ideally functioning self, in turn broadly affect our experiences of ourselves. And they are saturated with gender bias.

BIAS IN SCIENCE AND LANGUAGE

Evelyn Fox Keller delineates what I think are the consequences of this bias in the realm of science, pointing out that there are two basic approaches in science: the Baconian model, where knowledge leads to "power over" nature, and the Platonic approach, where knowledge occurs through entering into the world of the studied (Keller, 1985, p. 34). The former lauds the capacity to abstract and objectify, while the latter suggests a much more contextual orientation. The Baconian approach might be thought of as fitting the power–dominance mode, which I suggest is the ruling ethic for Western male socialization. It leads to what Belenky et al. (1986) refer to as "separate knowing." In contrast, the Platonic model represents the empathic mode or "connected knowing," encouraged in traditional female development.

In no science is the bias of the scientist about these issues more likely to affect the material she or he studies than in psychology. I submit that we are at all times, even in the most rigorous empirical studies, trying to learn something about ourselves; at worst, we are trying to "prove" something about or for ourselves. Our efforts at being objective are limited by our prejudices, needs, and conditioning. The enterprise is fraught with contradiction. If we could accept this contradiction and acknowledge it, perhaps we could come a step closer to the complex flow of life. But I think psychology as an enterprise has suffered from a sense of shame about the limits on its "objective powers" and therefore has become even more heavily invested in extolling the separation of subject and object, denying the subjective nature of its own being. This pressure can lead away from a study of human process as movement and mutual influence to celebration of the dualism implied in subject versus object and contributes heavily to the metaphor of "separate self." As Keller notes, "the relation between knower and known is one of distance and separation. It is that between a subject and an object radically divided, which is to say, no worldly relation" (Keller, 1985, p. 79). Belenky et al. (1986) point to the differences between knowledge and understanding, a difference which is familiar to clinicians. Knowledge "implies separation from the object and mastery over it," while "understanding involves intimacy and equality between self and object" (Belenky et al, 1986, p. 101).

Nevertheless, the tendency to objectify and "it-ify" or render into "thingdom" is powerful in psychological theory. As Robert Kegan notes: "We are greatly tempted and seduced by our language into experiencing ourselves and the world as *things* that move" (Kegan, 1982, p. 8 [emphasis mine]). I think this is in part because of our culturally induced need to control and predict. The material world, the person as discrete body in space, is a compelling reality. And language is used to both express and create this reality. Unfortunately, the effort to transcend these biases often fails, particularly with language. Thus, even in Kegan's very fine attempt to move psychology out of this bind ("This book is about human being as activity" [1982, p. 8]), his ultimate definition of subjectivity relies on "having" rather than "being," whether actions, sensations, impulses, and so on. "Having," again, falls into the old paradigm of things that are possessed by a possessor, that is, structured, "owning" self. In his approach, "having" is a more mature mode than "being."

Our language, so neatly split into discrete words, nouns, and verbs, further makes discussion of this material almost impossible. The drift toward abstracted entities occurs again and again as I struggle with these ideas. Nevertheless, in shifting from a study of separate knowledge to connected knowing (Belenky et al., 1986) or from "self-development" to "relational development" (Jordan, 1989), I attempt to leave a language of structure and dualism for one of process. I look beyond the polarities of egoism versus altruism, self versus other. Concretely, I see that people move into relationship, not just as a means towards self-development or to acquire something for the self (be it love, money, or sex) but to contribute to the growth of something that is of the self but beyond the self. . . the relationship.

Self, other, and the relationship—no longer clearly separated entities but mutually forming—are interconnected rather than in competition in a model of relational movement. Growth occurs in becoming a part of relationship rather than apart from relationship (Jordan, 1990). The enhancement of the relationship may constitute a greater goal than individual gratification and ironically may lead to greater individual fulfillment (Jordan, 1987). Stated more strongly, perhaps the most basic human need is the need to participate in relationship (Kaplan, 1984). It is movement, growth in connection, differentiation and integration in the evolving context that characterize this view of Life.

Central to any discussion of self is the dilemma of process and structure. Our language does impose limits on our ability to delineate modes of being, to trace continuities of intention, memory, energy, and sensation; we quickly resort to reifications, making solid that which is fluid, changing and ongoing. One reason I prefer the term *relational being* to *relational self* or *self-in-relation* is that it is purposely true to the process nature of experience. The ambiguity of the term *being* (noun or verb, structure or process?) nicely captures the paradox of the process–structure–interface. The experience of being "real," central to the sense of self, then emerges in an ongoing relational context. The metaphor of "voice" so often used to characterize the experience of self, is apt, for one's voice is vividly shaped by the quality of listening provided, whether with a real audience or an imagined one.

In Hazel Markus's terms, "the dynamic interpretive structure," it seems to me, is shaped importantly in relational contexts. Markus notes "the self concept can no longer be explored as if it were a unitary, monolithic entity" (Markus & Wurf, 1987, p. 300). Some have gone so far as to argue that there is no integrative self-process but that the individual is a separate and new self in each context in which he or she participates (Sorokin, 1947), or as Goffman notes, the individual can be thought of as a constant "mummer" (Goffman, 1959). If we posit a model of contextual, dialogic movement, the constancies and patterns of interpersonal interactions and the ways they shape our sense of ourselves become the focus for understanding personal integration. Study of relationality is needed to supplement intrapsychic investigation.

To summarize, from a relational perspective, human beings are seen as experiencing a primary need for connection and essential emotional joining. This need is served by empathy, which in authentic relatedness, is characterized by mutuality. Further, in relationships one comes to experience: clarity about one's own experience and the other's; the capacity for creating meaningful action; an increased sense of vitality; and capacity for further connection (Jordan, 1987; Miller, 1986). Relational capabilities and processes exist from the time of birth and develop over the course of one's life. In our culture, there has been a split along gender lines between the ideal of a separate, autonomous, objective male self and a relational, connected, and empathic female self. Notably, different values, motivational patterns, ways of knowing (Belenky et al., 1986), moral systems (Gilligan, 1982), primary ways of organizing interpersonal experience (Jordan, 1987), and spheres of influence have been delineated by gender. Scientific inquiry itself has been aimed toward "objective truth," mastery over nature; as such, it represents a masculine ideal (Keller, 1985). Despite the revelations of modern physics of the interpenetrability of all movement and structure, the myth, and possibly the arrogance, of this notion of impersonal, objective truth perseveres. In psychology, we must be very cautious with our language, for in naming, we give form. We shape areas of study; we eliminate others. Needed is a move toward a psychology of relationship and exploration of intersubjective reality, expressed by a relational language that supports relational understanding. Although we can most easily see the importance of this in the depiction of women's lives, the exploration of "relational being" should not stop with women. A larger paradigm shift from the primacy of separate self to relational being must be considered to further our understanding of all human experience.

REFERENCES

Baldwin, J. (1968). The self-conscious person. In C. Gordon & K. Gergen (Eds.), *The self in social interaction* (pp. 161–171). New York: Wiley. (Original work published 1897)

Basseches, M. (1980). Dialectical schemata: A framework for the empirical study of the development of dialectical thinking. *Human Development, 23,* 400–421.

Belenky, M., Clinchy, B., Goldberger, N., & Tarule, J. (1986). *Women's ways of knowing: The development of self, voice, and mind.* New York: Basic Books.

Broverman, I., Broverman, D., Clarkson, F., Rosenkrantz, P., & Vogel, S. (1970). Sex role stereotype and clinical judgments of mental health. *Journal of Consulting and Counseling Psychology, 43,* 1–7.

Chodorow, N. (1978). *The reproduction of mothering: Psychoanalysis and the sociology of gender.* Berkeley: University of California Press.

Cooley, C. H. (1968). The social self: on the meanings of "I." In C. Gordon & K. Gergen (Eds.), *The self in social interaction*, (pp. 87–93). New York: Wiley. (Original work published 1902)

Erikson, E. (1963). *Childhood and society* (2nd ed.). New York: Norton.

Fairbairn, W. (1952). *An object relations theory of personality* New York: Basic Books. (Original work published 1946)

Fliess, R. (1942). The metapsychology of the analyst. *Psychoanalytic Quarterly, 11*, 211–227.

Freud, S. (1955). Beyond the pleasure principle. In J. Strachey (Ed. and Trans.), *The standard edition of the complete psychological works of Sigmund Freud* (Vol. 18, pp. 3–64). London: Hogarth Press. (Original work published 1920)

Gergen, M. (1988). *Feminist thought and the structure of knowledge.* New York: New York University Press.

Gilligan, C. (1982). *In a different voice.* Cambridge, MA: Harvard University Press.

Goffman, E. (1959). *The presentation of self in everyday life.* Garden City, NY: Doubleday Anchor.

Guntrip, H. (1973). *Psychoanalytic theory, therapy and the self.* New York: Basic Books.

Hoffman, M. (1977). Sex differences in empathy and related behaviors. *Psychological Bulletin, 84*(4), 712–722.

Horney, K. (1967). The flight from womanhood. In H. Kelman (Ed.), *Feminine psychology* (pp. 54–70). New York: Norton. (Original work published 1926)

James, W. (1968). The self. In C. Gordon & K. Gergen (Eds.), *The self in social interaction* (pp. 41–51). New York: Wiley. (Original work published 1890)

Jordan, J. (1984). *Empathy and self boundaries.* (Work in Progress No. 16.) Wellesley, MA: Stone Center Working Paper Series.

Jordan, J. (1985). *The meaning of mutuality.* (Work in Progress No. 23.) Wellesley, MA: Stone Center Working Paper Series.

Jordan, J. (1987). *Clarity in connection: Empathic knowing, desire and sexuality.* (Work in Progress No. 29.) Wellesley, MA: Stone Center Working Paper Series. (Reprinted as Chapter 3, this volume)

Jordan, J. (1989). *Relational development: Therapeutic implications of empathy and shame.* (Work in Progress No. 39.) Wellesley, MA: Stone Center Working Paper Series. (Reprinted as Chapter 7, this volume)

Jordan, J. (1990). *Relational development through empathy: Therapeutic applications.* (Work in Progress No. 40.) Wellesley, MA: Stone Center Working Paper Series.

Jordan, J. & Surrey, J. (1986). The self-in-relation: Empathy and the mother-daughter relationship. In T. Bernay and D. Cantor. *The psychology of today's woman: New psychoanalytic visions.* New York: Analytic Press.

Kaplan, A. (1983). *Women and empathy.* (Work in Progress No. 2.) Wellesley, MA: Stone Center Working Paper Series.

Kaplan, A. (1984). *The "self-in-relation": Implications for depression in women.* (Work in Progress No. 14.) Wellesley, MA: Stone Center Working Paper Series.

Kegan, R. (1982). *The evolving self: Problem and process in human development.* Cambridge, MA: Harvard University Press.

Keller, E. (1985). *Reflections on gender and science.* New Haven, CT: Yale University Press. (Reprinted as Chapter 7, this volume.)

Kohlberg, L. (1989). *The psychology of moral development: The nature and validity of moral stages.* San Francisco, CA: Harper & Row.

Klein, G. (1976). *Psychoanalytic theory: An explanation of essentials.* New York: International Universities Press.

Klein, M. (1953). *Love, hate and reparation,* with Joan Riviere. London: Hogarth Press.

Kohut, H. (1984). *How does analysis cure?* Chicago: University of Chicago Press.

Lynd, H. (1958). *On shame and the search for identity.* New York: Wiley.

Lynn, D. (1962). Sex role and parental identification. *Child Development, 33*(3), 555–564.

Mahler, M. S., Pine, F., & Bergman, A. (1975). *The psychological birth of the human infant: Symbiosis and individuation.* New York: Basic Books.

Markus, H., & Wurf, E. (1987). The dynamic self-concept: A social psychological perspective. *Annual Review of Psychology, 38,* 299–337.

Mead, G. H. (1968). The genesis of the self. In C. Gordon & K. Gergen (Eds.), *The self in social interaction* (pp. 51–61). New York: Wiley. (Original work published 1925)

Miller, J. B. (1976). *Toward a new psychology of women.* Boston: Beacon Press.

Miller, J. B. (1984). *The development of women's sense of self.* (Work in Progress No. 12.) Wellesley, MA: Stone Center Working Paper Series.

Miller, J. B, (1986). *What do we mean by relationships?* (Work in Progress No. 22.) Wellesley, MA: Stone Center Working Paper Series.

Piaget, J. (1952). *The origins of intelligence in children.* New York: Norton.

Pollak, S. & Gilligan, C. (1982). Images of violence in thematic apperception test stories. *Journal of Personality and Social Psychology, 42*(1), 159–167.

Sagi, A., & Hoffman, M. (1976). Empathic distress in newborns. *Development Psychology, 12,* 175–176.

Sanday, P. R. (1988). The reproduction of patriarchy in feminist anthropology. In M. Gergen (Ed.), *Feminist thought and the structure of knowledge.* (pp. 49–69 New York: New York Universities Press.

Schafer, R. (1959). Generative empathy in the treatment situation. *Psychoanalytic Quarterly, 28,* 342–373.

Shotter, J., & Logan, J. (1988). The pervasiveness of patriarchy: On finding different voice. In M. Gergen (Ed.), *Feminist thought and the structure knowledge* (pp. 69–87). New York: New York University.

Simmer, M. (1971). Newborn's response to the cry of another infant. *Developmental Psychology, 5,* 135–150.

Sorokin, P. (1947). *Society, culture and personality: Their structure and dynamics.* New York: Harper.

Stern, D. (1986). *The interpersonal world of the infant.* New York: Basic Books.

Stiver, I. (1984). *The meanings of "dependency" in female–male relationships.* (Work in Progress No. 11.) Wellesley, MA: Stone Center Working paper Series.

Sullivan, H. S. (1953). *The interpersonal theory of psychiatry.* New York: Norton.

Surrey, J. (1985). *Self-in-relation: A theory of women's development.* (Work Progress No. 13.) Wellesley, MA: Stone Center Working Paper Series.

Thompson, C. (1941). Cultural processes in the psychology of women. *Psychiatry 4,* 331–339.

Tiryakian, E. (1968). The existential self and the person. In C. Gordon & K. Gergen (Eds.), *The self in social interaction* (pp. 75–87). New York: Wiley.

Trevarthan, C. (1979). Communication and cooperation in early infancy: description of primary intersubjectivity. In J. M. Bullower (Ed.), *Before speech: The beginning of interpersonal communication.* New York: Cambridge University Press.

Turner, R. (1968). The self-conception in social interaction. In C. Gordon & K Gergen (Eds.), *The self in social interaction* (pp. 93–107). New York: Wiley.

This chapter is reprinted from *The Self: Interdisciplinary Approaches* (J. Strauss & G. R. Boethals, Eds.), New York: Springer-Verlag, 1991. © 1991 Springer-Verlag. Reprinted by permission.

2

Some Misconceptions and Reconceptions of a Relational Approach

JEAN BAKER MILLER
JUDITH V. JORDAN
ALEXANDRA G. KAPLAN
IRENE P. STIVER
JANET L. SURREY

Aren't You Idealizing Women? Aren't You Idealizing Relationships?

JEAN BAKER MILLER

In recent years several groups of workers have been building a relational approach to understanding psychological development (for example, Belenky, Clinchy, Goldberger, & Tarule, 1986; Gilligan, 1982; Gilligan, Brown, & Rogers, 1990; Gilligan, Lyons, & Hanmer, 1989; Miller, 1976; *Work in Progress*, 1982–1990; and others). Many people have been involved in this work, and we certainly cannot speak for all of them. We will try to discuss some questions as we each see them.

Over the years, those who have read or heard presentations of the relational approach have raised cogent comments or questions about it. We will cover some of the most frequent ones. We suspect that this discussion will lead to more questions, but that is what is valuable. An ongoing dialogue creates the best hope for further clarifying and enlarging everyone's work. We will each briefly discuss one or two topics. I will begin with perhaps the most general questions.

Several sub-topics come under the question about idealizing relationships, for example: You don't see the bad or destructive aspects of relationships or that turning to relationships is basically defensive. It is defensive because it results from fear of, or from inability to, develop or advance oneself. From the perspective of some feminists, focusing on relationships represents a continuation of the old condition of women serving men or serving the patriarchy as opposed to finding full selfhood and liberation through autonomy, independence, and the like. That is, doesn't this perspective lead to sending women back to their old place making relationships for others, especially men and children? Some clinicians comment that this relational approach means "being nice" as opposed to being analytical or therapeutic.

IDEALIZING WOMEN

First, about idealizing women—some of these comments may follow from our history. We concentrated in the first few years on working very hard to "depathologize" many aspects of women's behavior and characteristics, and to emphasize that what this culture and prevalent psychological theories have seen as weaknesses or symptoms of pathology can be seen more accurately as strengths or the seeds of strengths. Examples are such features as emotionality" or the centrality of relationships.

We believed it was important to try to shift this groundwork before talking about so-called "pathology." By contrast, all traditional models in the psychodynamic field have begun from a base in pathology or deficiency. Although we did talk about some problems earlier, only in the last four years or so have we turned to more concerted attempts to try to explain various kinds of psychological troubles.

I believe that more people should continue to work on emphasizing women's strengths and women's values because powerful forces still act upon us to lead us to ignore or diminish these valuable characteristics. While some changes have occurred, it still takes extra effort because most of us have internalized a deficiency model of women. Indeed, I believe that some of the comments may come from the fact that women, ourselves, still have trouble claiming our own strengths and values enough. We can still find it hard to believe that how we tend to think or feel, or what we tend to want or like is valuable and important—as compared to some of the things we supposedly should be striving for which often don't feel as congenial.

All of this, of course, doesn't mean that women are all good. And an empathic approach, by definition, does not mean idealizing. Idealizing is creating a falsity. Nor does an empathic approach mean being a "nice person." An empathic approach means the attempt to be with the truth of the other person's experience in all of its aspects. Thus, for all women—and all men—it has to mean to be with the difficult, conflictual, and destructive feelings and thoughts that we all experience. But it also means being with the strengths and potential strengths as well.

IDEALIZING RELATIONSHIPS

One approach to this question is to say it concerns a basic belief system about the human condition. Once we examine women's lives without accepting prior assumptions if they do not apply, we begin to see that certain generally accepted propositions are not necessarily true. They follow from certain beliefs. So, for example, the notion that the goal of human growth is to develop a separate, individuated, well-bounded self, as is said to be exemplified by white middle class men, follows from certain assumptions. From another perspective, we have proposed that the goal of development is to participate in increasingly empowering relationships. It is probably impossible to prove that either of these sweeping statements is "true." However, we can look at the social as well as the gender origins of each notion. We can also ask whose purposes each proposition serves and what evidence we can bring to bear on each.

To deal with only the last point at this time, it seems apparent that the human condition is to grow and live in groups. That is, human beings can develop only within relationships with other people, more specifically, other people who can engage in relationships in a way which fosters the development of the people in them. However, once we have a societal system in which one group has made itself a dominant group, that group obviously cannot create a system of relationships based on fostering the full development of all people. By definition, a dominant group cannot build a system based on empathy for, and empowerment of, others. But all societies must provide such relationships to some extent, otherwise no one could develop at all. This whole realm of activity has been delegated to women to fill in for everyone. Once so delegated, it has not been truly valued, or even well recognized.

By contrast, we can look upon this growth-fostering activity as the most valuable of human abilities, an activity in which everyone can participate. This form of activity differs from the models we've had so far. It seems increasingly obvious that our societal models inevitably cannot be models of what it is to be fully human but models of what you should be in order to be a member of a dominant group.

If we turn to thinking of a model based on the strengths women have demonstrated, we can begin to envision another model for all. Certainly we are not suggesting a model based on serving others from a subordinate position, but a model in which everyone learns to participate in relationships which are growth-fostering for all the people involved, that is, mutually empathic and mutually empowering relationships. The essential concepts are mutuality and movement in relationship. Growth-fostering relationships have to be mutual, or more accurately, moving toward mutuality.

We are certainly aware of the problematic aspects of relationships, but we believe they can be understood in this context. No one has attained the ability to engage fully and well in mutually empathic and mutually empowering ways. We all have the potential, but we all have limitations because of the nonmutual background from which we all come and in which we still live.

To put all this another way, many people are trying to understand why they feel so miserable, or why relationships often can be so hurtful and destructive. Our obligation in the mental health field is to search for the origins of such problems and to try to discover what to do about them. In general, we are suggesting that all growth takes place within mutually empathic and mutually empowering relationships, and problems follow from the disconnections that occur in nonmutual relationships. Because our society's historical tradition and our formative relationships have been nonmutual, all of us are still caught—to varying degrees—in the problematic consequences of this nonmutuality and these disconnections.

At present, we're trying to describe more thoroughly what tends to go wrong in many relationships—between women, between women and men, in families as a whole, and in larger contexts. In all of these situations, we believe the important concept on which to focus is the "movement of relationship." That is, it is not a question of characterizing individuals as static entities but instead a focus on whether relationships are moving toward mutual empathy and mutual empowerment, and if not, what is preventing the movement.

REFERENCES

Belenky, M., Clinchy, B., Goldberger, N., & Tarule, J. (1986). *Women's ways of knowing.* New York: Basic Books.

Gilligan, C. (1982). *In a different voice.* Cambridge: Harvard University Press.

Gilligan, C., Brown, L. M., & Rogers, A. (1990). Psyche embedded: A place for body, relationships and culture in personality theory. In A. I. Rabin et al. (Eds.), *Studying persons and lives.* New York: Springer.

Gilligan, C., Lyons, N., & Hanmer, T. (1989). *Making connections.* Cambridge: Harvard University Press

Miller, J. B. (1976). *Toward a new psychology of women.* Boston: Beacon Press.

Work in Progress. (1982–1990). Wellesley, MA: Stone Center Working Paper Series.

Do You Believe That the Concepts of Self and Autonomy Are Useful in Understanding Women?

JUDITH V. JORDAN

Or as a woman at our Cape Cod seminar asked, "What is the Self and where is it located?" In traditional psychology the concept of self has been heavily objectified, spatialized, and reified. Further, psychological theories have viewed the self as primarily agentic, that is, acting on its surround from a place of relative independence and as using supplies from others to support its well-being and growth. This conceptualization portrays the self as a bounded, separate, and self-sustaining entity organized around self-development. This paradigm emphasizes its abstract, de-contextualized, and molecular nature. In contrast, the relational perspective stresses "being in relation," an interactional, ongoing "process of being" rather than a static structure dedicated to increasing self-sufficient functioning. Instead of self-development, we stress the importance of relational development.

The prevailing concept of self is modeled on the now outdated Newtonian physics, a paradigm which posited separate objects possessing clear identities whose interactions were secondary to their atomistic and bounded structures. The philosophical, socio-political context, which supported the development of this notion of self in Western culture, celebrated the sanctity of the individual and the importance of individual rights and entitlements; the individual was seen as needing protection from the presumed aggressive self-interest of others and from the impinging community. In this world-view, a pessimistic expectation of individual selfishness led to overvaluing the separate self at the expense of connectedness and community. Self-sufficiency and self-control, then, constituted an important part of the definition of the "ideal man"; self-interest became equated with health, while interest in others' well-being became equated with self-sacrifice or the devalued work of caretakers, i.e., women.

Related to this traditional image of self as separate and relationships as impinging, was the emphasis on autonomy. "Autonomous" literally means "self-governing." In many models of separation and autonomy, there has been a heavy focus on freedom from restraint by others and from having to attend carefully to the effects of one's actions on others. But is such a state really desirable or possible in any but the most abstracted, nonmutual, nonempathic situations?

In a paradigm that recognizes the relational and interdependent nature of our lives, we might replace "autonomy" with the capacity to be clear in our thoughts, feelings, and actions; to act with intention; to be creative and effective, but always with awareness of the source of our energy in relationships and with recognition of the impact of our actions on others. The capacity to integrate individual and relational goals and to deal with conflict within relationship becomes essential. I have referred to this as "clarity in connection" (Jordan, 1987). An appreciation of relational responsibility and context does not impair our effectiveness in the world; rather, it can positively influence and support the direction that our creative and productive energies will take.

The notion that one achieves safety in bounded separation, and strength in "power over" others, contributes to, and derives from, a view of the self as territorial, in control, mastering nature, and guarding itself against what is thought to be an inevitably predatory and competitive spirit in others. The need to connect and to make contact becomes subjugated to, and distorted by, the need to defend oneself from others. "Boundaries," then, are defined as means of protection rather than as channels of meeting, exchange, and communication. In protecting itself from others, the bounded self is restricted in its openness, disclosure, and emotional responsiveness. Traditional theories have fostered an overemphasis on static and self-preserving structure, rather than on lively initiative and responsiveness in interactions. Given this emphasis, Jean Baker Miller's (1984) statement seems apt: "As we have inherited it, the notion of 'a self' does not appear to fit women's experience."

Where, then, are we on this question? Some of us first modified the isolation of "the self" with hyphens, hoping that the term "self-in-relation" would emphasize the primary connectedness of the individual. With this phrase we tried to convey the sense of a being always developing with, and in relation to, others. But even this term begins to feel like a distortion, something too easily objectified, losing the fluidity and movement that we feel is essential to women's experience. Jean Baker Miller suggested an alternative term, "being in relation," which nicely captures the ambiguity of the noun/verb, structure/process quality of what I think we try to portray as women's sense of self.

Our perspective appreciates, along with traditional models of self, that people experience a sense of personal history, continuity, and coherence; that we demonstrate initiative and responsiveness; that we feel body sensations and limits; that we are aware of emotions and organize our experience in meaningful ways. We also view solitude, feeling effective in work, and relating to the whole nonhuman environment as essential human experiences. But our perspective stresses that we thrive in being in connection. We acknowledge intrapsychic reality, but we see the context, the ongoing relational interplay between self and other, as primary to real growth and vitality. We are suggesting a shift from a psychology of "entities" to a psychology of movement and dialogue. The goal of development is not the creation of a bounded entity with independent internal psychic structure that turns to the outside world only in a state of need or deficiency. On the contrary, in the ideal pattern of development, we move toward participation in relational growth rather than toward simple attainment of personal gratification.

The full realization of relational development depends on the flow of mutuality. An individual must be able to represent her or his own experience in a relationship, to act in a way which is congruent with an "inner truth" and with the context, and to respond to and encourage authenticity in the other person. Participation with another person(s) leads to a jointly created "feeling-milieu" and contributes to effective action for both (or all) people. In an authentic and mutual relationship, one will not be too accommodating (i.e., self-sacrificing) or egocentric (other-sacrificing). Often what people refer to as difficulties in "self-function" (so-called "co-dependence," "masochism," or "self-defeating behaviors") are really failures of mutuality in the relationship. Importantly, mutuality involves commitment to engage in the development and support of both people; it involves respectfully building a relationship together that both sustains and transcends the individuals engaged in it.

In fact, self, other, and the relationship are no longer clearly separated entities in this perspective but are seen as *mutually forming processes*. We are suggesting a profound rearrangement of traditional theories of "self-development" when we propose a model of "relational development" where "the enhancement of the relationship may constitute a greater goal than individual gratification and ironically may lead to greater individual fulfillment" (Jordan, 1987).

REFERENCES

Jordan, J. (1987). *Clarity in connection: Empathic knowing, desire and sexuality.* (Work in Progress No. 29.) (Reprinted as Chapter 3, this volume) Wellesley, MA: Stone Center Working Paper Series.

Miller, J. B. (1984). The development of a woman's sense of self. (Work in Progress No. 12.) Wellesley, MA: Stone Center Working Paper Series.

How Can a Group of White, Heterosexual, Privileged Women Claim to Speak of "Women's" Experience?

ALEXANDRA G. KAPLAN

Our work over the past 12 years has centered on ways that mutual relational processes enhance and empower women. We wanted to offer an alternative to the common tendency in developmental theory to define women's experience without identifying or exploring gender as one aspect that might profoundly affect the nature, course, and outcome of a developmental pathway. We therefore began by building on our own experiences, probing the interwoven nuances of our own lives, our clinical work, readings, our own group processes, and, implicitly, the different perspectives and frameworks we each brought to the encounter.

As a group of white, heterosexual, privileged women, or indeed as for any group of women, it is impossible to generalize from one's own work to assumptions about generic "women." Being conscious of these limits, we tried to use our own viewpoints as validly as we could as a basic frame, or template, from which to expand on the scope of women's development in range, nuance, breadth, and specificity. In doing so, we recognized that we were speaking, at different times and in different ways, about "some women," or "most women," leaving implicit room for the impact of diversity, but not addressing it directly.

At best, we might enlarge our understanding of women like ourselves, but should approach with great caution any attempt to represent the lives of a broader range of women. We needed in particular to focus on what was "experientially near," and to look to others to speak to their particular frame and perspective. Thus, in part, we turned to writings and presentations by women from a range of cultural, political, spiritual, or racial backgrounds. These women included Rich (1980), Gartrell (1984), Turner (1987), MacIntosh (1988), Spelman (1988), Cook-Nobles (1989), Heyward (1989), Mencher (1990), and others. Each, in her own way, pointed both to the ways that women's experiences are marginalized and devalued in patriarchal culture, and the ways that women find strength through connection and community, creating, in Lewis' words, "vital arenas of political survival and cultural resistance" (Lewis, 1981). In their consciousness of culture they reminded us that we all have a culture, even though, as hooks (1981) notes, in a racist society, the dominant group has the freedom to include or dismiss racial or other cultural identities as a consideration. Importantly, they also reminded us that those who label themselves the so-called "mainstream" represent but one small segment of a broad and diverse melange, and in fact, as privileged women within the world community, constitute a decided minority.

As such, we as a group have some particular considerations to bear in mind. One of the most important is that each woman should have the right to determine the qualities by which she chooses to define herself. No one should presume to label for another what factors comprise her selfhood, or into which of a range of possible categories (just for example—working class, musician, student, parent, homeowner, athlete, Catholic—the list is endless) she would define herself. Patriarchal culture has provided us with deceptively convenient, and therefore, all the more dangerous and oppressive, structures for categorizing groups of people (usually by social class, race, ethnicity, religion, or sexual preference). This categorization, then, becomes a vehicle by which those who claim a dominant position can presume the right to determine which aspects of identities are core, and by which aspects others will be known. Further, as H. Sussman (personal communication, 1990) notes, such arbitrary labeling also belies the richness and diversity that resides within each of us. Instead, people are known only in terms of where they fit in an arbitrary hierarchy of worth as defined by the dominant culture. The phrase "person of difference," for example, is in fact a meaningless term. It implies that there exists a larger, homogeneous body of people, whom one would have to call "normal" or "standard" people from which to cull out those who would be called "people of difference." In reality however, we are all different—from one another. As Spelman (1988) makes clear, there is no "essence" of women that serves as a "core" which we can then "expand upon." There is only the particularity of each woman's life as she understands it, an experience that is fluid, complex, and multiply layered.

One aspect of oppression, then, is to label someone with an "identity" that belies her vision, or to treat someone as a part of a category, not as a unique individual. But there are many times when others claim the right to define our core being or identity in contradiction to our own sense of ourselves. A child from a wealthy family, for example, may be considered privileged by her poorer classmates, but herself feel shame and isolation because of her status and the material possessions which surround her life. While her classmates might consider her lucky, she herself might feel most poignantly the fact that she had never learned the games that the others played, and was not allowed to go home with friends after school. Her struggle involves not only isolation from her peers, but more importantly, being placed in a category and an identity which completely denied her authentic way of being. If she had had an opportunity to share her discomfort with others, and the means to act in a way more consistent with who she was, she could have created a process for engagement through difference, rather than an experience of isolation and shame. As Keller (1985) notes, acknowledged difference between self and other can create the opportunity for a deeper knowledge of self and other and a deeper sense of the capacity for growth through connection.

From this starting point one can build towards connection. In doing so, we each need to speak for ourselves and our own realities. This entails examining our beliefs and assumptions, so as to be aware of our particular pathways towards engagement and the potential fears or inhibitions that may curtail our openness to understanding and trust. It may also mean listening to others for areas of misunderstanding, or for common but unacknowledged threads that are discovered through dialogue. Movement towards mutual connection and mutual enrichment, then, provide an opportunity for evolving, changing, and growing understanding of one another in terms of the particular contexts that each brings to an encounter. Through openness to one another's experience, each can expand her awareness of the other's context, feeling a greater sense of engagement through both similarities and differences, valuing what feels familiar and what feels new and challenging. There is an appreciation of the power and the vulnerability that each contributes, and a growing awareness of what processes for each are empowering or diminishing. Through their shared engagement, each comes to feel more connected to the other, more able to appreciate and value the other's frame, more open to exposure and risk, and more motivated towards continued engagement.

Jordan (1989) notes the paradox of empathy—that by joining with another, self and other (and the relational process) are enhanced. In an empathically grounded relational process, difference becomes a source of enlargement if each person can expand the boundaries of her experiences and if each can speak where she might otherwise have been silenced by shame or uncertainty. In a Western culture which, despite many changes, still operates in hierarchies of power and control, one may well hesitate to engage with full honesty, or reveal aspects of oneself that may not coincide with the experience of the other. It is hard to openly and honestly engage if one has been taught to fear or dismiss the other. Sometimes, it is useful to simulate a cross-cultural engagement in the form of an exercise, or lead people through a guided fantasy in which people are asked to imagine that they are outsiders within a cohesive and more powerful group. Such exercises can alert those involved to potentially new feelings of fear and alienation, but also of empathy and compassion. From there, one can then begin to envision ways to engage across cultures such that everyone's experience is affirmed.

As noted above, women, whom the prevailing culture marginalizes or oppresses, may need to suppress feelings or inhibit reactions to others, because of potential shame or alienation (Miller, 1988). They may also have internalized racism, sexism, or homophobia, thereby doubting the truth of their own perceptions, or feeling responsible for relational breaches. Further, women in the dominant group are all vulnerable to what Bernardez (1988) has called "cultural countertransference, the insidious ways that unconscious, culturally embedded assumptions about others distort one's ability to see others as they would like to be seen, to know them as they would want to be known." These layers of assumption or uncertainty can obscure paths to more open and honest interchange.

As a particular group of women engaged in the study of women's relational processes, we began by probing our own contexts as individuals and as a group, searching for greater clarity about the specifics of our own experiences. Simultaneously, we built on the particular realities brought to our work by women with a wider range of backgrounds, who enriched and challenged our own perceptions. Through these encounters, we could more clearly understand the processes by which differences serve as pathways toward a more complex and multi-layered engagement. Each of us here tonight can attend to the multiple realities to be discovered through trust in connection, and can gain the humility to recognize that one's assumptions always need further examination.

REFERENCES

Bernardez, T. (1988). *Women and anger—cultural prohibitions and feminine ideal.* (Work in Progress No. 31.) Wellesley, MA: Stone Center Working Paper Series.

Cook-Nobles, R. (I 989). *Social and psychological factors in the career development of the professional Black female.* Unpublished doctoral dissertation, Boston University, Boston.

Gartrell, N. (1984). *Issues in psychotherapy with lesbian women.* (Work in Progress No. 10.) Wellesley, MA: Stone Center Working Paper Series.

Heyward, C. (1989). *Coming out and relational empowerment: A lesbian, feminist, theological perspective.* (Work in Progress No. 38.) Wellesley, MA: Stone Center Working Paper Series.

hooks, b. (1981). *Ain't I a Woman.* Boston, MA: South End Press.

Jordan, J. V. (1989). *Relational development: Therapeutic implications of empathy and shame.* (Work in Progress No. 39.) Wellesley, MA: Stone Center Working Paper Series.

Keller, E. (1985). *Reflections on gender and science.* New Haven: Yale University Press. (Reprinted as Chapter 7, this volume)

Lewis, J. (1981). Mothers, daughters, and feminism. In C. 1. Joseph & J. Lewis (Eds.), *Common differences: Conflicts in black and white feminist perspectives.* New York: Anchor Books.

MacIntosh, P. (1988). *White privilege and male privilege: A personal account of coming to see the correspondences through work in women's studies.* (Work in Progress No. 189.) Wellesley, MA: Center for Research on Women.

Mencher, J. (1990). *Intimacy in lesbian relationships: A critical re-examination of fusion.* (Work in Progress No. 42.) Wellesley, MA: Stone Center Working Paper Series.

Miller, J. B. (1988). *Connections, disconnections, and violations.* (Work in Progress No. 33.) Wellesley, MA: Stone Center Working Paper Series.

Rich, A. (1980). Compulsive heterosexuality and lesbian existence. *Signs, 5,* 631–660.

Spelman V. (1988). *Inessential woman: Problems of exclusion in feminist thought.* Boston: Beacon Press.

Turner, C. W. (1987). *Clinical applications of the Stone Center theoretical approach to minority women.* (Work in Progress No. 28.) Wellesley, MA: Stone Center Working Paper Series. (Reprinted as Chapter 4, this volume)

What Is the Role of Transference and the Unconscious in the Relational Model?

IRENE P. STIVER

I will begin with a question contained in a letter to me, after I presented a paper on "The Meaning of Care: Reframing Treatment Models" (1985). In that paper, I proposed that the traditional model of therapy which required that the therapist be relatively neutral and guard against more open expression of feelings toward the patient, was in fact not very therapeutic for women, for whom relational connections are so vital.

The writer asks: "Isn't it necessary to include in the treatment relationship, the transference relationship?" She is concerned that attention to the "real relationship," which she feels is important, results in leaving out the significance of transference phenomena. She writes: "Developing a model of treatment which is based on a caring relationship still requires attention to the transference relationship; otherwise treatment may not reach it's goal. Caring alone is not sufficient."

This question reflects a significant misunderstanding of the concepts of mutuality and empathy, and it assumes that attention to those aspects of therapy which have not been adequately addressed by traditional theories must necessarily preclude attention to other therapeutic phenomena, such as transference, countertransference, the role of the unconscious, dreams, and the like.

TRANSFERENCE

Indeed, we believe that if the therapist is authentic and caring, she creates a more fertile ground for the essentials of transference to occur.

Because we are all replaying all significant relational dynamics in our lives in all relationships, we cannot avoid doing at least that in the therapeutic relationship. So, we do attend to "transference phenomena," but we are also refraining our understanding of transference and countertransference and the ways we work with these processes in therapy.

In fact, transference is very much a relational phenomenon; memories of one's past relationships, with their connections and disconnections, are expressed in many ways, in "a playing out," often symbolically and without awareness. Contrary to the traditional notion that it is the "blank screen" of the therapist that allows the transference to emerge and be "worked through," we believe that a genuine relational context provides *the safety* and conducive setting to attend to representations of old relational images in the transference, in a way that can be most helpful.

A short vignette will best illustrate the power of the transference in the setting of an ongoing "real" therapeutic relationship. I had had a minor accident which resulted in a bad foot sprain and could walk only in my Nike sports shoes. A client whom I had been seeing for more than three years, and with whom I felt comfortable and authentic, entered therapy the first day after my accident and saw me walk ahead of her with a decided limp. Clearly very angry, she sarcastically began the session, saying, "So, now in addition to everything else you do, you're out there running with your friends every morning." This reaction was perfectly meaningful to me. I understood it as her expression of the kinds of feelings of inadequacy and envy, which characterized her early relationship with her mother, who displayed enormous activity and energy and expected her daughter to perform and achieve for her.

Lack of neutrality, thus, does not seem to ward off the development of transference. Yet I was taught that it was both the therapist's neutrality and her/his "nongratification" of the client which facilitated the emergence of the "negative transference." That is, these conditions allowed for the release of angry feelings toward significant early figures (mostly mothers) and their projection onto the therapist. But a large part of these angry outbursts toward the therapist may be more an artifact of this therapy model itself, rather than an expression of "negative" transference. The therapist's withholding and "nongratifying" stance and the consequent lack of responsiveness may be enormously frustrating and alienating for the client, who responds with anger, despair, and other negative reactions.

We believe that focused attention to transference phenomena provides the central work of the therapy. By working with the relational images which emerge in the transference, client and therapist can gain greater understanding of past relationships, which have resulted in disconnections and distancing from others. They can then explore together those disconnections in past relationships, which lead to distorted expectations of self and others and are projected onto new situations, such as the therapeutic relationship.

Let me share a brief vignette which illustrates the ways in which transference images can be addressed productively with a relational perspective. A therapist I supervise told me about a client she has been seeing for almost a year who expressed great difficulty in talking and is often mute. As we explored this problem, I learned: (1) that the client's ostensible reason for coming into therapy was that her mother didn't want her to, and (2) that over time the client has been able to state that she is afraid that if she does talk about herself, the therapist will tell her to leave. The transference issue that is most apparent is her replication in the therapy of her struggle with her mother, e.g., how to stay connected with her, but also how to be out of relationship with her and defy her because of past hurts and anger.

To come to therapy and not talk allows her to ward off her mother by defying her; but she also stays in connection with her by complying with her through not truly engaging in the therapy, i.e., not talking. With her therapist, she replays the same dilemma, and distances and disconnects from her. This seems to be an expression of her expectation that the therapist, like her mother, will not want to hear what she has to say, nor respect her need to talk about herself and find help. She can then feel as conflicted with her therapist as with her mother, and as isolated and disconnected. Her therapist can talk about this by beginning to name the dilemma, to see it not *as resistance*, but rather as the client's intense efforts to *maintain connection* with her mother while she tries to protect herself from being wounded again. When the therapist takes this perspective, which is also nonjudgmental and uncritical of her mother, she empowers the client to see that she can be connected with both her mother and her therapist.

In reframing the understanding of transference phenomena and the ways of using these phenomena therapeutically, I would like to focus on two of the differences between the relational model and traditional approaches: One is the need for neutrality of the therapist in order for the transference to emerge, and the other is the usefulness of "interpreting" the transference as the major work of the therapy.

The first point about the neutrality of the therapist, I have already addressed in part. That is, transference phenomena emerge in all relational settings, and it is important to know that and to recognize and respect their importance in the treatment. But, in addition, we believe that the very neutrality and distancing by the therapist impede the ways in which therapy can provide a "corrective relational experience"—i.e., a new and different relational experience. As long as the therapist remains "neutral" or relatively noncommunicative, the client does not experience as effectively as she could the significant *differences* between the client's real relationship with the therapist and those relational images from the past which the client re-experiences in the therapy.

The next point is about the interpretation of the transference. I am not at all persuaded that the therapist offering formulations about the transference to the client is necessarily as effective as we were taught it would be. Clients can often experience these formulations as highly intellectualized, not very meaningful, and often as criticisms.

In the relational model, as two people struggle to establish a relationship of trust and mutuality, the therapist needs to be keenly aware of how she feels *she* may be misunderstood in the light of the transference projections. As she begins to understand more and more, she can become more aware of her own experience of difference, as well as some similarities, between her and these projections on her which she experiences from the client. She can then begin to modify her inner attitudes and overt behaviors in a way which will consistently and regularly highlight to the client the significant differences between her and those disconnecting relationships in the past. All of this need not necessarily be verbalized.

Perhaps in some instances it may be best not to verbalize about transference until enough trust and mutual participation in the therapeutic process has evolved. I do not mean that the therapist should role-play, nor behave in some contrived fashion to "look" different from past important people in the client's life; rather I mean that the therapist needs to become more aware of *who she is* and how she sincerely does want to relate to the client more constructively than the client experienced in the past.

If the interpretation occurs *without living out* this difference in the therapy, a client may experience it only cognitively—as an intellectual exercise, making little difference in reorganizing her experience. It may also be too threatening to call attention to the destructive aspects of past relationships before the client has established a solid sense of connection and mutual understanding with the therapist.

COUNTERTRANSFERENCE

A few words about countertransference as another vehicle for mutual growth and change: As the therapist attends to those countertransference reactions which help her understand more about the client's experience, she can more empathically engage with her. By sharing in carefully timed fashion her own reactions and their meanings, a newer level of connection will emerge in the relationship. There is not sufficient time to explore other complicated issues involved in the countertransference, but Janet Surrey will be taking up some of these issues in her discussion of mutuality.

THE UNCONSCIOUS

Some brief comments about the unconscious: If the relational context develops so that the client feels safer and safer over time and experiences the therapist as real, accessible, and truly participating in the therapeutic work, then memories do begin to emerge which were previously "repressed," split off, or robbed of their meanings and importance. The notion that a "correct" interpretation with perfect timing lifts the repression, and the unconscious becomes conscious, and dramatic change occurs, has not been part of my clinical experience. Rather, as the sense of connection between therapist and client grows, the client becomes able to know and understand those parts of her experience which had been too painful to encompass.

In the same way, relational distortions and destructive relational experiences, which may have been too threatening to even look at before, can begin to emerge when the client can trust that the therapist will be able to tolerate these experiences, responding genuinely and effectively to them. As the person feels more accepted, she can bring more and more of her whole person into the relationship, which we believe is the way she will gain access to unconscious or previously split-off experiences.

REFERENCE

Stiver, I. P. (1985). *The meaning of care: Reframing treatment models.* (Work in Progress No. 20.) Wellesley, MA: Stone Center Working Paper Series.

What Do You Mean by Mutuality in Therapy?

JANET L. SURREY

Mutuality is the fundamental property of healthy, growth-enhancing connections. In these connections both or all participants are engaged in creating mutual, interactional growth, learning, and empowerment. In relationships based on the search for mutuality, each participant can represent increasingly her feelings, thoughts, and perceptions in the relationship, can have an impact on the other(s) and on the relationship, and can be moved by or move with the other(s). Mutual empathy and authenticity suggest a way of being "present" or joining together in which each person is emotionally available, attentive, and responsive to the other(s) and to the relationship. Mutuality describes a creative process, in which openness to change allows something new to happen, building on the different contributions of each person.

This forward movement towards enlarged connection, clarity, vitality, and awareness is the movement of mutual relationship. We believe that these qualities are fundamental to the therapy relationship, i.e., that the movement toward mutuality is central to healing and empowerment. We have just begun to try to articulate the specifics of these notions for the therapy relationship. We have described the capacity to engage in mutual relationships as the goal of psychological development, and we see the growth of mutuality and enlarged connection in the therapy relationship as the core of therapy, not the ground or context within which the real work occurs, e.g., interpretations or transmuting internalizations.

Clearly, the therapy relationship has unique properties. It has a specific purpose and primary focus on the growth and healing of the client through elucidation of the client's experience. The therapist brings herself and her experience to the relationship with this purpose and responsibility. The relationship has a relatively fixed structure, an economic basis, certain power inequities, and legal constraints that must be acknowledged. However, when the therapy relationship is working well, client and therapist come to a sense of shared purpose, a "working together" which implies commitment and emotional investment in the relationship as an arena for growth and change. Initially, the therapist may assume more responsibility for the relationship, but as therapy proceeds, the client takes on an increasingly shared responsibility for the relationship.

For the therapist, mutuality refers to this way of being in relationship: empathically attuned, emotionally responsive, authentically present, and open to change. The therapist's growth in the relationship involves enhanced empathic possibilities, capacities to stay present with a range of complex and difficult feelings in herself and others, and greater freedom to "stay in" the process and bring more and more of herself into the relationship. With increasing clinical experience, I have developed much more trust in the process and feel far less concerned about following an externally defined standard of how to "be" or how to "do" therapy. I am also aware of the energy, investment, and vulnerability necessary for engaging well in the therapy; I have come to see my own limits of energy and openness. The complexity and creativity of this relational stance require much more attention and study.

It is essential to emphasize what we do *not* mean by mutuality in therapy. We certainly do not mean disclosing anything and everything with no sense of purpose, impact, timing, or responsibility, nor do we suggest inattention to the complex power dynamics of this relationship. Some clinicians have expressed concern about the notion of therapist's authentic engagement. They relate it to the loss of neutrality and therefore loss of opportunity for the patient's projection and transference. (Irene has just discussed the hardiness of transference!) The concern also appears to be that speaking about the involvement or growth of the therapist suggests a possible loss of boundaries, "gratification" of therapists' needs, or clients "taking care of therapists." This notion is based on a zero-sum model of gratification based on a separate-self paradigm of self-interest: If I get, you lose. In fact, standards of distance and detachment have not precluded gratification of inappropriate needs on the part of some therapists. An ethic of mutuality and authenticity is far more likely to keep the therapist empathically grounded in the realities of the client's experience and well-being.

It is striking that the traditional emphasis in our field has been on the potential negative impact of therapist involvement. It seems more likely that *lack* of authenticity, openness, and responsiveness paves the way for abuse and suggests whole new definitions of "relational abuse." I suggest we need to attend to both sides of the question in any clinical situation. What is the potential impact on the relationship of involvement of the therapist and what is the potential impact of therapist noninvolvement, detachment, or neutrality? Jordan (1990) has discussed the negative impact of emotional neutrality and nonresponsiveness in therapy with sexually abused women and incest survivors.

Mutuality does not mean equality, sameness, or a simplistic notion of mutual, personal disclosure. Since the therapist is always there and always participating to some degree in the relationship, it is odd to think that disclosure can be avoided. Our clients, in fact, know us very deeply in some ways, even if they don't know particular facts. (I remember one man I saw who actually sympathized with my vulnerability around disclosure. He came to my office, saw my messy desk and the like, and he could hide these physical realities of his life!) An ethic of mutuality does not mandate disclosing facts or answering questions. Therapists make decisions about disclosure depending on the situational, personal, and relational aspects of the therapy at any given time. Mutuality in therapy would suggest engaging with the client around such decisions, giving clear and honest explanations about why one may not be disclosing. Opening to an interchange around the decision may lead us to more possibilities for productive change.

When I think about the criteria I use to decide about verbal or conscious disclosure, they center around the potential impact on the client, myself, and the relationship. Will this help move the relationship toward expanded connection? Will it enhance the possibilities of empathic joining, either through my reaching out to join with the client or, sometimes, by asking the client to stretch to encompass something difficult to hear from me? Also important are: my assessment of how well I know the person, how strong or fragile the relationship is, how much might the material effect the client's freedom to be spontaneous without fear of burdening me; or how much will *not* sharing something have a negative impact on my being present and responsive in the relationship.

Working within the relational model has moved me to be much more open about my own thinking and processing in the therapy relationship. Similarly, supervising therapists, I often suggest the value of letting the client hear you think out loud about your own thought processes, almost as they occur—e.g., "I'm aware that it's very important for you to know X, but I'm also considering what opportunities we might lose for exploration if I told you now," or "I'm aware of how important this is for you because of your past experience with therapists, *and* I'm thinking about my own sense of comfort, too." The therapist can work to expand this process, thus building the sense of *We*— of working together, which we call relational empowerment—e.g., "Let's think about how *we* can work with this now."

The therapist's use of I and We language is very significant. I am here as therapist and I share (this word has such a different feeling than disclose!) my thoughts, perceptions, feelings, and insights about what is being discussed. I am also here as therapist with a personal history or current reality you may want or need to know about (e.g., I am pregnant). The therapist is here as part of the We of the relationship, and she may also use the We to include herself in other aspects of the patient's experience, e.g., the We as women, or as lesbians, human beings, or cat lovers. I often find myself sharing very different aspects of my own life and experience with different clients, depending on what we're talking about, or where they feel most isolated or alone in their experience, or with what particular struggles they are grappling.

Indeed in reviewing my experience, I'm amazed at the very different parts of my life I have shared with particular clients. Sometimes it is these moments of sharing that feel most memorable or healing, yet it is likely the longer ongoing work in the relationship that makes these moments possible. Clients frequently recall the therapist's risking vulnerability and openness as deepening their sense of themselves as trustable and reliable relational beings and as enhancing their sense of the power and meaning of the therapy relationship.

In the classical sense, "countertransference" reactions come from the therapist's past unresolved experiences. Clearly, we would emphasize the importance of the therapist having a relational context which helps her to understand her own past and present life experiences. Especially when a particular therapy relationship is difficult or confusing, the therapist needs to make certain she has a growthful relational context for herself. We also emphasize the importance of an enlarged relational context for client and therapist together—through adding other therapists, groups, or consultation—not as signs of failure but often as necessary arenas for growth and relational movement.

In an ongoing therapy relationship, unusually strong or atypical responses of fear, anger, boredom, etc. in the therapist may signify countertransference phenomena in the relationship. They can be most relevant for expanding empathic connection when shared in a nondestructive way. The concept of countertransference to describe the emotional reactions of the therapist is only a small subset of what we mean by mutuality; mutuality involves the whole movement and development of the relationship.

To deepen our clinical work in a relational model, we all need an empowering community which facilitates our growth and confidence in the relational mode, helps us to heighten our sensitivity and articulateness about the nuances of relational phenomena, and helps us work with our own personal and professional mutuality.

I realize in saying this that I am still saying that the therapist is not totally spontaneous, that she is still taking major responsibility for the relationship and is making many one-sided decisions based on her view of what will further the relationship. As therapy proceeds, she should move into greater spontaneity and openness. Some of this process would be true in any relationship. We become more spontaneous, open, and trusting as we learn more about each other. The movement from major responsibility for the relationship to more mutual responsibility, however, is a characteristic more specific to the therapy relationship. We are still struggling with this issue. It is possible that we are still too caught up in traditional views which arise in a nonrelational framework and that we don't see the ways in which mutuality can occur earlier and more fully.

I hope we all will be working together to grow into an empowering community and to deepen our understanding of these central issues.

REFERENCE

Jordan, J. (1990). Empathy and mutuality essential to effective therapeutic relationships. *The Psychiatric Times*, Vol. VII, No. 4.

DISCUSSION SUMMARY

A discussion was held after each colloquium presentation. Selected portions of the discussion are summarized here.

Question: There are some groups in society that are more dominant than others, and implicit in some relationships is the power differential. If there is a power differential, it would seem that mutual empathy and mutual empowerment cannot be achieved. Isn't there then a need for a sense of individual autonomy based on the old definition, because the more dominant individuals and groups do impinge upon other individuals (e.g., minority group members, women, and others)?

Jordan: That's an excellent and difficult question. There certainly are power differentials which interfere with the development of mutuality. Dominant groups do not want to hear the authentic experience of the subordinate group if it conflicts with their needs. They find all sorts of ways to silence that group. It is very difficult but very important for the less powerful groups or persons to try to gain clarity and to find a way to represent their truth in the relationship and to continue to function effectively outside the relationship. Some might call this autonomy. Where there is a power differential, there is a suppression of real conflict and of the authentic voice. That's an incredible problem. In such a situation, where a more powerful person is destructively impinging on you, you will often have to move out of connection. This takes a lot of courage and confidence, which is most often engendered and encouraged by having other connections.

Stiver: I would like to elaborate on that a little bit. I think, as Judy has said, the concept of autonomy can be translated in various ways, in terms of the relational model. Finding one's own voice, to use Gilligan's words, feels to me like another way of talking about autonomy. I think we find our own voice only when we have a network of support. When faced with that power differential, the more we can find others who are also in subordinate positions, who are able to join together to validate our experiences, the stronger our voices become. In the face of power imbalances, we do feel in some degree of isolation, but it can be countered by a relationship to a network of support. That's how empowerment happens, which makes for the possibility of bringing about some changes in that imbalance.

Question: Another related question: Is, or how is, mutuality possible in a relationship in which there is a gross power differential? (For instance in the therapeutic relationship and also in heterosexual couples.)

Jordan: I find this very problematic and I have been struggling with it a lot lately. One thing I think is important in therapy is that there is the hope of empowering the client *and* the relationship. This is not a permanent power imbalance and the therapist should not use the power to exploit the client but to try to serve the client's needs.

Surrey: There are structural power factors in all of our relationships based on sex, class, race, age, and other factors. On another basis, we hear men say that women have so much power in relationships because that is how they often experience it. There are times when we can feel that our clients have power or that parents feel that their children have. In all situations, the search for mutuality is the emphasis.

Stiver: In therapy, the attempt to move toward mutuality is a goal that two people can try to reach together. Even if it is not yet all that we might wish, this is more true for the relational model than in the more traditional models where silence and prohibitions against therapists' emotional responsivity prevail.

Miller: The oppressed or socially unequal person does have some kinds of power, as Jan suggests, but there is no question as to who has the structural power in the two situations you raise. So far, the best way that we've reached to talk about it is to think of moving towards more mutuality or engaging in the search for mutuality. In the woman-man relationship, there can be a search for mutuality. Some of it is happening in individual relationships but in society we still have a long way to go to bring about the structural changes in power.

Question: Where does creative activity or relationship to nature fit into all of this relational stuff?

Jordan: I think that often in solitude we are in active relationship with internal images of other people and memories that involve people. There are frequently internal dialogues with others. There is also something wonderfully important about being in relationship with nature and with the largeness of nature. We respond to it and are moved by it. These relationships can feel very expansive and sustaining. The openness and vulnerability we experience in being in some unspoiled and compelling place in nature are very important to our growth and well-being. This is different from trying to dominate or "conquer" nature.

Miller: We don't mean at all that people have to be with other people all the time. We are talking about developing psychologically within a sense of connection to others and with the world as opposed to a sense of isolation. Many people who are engaged in creative activities need the time and space to be alone; sometimes they need to move in and out of time spent with others in creative ways.

Surrey: I think the creative process is very much about the ability and freedom to move in new ways, to "move with," to receive "the new," to be spontaneously responsive. We're trying to suggest the kind of development which can lead to those possibilities.

Question: I am wondering whether you are now creating something of a deficiency model for men's experience. Men are also part of a patriarchal context, but it seems that we are creating a model that fits for women, but that negates the self-differentiated model that has been true for men.

Miller: I believe that a relational model is more true to the necessities of the human condition. Being forced to develop within a model that deprives you of that does leave you deficient. I really think that there are ways that men are forced to be deprived and distorted, as we discussed at our last colloquium. Women are, too, but in the different ways that we are discussing tonight.

Kaplan: Building on Jean's comment, I believe that there are ways that men can grow in awareness of and attention to their experience, by building on the relational framework. Clearly men's and women's experiences differ in many basic ways, but the underlying process of discovery can be similar. We would strongly encourage, support, and applaud men who choose to really examine their experience in the long-term and probing way that we and others are doing with women's experience. This process may be harder for men, but therefore all the more necessary, because large numbers of men may not feel it as necessary to face the task of ferreting out their own authentic ways of being from the layers of assumptions and distortions placed on their realities. The question is whether and how men will choose to engage in the process; some have already done so. One of the problems that men face in this task is that Western patriarchal culture has created a false illusion of power and authority which can leave men with little motivation for change.

Question: While I agree with the revaluing, even reverencing, of relationship, there does seem to be something missing in terms of "exit" in the way Carol Gilligan talks about "exit" and "voice." Isn't there a place for reverencing the breaking of relationships? Isn't exit also an empowering and valuable option?

Miller: I think you're absolutely right. There has to be a place for exit. That is very different from the whole question of trying to build a separate self. There are certain relationships that are very destructive, and the best thing is that they be ended. Carolyn Swift's Working Paper on battered women, "Women and Violence: Breaking the Connection," brings evidence to show that the way to break connections is to make connections, that the women who have found a way out of very destructive relationships are the women who have been able to find new connections. They don't do it by becoming isolated and independent, but rather by finding valuable connections—in this instance, through the battered women's shelters.

Stiver: For battered women in a shelter, for example, having the opportunity for validation of the destructive aspects of these relationships is what empowers women to move.

Jordan: In the old theory, "exit" used to mean self-sufficiency and separation. We would suggest that optimal movement in "exit" is to move into a context where mutuality can be created. Mutuality is a goal that is clearly not always attainable at all times, but it is always the goal.

Surrey: Growing into connection involves many forms of relationship, and time and space for solitude. The capacity for aloneness or solitude is very different from going into isolation. Isolation is a form of unchosen disconnection—an outcome of unhealthy relationships.

This chapter was presented at a Stone Center Colloquium on December 6, 1990. © 1990 Jean Baker Miller, Judith V. Jordan, Alexandra G. Kaplan, Irene P. Stiver, and Janet L. Surrey.

3

Clarity in Connection: Empathic Knowing, Desire, and Sexuality

JUDITH V. JORDAN

> There are two great tragedies in life. One is not to get
> your heart's desire. The other is to get it.
>
> G. B. Shaw

This chapter is about desire—how we know it and how we act on it. The notion of a contained and separate self, basic to most of Western psychology, contributes (in practice if not intent) to the idea that there can be clarity about the self separated out from context and that one can be aware of and true to one's values, desires, motives, feelings, and thoughts as if in a vacuum. Acting in a "self-determined" way out of this clarity is often what is meant by "individual freedom" or autonomy.

Pivotal to this individualistic picture of human beings is the pleasure principle (Freud, 1920; Mill, 1861). This principle is profoundly engrained in Western psychology in both the Freudian and behavioristic traditions: attainment of satisfaction, motivated by desire, is the supreme goal of conduct and therefore serves to shape the self. In this tradition "the self" *is* the personal history of gratifications and frustrations of desire and the projection of these into the future in the form of intention.

By contrast with this basic mode, I will examine some implications of a different view of the self (Jordan, 1984; Kaplan, 1987; Miller, 1986; Stiver, 1986; Surrey, 1984); this view suggests other routes to attaining a sense of clarity in knowing ourselves. I will look at the part desire plays in this process and I will illustrate it by discussing women's and men's expression of sexuality in adolescence.

I suggest we achieve a sense of personal integration through relatedness with others and that this integration, not a state of separate homeostasis of drives (Freud, 1920), provides a sense of well-being. An intrinsic interest in and movement towards connection is a basic organizing and motivating force in psychological growth. This statement does not fit neatly into either a self-centered drive theory nor altruistic explanations of motivation. Further, a sense of uniqueness does not depend on separateness or comparative, hierarchical measuring. The espousal of self-containment, self-sufficiency, and self-assertion as a model for self-development contributes to the illusion of separateness and leads paradoxically to an experience of self as endangered and fragmented. When disconnected from you, I feel less confident that you will be responsive to my needs; a system of power, rights and entitlement then develops to try to ensure that my wants will be met.

HOW DO WOMEN WANT?

The question, "What do women want?" has been posed repeatedly, most notably by Freud ("Was will das Weib?" Jones, 1958, p. 421). Often there is an edge of impatience to it, as if to say, "When are these women going to get clear and tell us what they want!!!?" Two responses occur to me. First, before we address the question *what* do women want, we might ask: "*How* do women want?" And related to this is: "Who is listening to what women want? And do the people who pose this question really want to hear?"

Several authors have addressed the nature of woman's voice (e.g., Gilligan, 1982; Belenky et al., 1986), and some have begun to explore further the importance of the listener to the quality of the voice that emerges (Miller, 1986). The expectation that someone will listen and make an effort to understand greatly enhances the clarity and sureness of the message presented.

A vignette from a psychotherapy session may capture this dynamic. Ann, an artist, started off her session talking about the importance of a friend's responsiveness to one of her paintings in helping her to move forward with it. She then spoke of not liking to write in her journal anymore because it felt lonely, a dead-end. She was making a lot of sense but I was preoccupied—with this chapter, as a matter of fact. She fell into more silences and disjointed utterances, and finally said "I feel lost, like I'm in a fog today. I don't know what I want to talk about." More silence, as I ruminated about how to get this chapter done and struggled with my own drifting, confused thoughts. I indicated things did not seem clear. Thankfully, she helped me by saying, "With you or me?" Suddenly, becoming clearer myself, I could tell her that I felt preoccupied and that I thought I had left her alone, as with her journal, in the session. I had been unable to be fully attentive, and we both now felt confused. With this, she looked relieved and talked about the importance of my being more present and about what she wanted from me; both of us came back into focus.

If the other person does not really wish to know my experience, or does not wish her/his experience known, I may become confused about my desires. This happens routinely to another woman, Cynthia: she approaches her husband with a concern; he impatiently lets her know he is much too busy for this; she withdraws and comes back later, upset now; he criticizes her "overemotionality"; she collapses in tears and feels confused about her original concern. The invalidation that Cynthia experiences is enormous. Cynthia's lack of clarity then becomes the *condition* for the continuation of the relationship.

Thus, when I hear women patients struggling with a sense of inadequacy or despair that they do not know what they want in important relationships, often with lovers or spouses, I explore the quality of the listening that the partner provides. Is the listener interested, curious? Is he or she empathically present?

If one person relies on empathy to know the other, there is often the expectation, not always conscious, that this will be mutual. If the other is not empathically attuned, disappointment and a sense of being unheard or invalidated results; one's sense of clarity diminishes. Also, because of our own sensitivity to the impact of our wishes on others, women often experience our wants as tentative and unformed. Such tentativeness, in the service of interpersonal sensitivity, could be viewed as *facilitating* relationship, rather than as a personal inadequacy.

Further, a woman's voice often will not be heard, even when it is quite clear, if the woman's reality is not congruent with dominant societal values. Those in a minority position (women, blacks, lesbians, gay men) often do not experience receptivity in the listener from the dominant culture. This failure to hear can, at its worst, lead to profound invalidation resulting in depressive withdrawal and/or outrage. Relationship as dialogue challenges a clear subject–object split (Kaplan,

1987). The "how" of wanting for women is tied to the relational context in which we experience the wish.

CLARITY

Our self awareness has varying degrees of clarity. Unlike the concept of identity (Erikson, 1968), the notion of clarity reduces our tendency to concretize "the self" as "body." When people talk about merging or experiencing "loss of self," they are likely talking about a decreasing clarity, distinctness, and focus about their experience: I cannot see myself clearly, my affect is not highly articulated or differentiated, intentions either become hazy or drop away altogether. An increase in clarity, sometimes expressed as "being more in one's truth" or in one's "real self," is often accompanied by a sense of relief or "fit." For instance, even when a person moves into a sharper, more distinct experience of sadness, she/he can experience relief, often moving from the more contaminated or complex state of depression. In a mutually empathic relationship each individual allows and assists the other to come with focused energy more fully into his or her own truth or reality and into relationship, what Jean Miller calls "representing your own experience in relationship" (1986).

A woman whom I'll call Susan is a highly successful, usually confident clinical psychologist. Yet she has difficulty in communicating her desires to her husband. "I get unclear about what I want. John feels so entitled that his wants are like *needs*. I felt terrible about something at work and wanted to talk to him. He was working on a paper; he said this work was life and death. Of course I said, 'Fine, O. K.' Besides, I wanted him to *want* to help me, to be with me. I didn't want to have to convince him. I wound up feeling too needy." Later, in discussing the ending of therapy, Susan commented, "I'm afraid I'll be a nonperson when we terminate." I asked, "How would that be?" and she responded, "Well, I connect with myself through connecting with you. I know myself partly through your knowing me." With an empathic response, her own experience comes into focus, and without it she fears the sense of her own reality will blur.

TWO MODES OF KNOWING AND RELATING

I would like now to delineate two modes of knowing and relating which influence our experience of relationship and, in turn, of desire: An objectifying/power/control mode, and an empathic/love mode.

These represent extremes, and all of us in this cultural tradition probably move to some extent in each of these ways.

The Objectifying/Power/Control Mode

The objectifying/power/control mode is the dominant mode of Western culture and its values are central to the socialization of males, in
particular, in our society. Mastery and individual autonomy are the
hallmarks of this developmental track. In operating out of a drive to
satisfy my own need for power, when I want to know you, it is not really to understand or delight in your particular way of being; it is so
that I can better get you to comply with what I believe I want or need
from you. Here we see the dilemma and paradox of viewing the other
as separate self but treating the other as part of one's need system. The
need for you to comply with my desire fires fears of being dependent
which conflict with the wish to appear autonomous; therefore we disavow these needs or meet them covertly (Stiver, 1983) as in having a
wife or mother whose role it is to take care of our desires.

A system of entitlement and belief in one's "rights" supports this
denial and need. My experience of being individually unique is transformed readily into "being better than" in order to justify and buttress
my entitlement. The projection of objectification (I make you into an
object and you do the same to me) and the hostility accompanying a
competitive spirit (I must be better than you, beat you, in order to
demonstrate to myself and others that I deserve "to get") lead us to believe it is a dog-eat-dog world. Domination is safety. Thus power is an
essential feature. Since life is seen as a zero-sum game in which my
gain is your loss, getting and being loved or admired are primary,
while giving or loving may seem draining or leading to a sense of dangerous vulnerability.

In this system, wanting to control the other relates to the emphasis on self-control. And isn't control at the center of the overemphasis
of the rational at the expense of the emotional (and contributing to the
dichotomous split between the two)? Isn't it the felt sense of feelings
happening to us, being beyond our will, that leads to devaluing and
fearing them rather than seeing them as powerful sources of knowledge, expression, communication and growth? We are seduced by an
illusion that thoughts are more subject to control and volition and
therefore are more trustworthy.

In the power mode, pride, which some think of as a sense of joy or
satisfaction in one's experiences, may instead be characterized by a
comparative and possessive spirit: "Look what I did" or "Look at
what I have that sets me apart from and above you." Fear then devel-

ops that someone else might take away that which we possess (either directly by taking away material goods or competitively by taking away the comparative advantage we enjoy in the possession of a "superior" trait). A need grows to buttress self and diminish others in order to perpetuate good feelings about the self. No wonder that pride is the first of the seven deadly sins! Pride, in this sense, can then constrict and separate, unlike joy or confidence which do not imply comparison or hierarchy. (The *Oxford English Dictionary*'s first definition of pride is: "A high or overweening opinion of one's own qualities, attainments, or estate, which gives rise to a feeling and attitude of superiority over and contempt for others; inordinate self esteem.")

The pathological variant of pride is arrogance, what, in psychological terms, we might call narcissistic encapsulation and entitlement. (Again, the OED suggests arrogance is "the assertion of unwarrantable claims in respect to one's own importance; the taking of too much upon oneself as one's right.") This is the ultimate defense against experiencing the need of the other and the fear of possible helplessness and isolation if the other does not provide.

The profoundly fragile and defensive nature of this posture creates severe limits to relating to others. A person functioning in this mode often seeks clarity in isolation. A patient described a very painful time following the death of her husband's mother. She knew that he was experiencing intense grief but as she said, "He did not want his sadness and vulnerability known"; so he withdrew. She was empathic to both his sadness and his need not to acknowledge it but could not find a way to bring this understanding into their relationship. She began to doubt her own feelings and her wish to help him; perhaps she was just "projecting." Maybe she needed to "mother" him for her own needs, not for him. Both people felt increasingly isolated; my patient began to feel very confused and depressed as her husband clung to his separate and hidden experience of grief. What could have been a time of real closeness and growth for both of them and a strengthening of their relationship led instead to alienation, confusion and stagnation.

The Empathic/Love Mode

Empathy leads to an understanding of the other as subject, not object. The sameness and commonality of self and other is as central to our well-being as the differentiating features that allow us a sense of uniqueness (Jordan, 1984). Mutuality is sought. I look for a sense of connection and relational expansion rather than control, domination, or satisfaction of individual wants. You are experienced as having your own subjective needs, values and intentions which may or may not be in harmony with mine. If they are not, the differences are acknowledged and some work on areas of conflict is necessary. In this mode, understanding of the self and other is achieved through interaction, not through separation and abstraction. One is responsive and listening. Feelings are valued as a means of knowing, as a basis for communication and action. Identification with the other is a source of clarity and joy rather than a reason to fear losing one's specialness.

The Oedipus complex (Freud, 1924). based on a Hobbesian notion of competition, power, aggression and possession of others as objects, is no longer accepted in this model as the central developmental milestone; rather, we can posit a continuous evolving relational elaboration with mutual empathy (Surrey, 1984) at its vital core.

Gilligan's notion of responsibility and caring is at the heart of the moral system here (Gilligan, 1982). Morality no longer centers on just containing basically self-serving interests, but includes the responsibility to care for others. It might also involve what Surrey refers to as "taking care of the relationship" (1984). Further, fostering another's growth sometimes demands protecting them and sometimes relies on stimulating them to do what is not immediately comfortable. (Historically, we have tended to overprotect girls, failing to help them to enlarge their experience, especially at adolescence, and overstimulate boys, failing to honor their need for protection and recognition of fear.)

An interest and curiosity in the other person's history, circumstances and full humanity expands the notion of empathy from a momentary state of knowing and experiencing with the other to an overarching sense of presence with and openness to the other person's experience and general point of view, a kind of "contextual empathy." It is as if we can understand more fully the scope of the necessity of their particular organization of experience.

Joy often accompanies clarity and characterizes the empathy / love mode. We feel a sense of well-being, pleasure, and delight in knowing and being known. Joy seems "contactful" and outreaching and not comparative. Other pathways to a sense of self-worth that are not competitive are: confidence in self and others, gratitude, courage, clarity, relational capacity and what Jean Miller refers to as zest (1986); all of these attributes can increase our sense of connection in contrast with competitive comparison which decreases it. Unlike entitlement, confidence does not involve a "right" or a "claim" to something because of one's achievements or inherent worth. It is trust or faith in oneself and/or others, a clearly relational concept. Both joy and confidence stand in marked contrast to narcissistic pride as a basis for good feelings about oneself.

TRADITIONAL POWER MODELS OF DESIRE

Traditionally, desire is defined as "The feeling or emotion which is directed to the attainment or possession of some object from which pleasure or satisfaction is expected; longing; craving." A secondary definition involves "physical or sensual appetite; lust" (*Oxford English Dictionary*). The noun "want" often suggests that something is lacking or missing or I experience a need for something more. I feel a longing, I perceive something to satisfy it, I act to get it. Here we have the presumed self-determining, autonomous, Western adult, and we also reinforce the subject–object split. Entitlement, a sense of having a *right* to gratification, supports active pursuit of the desired object. Pride often accompanies the attainment of the object.

Desire and the Need to Control

Because the inability to "get what one wants" leads to apprehension in a system where self-sufficiency and self-determination are so highly prized, the experience of desire typically has become intertwined with the need to control and exert "mastery" over or "to own."

Translated into psychological theory, the extended period of infantile dependency during which the baby cannot motorically or cognitively provide for his or her own needs is viewed often from the adult vantage point as a time of extreme helplessness and noxious vulnerability. The adult perception of this time has seemed to lead to a tremendous fear of being plunged back into such a state; therefore, the first order of business becomes the effort to control people from whom we need or want something, or to deny the needing altogether. Not to know what we want is sometimes a protection against the experience of helplessness as well.

In a power system, whatever I believe I need to satisfy my wants may readily become objectified; the other person's wholeness or subjectivity can become secondary to my desire. This is at the heart of an egoistic, individualistic system! And Western psychologies are almost without exception supportive of this image. Thus, in Kohut's system there is the implication that the self needs the illusion of control over the self-object in order to repair or supply structure lacking in the self (Basch, 1984; Kohut, 1984). The self-object is to be manipulated much as the breast in Melanie Klein's system (Klein, 1948) or the libidinal object in the Freudian model.

Any system that emphasizes the ascendancy of individual desire as the legitimate basis for definition of self and interpersonal relationship is fraught with the possibility of creating violent relationships

based on competition of need and the necessity for establishing hierarchies of dominance, entitlement, and power. Typically this is where
questions of morality come in: in Kant's (1957) system, carried forward by Kohlberg's work (1964), an action is moral if it is done out of
duty, based on reason, not on passion or feeling which are seen as un-
dependable, i.e., these systems are based on the prior assumption of a
power model. Thus one arrives at an abstract rule, the categorical imperative, to contain the violence inherent in a system of power and hierarchy. In a subtle way, abstract rather than contextual morality is
most needed in a system that rests on hierarchy and power; it follows
the logic and language of distance and control. Where empathy, non-
comparativeness, and mutuality prevail, an alternative path to moral
action would emerge, involving empathic responsiveness and a sense
of compassion in a context of caring for the well-being of others. Gilligan's (1982) morality of care and responsibility, however, is judged as
inferior by those who espouse the morality of duty and abstract law.

But isn't the notion of being in control, and self-sufficient, illuso-
ry? In this system, aren't instances of instrumental efficacy highlighted
as a means of supporting the myth? Isn't the dominant group (manag-
er, executives) seen as being in possession of the power and control to
effect predictable and controllable change while those outside of the
traditional power system are assigned to "the human arenas" in which
the "lack of control," according to this system, is more obvious, that is,
the "feeling realms," childcare, responsiveness to others. Then, these
people (those not in power) are blamed, as if the apparent lack of control in these situations indicates lesser ability, less moral dignity, less
reasoning ability, less will and lack of other so-called "higher virtues."
(Who eats the apple, opens Pandora's box?)

Another dilemma exists in such a system when the subgroup, i.e.,
women, who have been "assigned" to the so-called "uncontrollable arenas," actively value relationship and feelings and encourage the importance of subjectivity and the enhancement of others (Miller, 1976). The
need for acceptance (or even the "need for approval") and affiliation,
which is supportive of connection, is seen as infantile, while the need
for esteem, status and self-sufficiency, which is supportive of narcissism, is seen as mature. Rather than feeling ashamed of our wish to
please people and to get approval, as if it is a sign of some deficiency, we
might see it as one aspect of facilitating connection, a positive motivation. The "need for approval" seems to rely on a wish to be liked, an af-
filiative wish to draw near to another person while the wish for status
relies on a wish for position, i.e., power, which suggests movement into
hierarchy and objectification. Thus, although the need for approval
may at first appear to share the narcissism of the wish for status, it ac-

tually would seem to lead to more connection, unlike status-determined relationships, which are characterized by disconnection.

DESIRE WITH EMPATHIC AWARENESS: A NEW MODEL

An alternative way of conceptualizing desire suggests that our wishes or wants are always contextually embedded and arise from that interactive context. Acting on our "felt needs" has an impact on another person and occurs within connection. Further, we care about that impact. If I want something from or with you, an empathic awareness of you will alter the experience of how and what I want. You are not just an object to me. In a mutual and empathic relationship both people can be enhanced by the expression and satisfaction of a desire. My becoming clear about my wants in part allows you to become clearer as well; together we create more clarity. Basically, the enhancement of the relationship may constitute a greater goal than individual gratification and ironically may lead to greater individual fulfillment.

Our culture seems tragically lost in a system that views "real desire" as selfish by definition; any desire that takes into account another's wishes or needs is suspect as illegitimate. One patient reported telling a former therapist about her hopes for her mother's success with a new business venture. While acknowledging ambivalence towards her mother, she passionately cared for her mother's well-being, although in this instance it meant her mother would no longer babysit for her children. The therapist confronted this wish as if the patient could not possibly want what was best for her mother if it introduced stress into her life. That the patient could anticipate the pleasure of a fuller relationship with her mother as her mother grew and could take joy in her mother's joy was seen as defensive reaction-formation and self sacrificing.

Energy put into relational growth, rather than into pleasure narrowly defined as *for the self*, is judged often as masochistic or self sacrificing. But desire without appreciation of the other person's experience and without attention to the consequences of one's desire and actions for the other person becomes nondialogic, power-based and potentially abusive or violent.

Sexuality can serve as an example of the complex meshing of interpersonal and personal desire. My sexual pleasure is a function of my own intense sensate experiences, joy in joining with and exploring your experience, excitement in having fun, pleasing you and knowing you want to please me, feeling "abandoned with you"; but there is a larger, synergistic sense of the pleasure of both, the mutual surrender to a larger union, a diminished self-consciousness and decreased awareness of the other as a separate person. This is the heartbeat of passion. So the desire is not simply a desire of each self for its self pleasure. But what is it *for*? Possibly, if it is for anything, desire is for the experience of joining toward and joining in something that thereby becomes greater than the separate selves.

Typically defined, desire may shape the self and thus limit the self. But desire, like affect and passion, can be thought of as "something larger" that directs us to connection rather than separation. It is when we try to own and "control" the desire that we diminish the sense of something larger than us moving through us; in so doing, we reduce our opportunity to move out of narcissism. Desire in the larger sense affirms connection and being "a part of" rather than "apart from." It leads to *expansion* rather than *satisfaction*; the former suggests growth, life and openness; the latter suggests stasis.

SYSTEMS IN CONFLICT: SEXUAL DESIRE

The shaping of sexual desire and expression in heterosexual relationships in adolescence will illustrate some of the difficulties that ensue when the two modes of organizing knowing and desire meet. By its nature intensely private, hidden, and not given to public exchange or articulation, sexuality tends to become more and more a part of core self definition and less and less open to exchange and learning in relationship. Ironically, even in the sexual relationship itself there is reason to believe that many people, women especially, falsify their experience (according to the Hite report [1976] about 50% of women fake orgasm). Women do this in order to fit some fantasy of what should be—for the man and for their own definition of themselves as women (according to current standards. At other times, women were told other things about what their sexuality should be). Men likely distort their experience in different ways. Thus, an experience that could bring us intensely in touch with an integrated sense of self, other, and transcendence, the paradox of sexual abandon, leads to denial of one's own experience and distancing from the other.

Before turning to some of my speculations about sexuality in adolescence, let me say that I feel tentative and questioning and that feels clearly, strangely appropriate. What I am about to describe is far from an exhaustive account of adolescent sexuality. I want to emphasize, too, that I am speculating about *adolescent* sexuality. I think there are major shifts in sexuality for many men and women as they mature.

At a deep private level, both boys and girls probably experience intense curiosity, excitement, and apprehension about sexual activity. However, the two modes of knowing, and especially managing anxiety and desire, become socialized differently, by gender, particularly in adolescence. I'll address primarily the damaging and distorting consequences of these adolescent sexual rites of passage.

In my clinical practice, I have been struck by the difference in the fears that men and women typically express about their sexuality. When men recall adolescent sexuality they remember being anxious to have their first sexual intercourse; they remember the pressure to lose their "virginity." Less acceptable, was the general anxiety, confusion, and total urgency about sexuality; as one man said, "I just wanted to get it over with and hoped I wouldn't be too humiliated." Another man poignantly said, "After I had sex the first time, I said to myself, 'O.K., now I can die.'"

The Boy's Experience

In our society there are few rituals for entry into manhood; first heterosexual intercourse appears to be used as one of the primary signs of this transition. Fears of not being a man or not appearing like a man to one's peer group become very prominent. They can lead to treating the partner as a means to the end of accomplishing an important intrapsychic and social identity task: "I am now a man; I am now accepted into the club of those boys/men who have 'done it.'" The social task of "scoring," the need to disavow fear and disown the wish to please the partner, often leads to alienation from the wish to be known and loved in a sexual relationship. The wish to be known and loved becomes a secret, often hidden from the boy himself.

One patient spoke enthusiastically of telling his older brother and his brother's friends about "getting to third base" when he was ten; their disbelief in his "accomplishment" and his pride in their awe stood out as the most significant part of this story to him. But the objectification of the other can also be part of the objectification of the penis and the corresponding anxieties about "its" performance. Will "it" stay soft and fail to be willed to erection when I want "it" to or "it should"? Will "it come" too soon? On the other hand, will "it" become erect when it isn't appropriate and will I be embarrassed by "it"?

Sexuality then becomes subsumed into a system of achievement, competition, mastery, and performance (other men have bigger and better erections, are better lovers, have had more lovers). Satisfying the other becomes another way to perform, not an empathic attunement to the other's body and inner experience. Ironically, attention to one's own internal world also becomes narrowed and compartmentalized. If one is comfortable with disclosure and vulnerability, sexual intimacy, literally becoming naked physically and psychologically with one another, can provide the most incredible arena for exploration, discovery of self and other, and pleasure. Attempts to achieve status, and gender identity through early sexual performance, however, encourage self protection, separateness and egocentric preoccupation. There is another powerful irony: the sought after orgasm promises loss of control and loss of a sense of separateness, states quite at odds with those traits towards which males are socialized.

Further, the need to "conquer" or even "use" the other may involve an aspect of what is described as the male's active need to "disidentify" (Greenson, 1968) with the mother or escape the clutches of the "engulfing mother." Desire for sexual intercourse brings the boy into contact with a need for another human being, specifically female, as masturbation and homosexual activity do not qualify for the rite of passage to manhood in our culture. Because he needs the girl so much and this need conflicts with the pressure to be manly and super-independent, he must strongly repudiate this need. As a result, the girl is treated as a "sex object." Thus, the emphasis on power and independence does not allow the boy initially to experience the centrality of the relationship, the wholeness of the other, or vulnerability in his sexual explorations.

The Girl's Experience

For women remembering adolescent sexuality, the most frequent fears I have heard have to do with not being loved, being "used" and "being left." The fear of pregnancy is related to these in the sense of struggling with some sense of responsibility for limiting sexual involvement because of the possible consequences for the woman/girl and perhaps a child.

Unlike the boy's, the girl's confirmation of gender identity occurs dramatically with the appearance of the first menses. *Becoming a Woman* is the title of the pamphlet which the Kotex company has distributed to thousands of pubescent girls in high school hygiene classes over the years. Note the title is not *Menstruation* or *Reproductive Facts*, etc. A clear, definable event marks the movement from girl to woman.

Theorists often talk about the explosion of sexual impulses in adolescence, the powerfully reorganizing function of these changes, the peremptory quality of genital sensations pushing for discharge. While acknowledging the wide range of adolescent sexual experience, I have rarely heard women talk about their experience in this way.

Most women, in speaking about early sexual experiences or their first sexual intercourse, talk about the importance of the relationship and about the boy's initiative and excitement. Many women felt they "gave in" sexually in order to please the boyfriend or to maintain the relationship. I am not suggesting that girls don't become powerfully aroused in the early adolescent explorations of kissing and fond-ling—and women are clearly capable of powerful, intense orgasms. However, the push for intercourse specifically rarely seems to come from the girl; she is interested in closeness, tenderness, being loved. Hite reports, in answer to the question: "What is it about sex that gives you the greatest pleasure?" Many more of the women spoke about emotional intimacy, tenderness, sharing deep feelings with a loved one and other intense relational experiences than about orgasm *per se* (Hite, 1976). This evidence does not discount the real physical pleasure of sexual intercourse, of opening deeply to another, and the wonderful abandon of orgasm but does say that the relational con-text in which these acts and responses occur provides the meaning and joy.

Intercourse alone does not produce orgasmic release so reliably for women as for men, since clitoral stimulation occurs less satisfacto-rily from intercourse alone (of the 30% of women who achieve orgasm during intercourse, clitoral stimulation is quite important and "for most women, having orgasm during intercourse as a result of inter-course alone is the exceptional experience, not the usual one" [Hite, 1976, p. 229]). What happens, then, to our sense of reality when a cen-trally preoccupying interpersonal experience for both sexes is defined largely in terms of the experience of one sex?

What does it mean that "sex" is generally accepted as meaning sexual intercourse when that may be the primary route to pleasure for one sex but not the other (particularly in adolescence)? And what does it mean that sexual orgasm is defined as the most important thing hap-pening in that exchange? These are the kinds of constructions of reali-ty that lead to a profound sense of disempowerment and disenfran-chisement for women. And further, what are the consequences when a part of the developmental pathway for one sex (becoming a man in part through objectification of the other as sex object) directly conflicts with the primary needs of the other sex (the need not to be used, and to be empathically validated and "emotionally held")?

SEXUAL ENTITLEMENT

Sexual desire and passion are often described as "being carried away" by a compelling force. For the male adolescent especially, the intensification of sexual impulses at the same time that he wants to be, or is told he should be, more "in charge" of his own life, poses a real integrative dilemma. Hence, sexual desire becomes infused with a sense of sexual entitlement. The pressure for genital release, combined with the need to establish manhood, may then be experienced as peremptory ("I *need* to get laid"). Rather than experience it simply as being "taken over" by the feelings, boys and men often transform it into taking over the other. The inner urgency is directly communicated outwardly. He wants to "fuck" the woman, to *do to* the other. The other side of this appears in the expression to "get laid," perhaps expressing (in a covert manner) the split off desire to have one's striving, autonomous self laid to rest. It also expresses indirectly the wish to be cared for and cared about.

Both boys and girls learn to believe in the compelling and entitled quality of male sexuality. A patient, Diana, was sexually abused several times at age eight by a brother twelve years older. When she finally summoned the courage to tell her mother, who she knew favored this brother, mother said, "What do you expect when you parade around in your underwear!" This is another variant of all the horrible instances of blaming the rape victim for "asking for it," and even women are taught to think this way. A less extreme but frequent example was reported by another patient: "My mother told me, "If you get a boy too excited, it's your responsibility to stop him. They can't control themselves." Both women had incorporated the message society gives: Male sexuality is powerful and entitled to expression. The man cannot be expected to take responsibility for his actions in the face of these impulses. Herman (1987) cites data that indicates that this rationalization is acted out with frequency: 22% of men in a normal college sample admitted to having had intercourse with "unwilling partners" and 9.2% admitted using force to have intercourse.

The adolescent girl, then, must learn that she is in danger of becoming an object of this "peremptory urge," that she may need protection from it or need to learn to protect herself; managing the other's desire at the expense of her own becomes the developmental task. There is the further implication that the male ego, identified with masculine potency, is fragile and the girl must protect this as well; quite a balancing act! Female sexuality is seen as more subtle and malleable. What a complicated, familiar picture: not only responding to, but also managing, another's desire for sexual gratification, not being true to her own wishes, possibly for nonorgasmic physical and emotional intimacy or orgasmic nonintercourse, the girl then faces the possibility of the ultimate accommodation to other in the form of pregnancy (literally giving over one's body to another's growth). The message is reinforced heavily in adolescence: to be female is to learn to accommodate to another's wishes. In a mutually empathic relationship this might take the form of increasing delight for both. But when accommodation meets entitlement, the accommodating person may feel invalidated; as one patient put it, "I'm the one who doesn't count."

WOMEN'S DESIRE

But what about the girl's own sexual desire? Irigaray said, "Women's desire would not speak the same language as man's" (Irigaray, 1985, p. 25). But how can we learn this language? Recent writers, in demythologizing and discovering the special nature of the female orgasm have helped to relieve the sense of inadequacy many women felt at not experiencing their fullest sexual release through sexual intercourse alone. But I suspect we know next to nothing about the nature of the development of female sexuality. The picture of adolescent sexuality is still heavily colored by the male experience. Although many suggest the female experience would be the same as the male's if the overlay of excessive social restrictions were lifted, I think not.

Much self awareness grows from attunement to our bodies, our responses, our feelings; the validation of our responses by others helps form and crystallize this self knowledge. Being "talked out of one's experience of body sensation is invalidation at a profound level. In sexual joining, defined as it was in the past (as sexual intercourse, male orgasm), the woman could not expect to be known or have her own experience validated; rather it was often seen (by both the woman and society at large) as deficient or faulty. Ashamed of their "deficiency," many women denied their own experience, adopted male norms or, not surprisingly, withdrew interest in sexuality and lost further touch with their desire. Thus, it is difficult for women to say, "I want this."

When discussing sexuality, I often ask women if they can tell their partner what they want or what pleases them; few can. Some, depressively, have given up on trying; some are enraged at the men who don't seem to know what the women want; some try, and feel unheard or judged because their experience does not fit the stereotype of the male model. Some are content in giving their partners pleasure and this may be an important part of their general investment in relationship. When I ask about expressing what they want, I do not mean simply "touch me here or there"; I mean finding a way to convey what is most important to them in intimate, sexual relating. Men, also, are rarely able to address what they truly yearn for.

While grateful for the latest technical information about female sexual responses (Masters and Johnson, 1966), I wonder if the female sexual experience has not simply been molded recently to fit the goal oriented adolescent male sexual experience. The pleasure of orgasm is intense and dramatic. Orgasms are quantifiable. The danger inherent in this kind of sexuality is the objectification of the other and ultimately of the self. Entitlement to gratification highlights objectification of the other, and at its extreme leads to sexual violation. Performance anxiety captures the consequences of objectification of self, and at its extreme, leads to sexual inhibition.

SO, WHAT DO PEOPLE WANT?

Ironically, it would seem that adoption of a primarily pleasure principle notion of sexuality makes for violation of everyone involved. It places desire (in the power/control sense), gratification, and self-satisfaction at the center of an interpersonal experience which promises transcendence of separate self, relational connection, deep knowing of the other and self.

By openly exploring the true nature of their desire in relationship and sharing interest in the presence of the other, there is some possibility for both men and women to come to know their own wholeness. Without this, men become crippled by their disavowal of need and vulnerability and-women are disempowered by their lack of clarity of desire and difficulty affirming the importance of relationship to them. In full sexual expressiveness, desire is not limited by the need to perform or control; it involves surrender to the powerful feelings evoked by the other person and allowing oneself to be carried along by the feelings which belong to both and go beyond both.

Honoring each others realities and desires, not in technique but in the deepest sense of recognizing each others truth, is at the heart of sexuality. In particular, two different individuals can enjoy and take responsibility for having an impact on the other, rejoice in pleasing one another, can explore differentness and discover sameness, can be sensitive, tender, exciting, receptive, and active; in short, they can explore a wide range of interactions. Or they can be invalidated, alienated from self and other, unable to transcend egocentrism. Sexuality offers us the opportunity to learn to move gracefully between desire focused in intense body experience and desire infused with concern for the other.

In summary, in this rather far-ranging chapter I have tried to question a model of desire which rests on the need to control, own, or use another as an object of gratification. Western stereotypes of maturity assume the existence of a "clear" sense of separate self. This self is supposed to be based on awareness of one's desires and on effective strategies to master the environment. And one is to master the environment in order to meet one's needs self-sufficiently. I have suggested an alternative model, based on a clear awareness of the interpersonal nature of desire, contextual desire, which is informed by empathic knowing of the other. A sense of clarity for women often involves trying to integrate an appreciation of one's own reality and a concern about the other's well being. The pleasure in *being part of* (rather than *apart from*) and building something larger than ourselves is suspect in an individualistic culture but I think it is vital to women's reality; further, understanding women's reality can lead to new understanding of everyone's reality.

DISCUSSION SUMMARY

After each colloquium lecture, a discussion session was held so that students and visitors could exchange ideas with each other and with the speaker. Portions of the discussion are edited and presented here to expand and clarify the speaker's ideas. In this session, Drs. Jean Baker Miller and Irene Stiver joined Dr. Jordan in leading the discussion.

Jordan: While you're thinking of some comments, I'll mention a cartoon I saw in the *Boston Globe* this week about research on the differences in the way men and women speak. The cartoon shows a large imposing man with a very pointed nose and prominent teeth; there is an exclamation point coming out of his mouth. Facing him is a very thin and fragile looking woman who is hanging upside down; there is a question mark coming out of her mouth. The study reported that in couples the woman gave more active encouragement to her husband to talk about himself while the husband listened less well and was less likely to actively bring her out about herself and her own topics. I think the exclamation point versus the question mark captures succinctly the difference between the power mode and the empathic mode.

Stiver: Let us begin by congratulating Judy on many things but especially for talking about female sexuality in a very different way, particularly, Judy's many points about the lack of clarity in women's experience of their sexuality. I think this is in part because there has not been an arena or safe place for women to feel heard without feeling they have exposed themselves as deficient and devalued. There has been a fear of not living up to some set of expectations about being a woman and being a certain kind of woman. We still know very little precisely because women have not been able to truly share their experiences in the way Judy has suggested we might.

Question: Have you had any experience with lesbian adolescents and have you found any differences there?

Jordan: It is a very good question. I specifically chose the heterosexual arena because I think that's where the most painful distortions and the clash between these two systems (power and empathy modes) occur. I do not have enough specific information on the experience of adolescent lesbians. My sense is that most women experience a lot of the pressures during adolescence which I've described here, whether they eventually go on to choose a lesbian or heterosexual lifestyle. Being talked out of your experience is common to both groups in adolescence. I would be very interested in learning more about this.

Question: Do you think things are changing for the next generation? I have a daughter who's sixteen and I see her interacting with her boyfriend and it certainly seems very different from the way it was when I was her age. They do a lot of talking and seem genuinely caring. There doesn't seem to me a lot of macho, tough stuff going on.

Jordan: I hope there's been some change. But I have the feeling that things change ideationally so much faster than they change in our hearts. I think the socialization around the sexual rites of passage is so powerful that it's hard for boys not to be deeply affected by it. Later, many men actually experience profound changes in their sexuality; sometimes as they get involved with women who can help them become more fully present and caring in their sexuality.

Stiver: It can be more complicated. There is a difference between closeness between men and women at all ages, which certainly we know is very possible and the whole empathic mode Judy is discussing. Judy is saying that we really know very little about sexuality because of the mode in which it has been cast. We know so little about women's sexual experience, maybe men's too, but we certainly read much more about men's sexual experience. I think that the notion of clarity about experience is what is at stake. Without feeling one has a voice and an opportunity to explore, one feels in danger of exposing oneself; this keeps clarity from emerging. We wind up misunderstanding a great deal about female sexuality.

Question: I recently came across a book, written by a woman in 1986, that contains an essay called, "On Not Liking Sex." I have several female clients who are concerned about their level of satisfaction with their sexuality and everyone that I have told about this article got all excited and ran out to get this book because they feel at last someone is speaking to them. One of the observations the author makes is that she finds sexuality okay, she enjoys participating in it, but she is not really interested in "undertaking" it. When she gets into it, it's okay, but she is not interested in initiating it. I've heard this from a lot of my women clients.

Jordan: It certainly fits with what a lot of women report about their adolescent sexual experiences; it's rare that they're initiators of genital sexuality. But another point you make is how much people are looking for some fresh discussion of sexuality, something that resonates with their experience. What I feel is most important about this chapter is not that I'm saying women's sexuality is this or that. But what is more crucial is that both men and women begin to feel some freedom to start talking about what they are *actually experiencing with one another sexually.* I think that everybody feels hemmed in by all their fantasies of "what is expected of me," "what do I expect of him." The freedom to explore and *find out,* that's the important thing. When you have a literature that doesn't make room for that kind of exploration and it is difficult to talk about with others, you begin to feel all alone with these feelings. Many women who share a lot with close friends don't talk about their sexual experiences; and there is often the sense that "sex is better for her," "something's wrong with me." We're beginning to open up our discussion of actual sexual experience and it's wonderful because this is a very important part of life.

Question: There is some recent writing that men who are "into" power are very attentive at the beginning of the relationship and once they know they "have" the woman, married or whatever, the attention stops. This is very distressing for the woman.

Miller: Yes, I've heard women say that. Perhaps it's that the woman believes the attention indicates a real interest in her experience, but it isn't. Perhaps, it's part of the technique of how you conquer or acquire as Judy described that.

Comment: What strikes me about what you're saying is that I think we men have talked about sexuality as an exploration of physical space. When we talk about empathic relationships we usually think about it in terms of emotional space. And what I've heard you do tonight so beautifully is talk about the extension of that into physical space. It also strikes me that much of male sexuality is very much like a suspension bridge in which the orgasm is actually the whole big end. In fact, where there is empathic exploration of the physical and psychological space, orgasms are events on the landscape and they're by no means central. They are things to which one comes and one continues beyond in the empathic exploration. They're delightful events but not the whole landscape.

Stiver: I would like to follow that up because there is another common observation about the difference between male and female sexuality. It is the woman's wish for *continued connection* after orgasm and the man's *withdrawal* from connection after orgasm. I think this is part of the dissatisfaction many women feel; the orgasm is not the end goal, but is really a way of becoming more connected and, as Jean says, the more connected we become, the more connected we want to be. That kind of yearning to continue the connection is powerful. If there is an abrupt ending of an intense connection, that is sometimes worse than no connection at all, as we know.

Question: I do a lot of work with couples. One of the problems I come across is how to help men become more motivated to become empathic and connected, not just sexually but in all ways. I find myself at a loss as to how to convince somebody that this is a worthwhile thing to put energy into.

Jordan: That's difficult. Often the first thing that you need to do is to try to help the man stop the *doing*, because so often men feel they *must* jump in to "solve a problem" or to "fix it," particularly if the woman in the couple is having a lot of feelings. Then you need to explore with both of them what they want when they express distress. The man may begin to see that *listening well* is terribly important and it isn't a catastrophe if he can't "fix it" or if he feels a bit helpless with the feelings.

Increased tolerance for one's feelings and interest and curiosity in all feelings and in the other person's inner experience, and deepening awareness of the joy of feeling connected are all central to growth in relationships. I believe the joy of connection provides a great sense of well-being, and once experienced, is intrinsically rewarding, and hence, motivating.

Miller: I think we've all been influenced by the power mode; we've all lived under its sway. It often leads us to not want to know the other person's feelings and even to be afraid to know them, and our own feelings, too. But sometimes, I think if we feel we're even making a step toward what you've described, we feel a lot better, long before we've reached anything like full tolerance or curiosity for our own and the other person's experience. Sometimes, in couples work, I've seen men begin to enjoy this whole new "mode." It's almost like a new unknown world.

It's hard for women and men but in different ways for each, for the reasons you've described in the paper.

Comment: That issue makes me think about my own children and children I have taught. So much of what you're talking about can be approached through literature. There is so much in literature to help us raise children to be attentive to how people become clear about what they need, through what you call intersubjectivity, through the joining of two people who become clear about each individual's wants, but also paradoxically whole. So much of what you talk about can be seen in Shakespeare, Flannery O'Connor, even *Charlotte's Web*: Wilbur became whole through his love.

Comment: This is a problem of monumental proportions. As a man I can say it's our male problem and it didn't start ten years ago. We have a large number of men who have been conditioned in the way you describe. I work with couples a lot. I think you are right. Women are more connected. If the woman in the couple wants to grow she has to confront these issues a little at a time. So many men still devalue women in many areas: in the sexual area, around finances, and others. What works is if the woman confronts the man and he gets uncomfortable but gradually gets brought into the feeling world.

Question: I want to ask something about language. You talked about males describing their penis as "it." Are there males who do not describe their penis as an object? And are there women who describe their sexuality in objective ways?

Jordan: I may have overstated the objectification process for men. What I was trying to get at was the particular aspect of the male sexual rite of passage by which in adolescence he objectives the girl and his own body. For many men this does not persist into adult sexuality. I'm also sure that, particularly since there has been so much emphasis on the female orgasm, many women get quite caught in a similar kind of goal-oriented sexuality. I don't think it is either/or.

Comment: In working with a lot of teenagers, I hear girls talking about their bodies in a detached way. They "it-ify" their bodies. They believe the media that the only way to get close and to have tenderness or even to hold someone's hand is to first have intercourse. This is a profound reversal of the sequencing of getting to know anybody intimately, sexually. They cannot take a stand apart from the current dictates. In their wonderful desires for closeness and tenderness and the kind of thing you're talking about, they collude with the cultural image that holds for them an elusive hint of that kind of closeness through an objectification of their bodies and I think that's gotten worse in the last 20 years.

Jordan: That worries me a lot and I think I also see it. It may be a part of a larger cultural phenomenon which is the "quick fix" gratification culture we live in. You look at the advertising and the way we are encouraged to believe that something quick, physical, and easy is going to make it (anything) better; and sexual intercourse is going to bring intimacy. Something very important is going to be lost if that trend continues.

Miller: How can we say to these girls, "Come on, don't fall into this"? As you point out, it is particularly at that age that the girl wants so much to make connections. And then there is this awful paradox: you make the connection by first making yourself an object because it seems the only way.

Comment: It seems to me one of the problems with sexuality in our culture is that it is linked with touch and as we grow up, touch gets so distorted. Part of the objectification is that there is no way we can continue, as we do with children, to explore the environment through touch. In adolescence we want to be close to someone and where do you learn how to do that? Particularly around touch. The family doesn't do it, TV is sexualizing everything, and violence is the norm. There's little opportunity to learn how.

Jordan: That's another important point. We've begun on many points tonight. There's a lot more to be explored. I want to thank everyone for a stimulating discussion. The spirit of openness and curiosity here is what we all need to more fully understand desire and our experience of relationship and sexuality.

REFERENCES

Basch, M. (1981). Selfobjects and selfobject transference: Theoretical implications. In P. Stepansky & A. Goldberg (Eds.), *Kohut's legacy*. New Jersey: Analytic Press.

Belenky, M., Clinchy, B., Goldberger, N., & Tarule, J. (1986). *Women's ways of knowing*. New York: Basic Books.

Erikson, E. (1968). *Identity: Youth and crisis*. New York: Norton.

Freud, S. (1920). Beyond the pleasure principle. In J. Strachey, (Ed. and Trans.), *The standard edition of the complete psychological works of Sigmund Freud, Vol. 18*. London: Hogarth Press.

Freud, S. (1924). The dissolution of the Oedipus complex. In J. Strachey, (Ed. and Trans.), *The standard edition of the complete psychological works of Sigmund Freud, Vol. 19*. London: Hogarth Press.

Gilligan, C. (1982). *In a different voice*. Cambridge: Harvard University Press.

Greenson, R. (1968). Dis-identifying from the mother; Its special importance for the boy. International *Journal of Psychoanalysis, 49*, 370–374.

Herman, J. (1987). Sexual violence. Paper presented at Harvard Medical School/Cambridge Hospital-Stone Center Conference, *Learning From Women*, Boston, April 1987.

Hite, S. (1976). *The Hite report*. New York: Dell Publishing.

Irigaray, L. (1985). *This sex which is not one*. Ithaca, NY: Cornell University Press.

Jones, E. (1957). *Sigmund Freud: Life and work, Vol. 2*. p. 421. London: Hogarth Press.

Jordan, J. (1984). *Empathy and self boundaries.* (Work in Progress No. 16.) Wellesley, MA: Stone Center Working Paper Series.

Jordan, J. (1986). *The meaning of mutality.* (Work in Progress No. 23.) Wellesley, MA: Stone Center Working Paper Series.

Kaplan, A. (1987). Dichotomous thought and relational processes in psychotherapy. Stone Center Colloquium Series, Wellesley, MA, March 1987.

Kant, I. (1957). *Selections.* In T. M. Greene (Ed.). New York: Charles Scribner's.

Klein, M. (1948). *Contributions to psychoanalysis: 1921–1945.* London: Hogarth Press.

Kohlberg, L. (1964). Development of moral character and moral ideology. In M. Hoffman & L. Hoffman (Eds.). *Review of child development,* New York: Russell Sage.

Kohut, H. (1984). *How does analysis cure?* Chicago: University of Chicago Press.

Masters, W. & Johnson, V. (1966). *Human sexual response.* Boston: Little Brown.

Mill, J. S. (1861). *Utilitarianism.* London: J. M. Dent.

Miller, J. B. (1976). *Toward a new psychology of women.* Boston: Beacon Press.

Miller, J. B. (1986). *What do we mean by relationships?* (Work in Progress No. 22.) Wellesley, MA: Stone Center Working Paper Series.

Oxford English Dictionary, Compact Edition, 1971. Oxford: Clarendon Press.

Shaw, G. B. (1903). *Man and superman.* In *The complete works of George Bernard Shaw.* London: Paul Hamlyn.

Stiver, I. (1983). *The meanings of "dependency" in female-male relationships.* (Work in progress No. 11). Wellesley, MA: Stone Center Working Paper Series.

Stiver, I. (1986). *Beyond the Oedipus complex: Mothers and daughters.* (Work in Progress No. 26.) Wellesley, MA: Stone Center Working Paper Series.

Surrey, J. (1984). *The "self-in-relation": A theory of women's development.* (Work in Progress No. 13.) Wellesley, MA: Stone Center Working Paper Series.

This chapter was presented at a Stone Center Colloquium in May 1987. © 1987 Judith Jordan.

4

Clinical Applications of the Stone Center Theoretical Approach to Minority Women

CLEVONNE W. TURNER

INTRODUCTION

For purposes of clarity and focus, I will highlight my work with Black women only. There are far too many differences in traditions, family norms, beliefs, attitudes, styles, behaviors, and the like existing in various racial minority cultures in this country to try unfairly to lump them all together in this chapter. Please note, however, that racial oppression of one sort or another and being *bi-cultural* in this country increase the possibilities for connectedness of women within a particular culture and often to other minority cultures considered different from their own. There will then be some "common threads" in applying the "self-relation" theory to all women of color which can be learned from working with Black women. Also note that women in the same family within a particular culture vary greatly from one another in their individual traits, perceptions, personalities, and feelings, so do not anticipate a "pat formula" from this chapter that clinicians can go forth and apply! The intent of this chapter is to share my findings in a way that will encourage the reader to:

1. Become more fully aware of your own ethnicity.
2. Increase your capacity to care, listen, respect, mutually engage, and validate in your clinical work a cultural "world view" that may be different from your own.

The Stone Center theoretical approach to clinical work with women is about fifteen years old now. It focuses on "the centrality and continuity of relationships" in women's development. A basic premise in the work at the Center is the belief that a closer examination of women and their development can lead to a new understanding of both women and men.

In previous *Work In Progress* papers Jean Baker Miller, Alexandra Kaplan, Irene Stiver, Janet Surrey, and Judith Jordan, among others, have defined it in greater detail than I can go into now. To paraphrase them briefly, I'll highlight a few key points. Women's experiences of self appear to contradict most developmental theories which emphasize the importance of disconnection from early relationships in order to achieve a separate and bounded sense of self (Surrey, 1984). Miller (1984) has written about some of the ways this theory is currently evolving at the Stone Center to reflect more adequately the neglected complexities of human interconnection more commonly seen in women's experiences. The "relational self" concept is an evolutionary process which is seen as developing within (not outside of) mutually empathic relationships starting early in the mother-daughter dyad (Surrey, 1984).

Rather than moving through a series of separations from mother and other significant family members, women add on relationships as they redefine primary relationships in age-appropriate ways. We believe that this type of development leads to self-awareness and understanding while serving to validate the "felt need" of women to understand and become better aware of the other. This is a dynamic, interactive and flexible process rather than a static self construct. Self differentiation is promoted and encouraged without a series of losses, as it is occurring within the context of staying meaningfully connected to significant others. However, if the "relational" context in the family, the surrounding society, and within the therapeutic alliance has been destructive, restrictive, or not conducive to growth-promoting relationships, women will experience greater difficulty in feeling good about themselves and in building healthy connections to others. Kaplan (1984) has written in detail about some aspects of this phenomenon as she described the resulting depressive features of women's vulnerability to loss and inhibition of action and assertion, as well as internalized anger and low self-esteem.

HOW THE THEORY RELATES TO BLACK WOMEN

The "self-in-relation" theory represents, validates and legitimizes a large and important part of the Black woman's maturation process. This maturation occurs as she strives to develop a balanced sense of self together with ethnic pride, in conjunction with an internalized affective, cognitive connection to her family and the Black community. Too often this has been misconstrued as "deviant" or "dependent" and not valued for its growth-promoting qualities. The process of adding to and redefining significant relationships, instead of separating from them, in order to achieve autonomy can now be examined in a new light. Because this developmental process starts with the mother-daughter relationship before it spreads to others, we should take a closer look at Black mothers and daughters.

As Black women develop and grow, they simultaneously learn to redefine and differentiate their sense of self in relation to their concern and feelings for significant others (mothers, fathers, siblings, relatives, friends, authority figures, and the Black community-at-large.) Autonomy and separation *may* not be valued in the "traditional ways" psychologists have written and theorized about them. A Black woman's connectedness to family and ethnic identity usually have been a source of love, strength, coping power, and stability which is vital and necessary for psychological survival and health. She doesn't cut off those important parts of herself if they have helped her to stay sane and negotiate the complexities of living in two cultural worlds with all its mixed messages. She tends to see it as a base that she will augment over the course of time.

If Black mothers are appropriately aware of their ethnic roots, they are constantly working in a "relational" context to instill in their daughters deeper feelings of positive self-esteem, awareness of both how to nurture and how to achieve more self-confidence, resourcefulness, and racial pride. In addition, these mothers are working to build within their daughters a sound base of inner strengths and coping mechanisms which they hope will fit well with the minority and majority cultures. Values are taught and reinforced continually even though these daughters are being raised in a society that often devalues both them and their mothers in every stage of each others development. These daughters are usually taught very early in life to *rely on themselves* as well as to *care for others*.

Empathic attunement between mother and daughter usually is learned and developed early in these relationships, often out of necessity. Depending on the socioeconomic level of the family, young

Black women may become immersed quickly in the care-taking responsibilities in the home. Jordan (1982, 1984) has written some very useful papers about the complex cognitive and affective components of empathy and self boundaries and their centrality to the development of the self and of relational capacities. These papers shed further light here.

BLACK WOMEN REPRESENT CULTURAL VARIATIONS WITHIN THE MODEL

When Black mothers raise their daughters, they have additional burdens and responsibilities due to the intertwining of the double binds of *sexism* and *racism*. For many of these mothers there is also the added bind of *classism*. As Black women move through the various developmental stages of childhood, latency, adolescence and adulthood, the issues around closeness, trust, self-worth, caretaking, industry, achievement, and sexual intimacy are bound together in different ways than for their white counterparts. A distorted, devalued image of Black womanhood has been fostered too often via myths, stereotypes, misconceptions, the media and Westernized educational systems, as well as through legal, social and political sanctioning in our society. Yes, there are those within majority and minority cultures, males as well as females, who work on correcting this image. However, the damage is still there, like a cancer which continues to fester. Black women, as a result of this and other harsh realities, are raised to be much more cautious than women in the majority culture. Discipline around what is acceptable behavior is often and necessarily much stricter in Black families because the consequences of doing something "nonacceptable" in the majority culture are usually more severe. Many times this "nonacceptable" behavior can affect one's family, job, residence—or even one's life in certain environments. This reality creates a set-up for "tension" and sometimes bitter arguments between mothers and daughters. These daughters are taught and expected to perform many tasks at an earlier age than many of their white counterparts, and they therefore experience themselves to be more "streetwise" and "grown-up" than their biological ages imply.

It is, needless to say, difficult for these mothers to both protect and teach, while striving to be positive and loving in an overall atmosphere of being cautious. As they attempt to balance the realities of "living in two cultural worlds," they are also trying to maintain a calm, meaningful relationship with their daughters and signifi-

cant others. Some of these mothers have been mislabeled as matriarchal, dominating, overly intrusive and hysterical. Some of the
daughters then are labeled as aggressive, hostile, argumentative, and
controlling when they each try to juggle their roles and expectations. There are high probabilities that there will be some conflicts,
misunderstandings, and hurt feelings, along with hiding or cutting off
their most vulnerable parts from others via several kinds of defense
mechanisms. This will be evident as these women relate to each other
and on a wider scale to other men and women of various cultures.
There are already complex, difficult issues arising between Black
women and men, Black women who befriend and/or date inter-racial-
ly, Black women, and white women, and Black women working with
white men. There are also serious relational gaps among Black
women.

Developmentally, as has been implied earlier, Black women have
been socialized to integrate traditional *male roles* of achievement, autonomy and independence with the more traditional *female roles* of
caretaking and nurturing as a "norm." For the majority of white
women this had been viewed as "deviant" or nontraditional until the
women's movement helped to make it more acceptable. Black women
are affected by the remnants of racism in the Women's Movement and
sexism in the Civil Rights Movement, which often leaves them
"caught in the middle."

In a previous Stone Center paper on psychosocial barriers to
Black women's career development (Turner, 1984), several resulting
syndromes are high-lighted. One that is particularly relevant here is
what I have labeled the *Chameleon Syndrome*. It refers to Black women
"fine tuning" and "adapting" themselves as they rotate alliances between various groups of men and women in order to pay attention to
all the parts of themselves which are important. It is well to note clinically that it is normal for Black women to be conflicted about how to
resolve these "splits" within themselves and to foster a "healthy paranoia" in relating to these groups. The nurturing, relational side will
want to heal these splits while the assertive, achievement side will
want to demand equality and support.

As clinicians, we will need to listen to and validate these legitimate and conflicting realities rather than deny, ignore or just react to
them. These women will need your support (not your sympathy) and
a verbalized, interactive willingness to work on a mutually empathic,
"connecting" relationship with them. This will be a benefit in solidify-
ing the therapeutic alliance for both of you, *and* will help them to integrate the various sides of themselves whenever possible.

COMMON CLINICAL BLIND SPOTS
TO THE "RELATIONAL SELF"

Some therapists have misinterpreted the meaning of "relational" development as "dependent," "regressive," "symbiotic," "deficient," or "weak." Any resulting therapeutic intervention based on this kind of mislabeling is harmful, and can interfere with the traditional, acceptable and adaptive values of the Black family. It will also dilute and undermine the establishment of a healthy, productive alliance between the client and the therapist. A major task for the clinician is to learn to understand the client's functioning within her own cultural environment and value system (as well as how she functions within the majority culture) as a "norm." By doing so, with the client's help, the clinician is in a better position to determine mutually with the client the extent of conformity or deviation. To impose a traditional "Westernized, majority culture" set of norms on this client will increase not only probabilities of misdiagnosis, but also mistreatment and a counterproductive therapeutic encounter.

Self-reliance is highly valued and encouraged in Black families but in a way that will not cut people off from their families, their ethnicity and their culture. The more that Black families adapt and become upwardly mobile, the higher the probability that majority norms will be imitated. This can result in problematic issues around accommodation, homogenization, perfectionism, superiority, inferiority and even "passing for white." Black women will sometimes discriminate against each other based on skin color, hair type, facial contour, physical appearance, socioeconomic status, regional background, and the like. It is well to note that this discrimination is a reflection of "self-hatred," insecurity and sometimes "superiority." This pattern is often mimicked from the majority culture's way of treating particular ethnic groups, and some use it to elevate their "perceived" status in society.

Be aware of what I have labeled a "seesaw" phenomenon. This is a type of sibling-like rivalry between those inside of a culture as well as those in other cultures over *who* receives more "goodies" or favoritism at a given time from the majority culture. This phenomenon occurs among those in the majority culture and between the majority culture and various racial cultures. The rivalry often involves who gets accepted into schools, who gets government and state monies, or, more often, who gets the larger portion of whatever is valued by both. Meaningful relationships and their consequences are then placed at a high risk.

If there is mutual empathy and support from significant others, the related cultures and society at large, the Black woman's emotional development is greatly enhanced. A problem area exists, however, if support or validation does not come from these sources, causing internal self-doubts, putting one's self down, labeling one's self "too selfish," developing insecurities, anxieties, suicidal and/or homicidal ideation, anger, hostility, and self-hatred.

It is not only *good* to try to understand Black women in a relational and systemic context relative to their ethnicity, it is *vital*. If we can understand anything about the legacies of slavery, of Black families being forcefully and legally torn apart, of the dehumanizing abuses and myths, and of the subtle and pervasive forms of racism and sexism which are alive and well today, then we can appreciate more easily the necessity of developing and achieving in this "relational" context for our Black women clients.

A student in a support group for Black women which I facilitated a few years ago summed up her "relational self-awareness" this way:

> "Whether my family and I are getting along or not, I always carry with me their belief in me and my ability to be whatever I want to be, with the unqualified belief that I will also be successful. I guess I realize how invaluable and important this is to my self-esteem and to my belief in myself that I *will* have a successful, meaningful life and career. This inner belief bolsters me when I have a setback or encounter a putdown. I know that if I fail or bring shame in some way to myself, I also bring those negative behaviors onto my family and the Black race in general. If I succeed, they in some way succeed too."

SUGGESTED CLINICAL GUIDELINES

There will be significant times in the therapeutic relationship when it will become necessary and appropriate to acknowledge the pathology and sickness that exist in our society (as opposed to inside the client) which contribute to extra stress for the Black woman client. In doing so, you can be in a much more collaborative and pro-active stance with her. In general, there are six important areas to explore as they relate to the woman's identified presenting problem:

1. How she feels about and experiences her ethnicity, along with her perceptions about how others feel about and experience her ethnicity;
2. Her strengths and coping skills in negotiating the "two cultural worlds" she lives in;

3. Those parts of herself which are responding resourcefully to forces both within and without her control;
4. The parts of herself and her experiences which cause her pain, hurt, and frustration internally and externally;
5. The interactive parts of herself, family, work, and social environment which work beneficially for her in fostering healthy growth and change, as well as those that interfere with this healthy process;
6. An examination of the extent to which she has acquired internalized and external meaningful connections and bicultural support systems. These systems include the affective and therapeutic connection with the therapist as well as significant others, groups, organizations, religious affiliations, and the like.

These important areas can be missed easily if you don't ask about them. Self-disclosure about these areas usually won't come easily, or at all in many instances. The client is usually aware if there is not a genuine quality of caring and resilience in the clinician and an ability to tolerate learning about these often well-insulated private and conflicting experiences. So many times "bicultural stress" is so time consuming, that these women have to decide if it does any good to share these concerns and, if so, with whom. They also learn to set priorities about which issues to put aside and which ones to take a stand on as a basic survival technique. Some elect to distance themselves from their Blackness and try to "fit in," forgetting that others can still see them as "Black." The first case below is an example of this behavior.

EXAMPLES OF CLINICAL APPLICATIONS UTILIZING RELATIONAL THEORY

Ms. A.

Ms. A. is a young Black woman college student who is dark-complexioned, extremely bright and an only child raised from the age of four by her upwardly mobile mother alone in a large northern city. She did not seek me out because I was a Black female therapist, but admitted she was assigned to me against her wishes because she was in a hurry to be seen and my schedule was the only one that matched hers that particular day in the clinic.

She presented with relational problems resulting from an argument she had with her three best girlfriends, all of whom were white. They were reportedly "fed up with her arrogance, belittling of them and acting as if she were a Black princess" around them. In a nutshell, she was devastated that they dared to call her "Black" as she didn't consider or see herself as Black, but as a person just like them. They had then stopped speaking to each other. She believed that by denying her ethnicity, others would follow suit. She had no Black friends then, nor had she ever been close to any in the past. Not surprisingly, her mother also lived this way and had maintained minimal and perfunctory ties to relatives and no contact with her husband since the divorce.

I saw Ms. A. eight times that year and four times the following year in the counseling clinic before she graduated. She elected not to have long term therapy and was seen using the Stone Center short term psychodynamic, interactive approach. Our time together was focused on not only reconnecting her to her friends, but also on reconnecting her to her ethnic sense of self in a way she had not valued or taken time for before. The interchange between us was critical in terms of increasing her ability to connect effectively with me, with other Black women around her, and with other white women on her dormitory floor, in a more appropriate manner. She and I created space in the therapy for her to express hostility directly at me, which she began to see was aimed also at herself. She was pleasantly surprised that I could both empathize with her experience and express my sadness around her ethnic denial without criticizing her. This experience led to a deeper awareness of the parts of herself she had cut off, and prompted her to call her mother one night to share this revelation. She was able to express directly to her mother the realization that her supercritical behavior of others was due in great part to "not liking herself for being Black." She and her mother cried together on the phone, and I believe this was a turning point for them *both* to use their new "affective connection" to each other (as well as to me) as a "lever for change."

In this case, a white clinician could have connected more easily to Ms. A. initially, and no doubt would have been seen as a more powerful and desirable person to engage with. I was more of an unwanted curiosity, but because I didn't appear angry, nervous or defensive, Ms. A. began to engage with me. At the time she perceived herself as "saving me the agony of rejection in front of my white co-workers at the clinic." She had the ability to be humorous as well as hostile, but more importantly she could express a wide range of meaningful affect with which I could begin to connect. I do believe the therapy could have proceeded with similar benefits with a white clinician who chose to deal with the ambiguities and self-hatred rather than ignore them. It might have been more tempting (and comfortable) to collude with the client and just treat the relationship issue, but the client would not have had the opportunity to engage the cut off parts of her reality. As this therapy progressed, it became clear to both of us that the early and unwanted loss of her father to a white woman contributed to a dynamic for her mother of being left for "someone perceived to be better than the mother." It further led to her mother feeling angry, vulnerable and "blamed" by her family because she could not hold onto her husband.

I would like to note that Black women of many hues from light to dark can suffer from self-hatred and identify more strongly with the majority culture than with their own for a variety of reasons.

Ms. B.

Ms. B. is a young Black woman in her twenties pursuing an advanced graduate degree. She had not had previous counseling and, until recently, had not experienced any serious setbacks or difficulties. She is one of several siblings, the younger daughter of a low-income intact family. One of her brothers has an advanced professional degree, but she will be the first woman in her family to do so. She presented with issues of deflated self-esteem, low grades and "hot off the press" news from her dean that the school wanted to "counsel her out of the program" by the end of the current semester. She had failed all of her tests and didn't seem to be making a good fit at the school, according to most of her teachers. She was shocked in light of her past high achievement in college and her motivation to succeed. She appeared not only deflated but depressed and agitated. She was not suicidal, but very down on herself and very frustrated. She told me that she studied religiously, knew the material, but just couldn't perform when she was expected to.

At closer look, I discovered that she was cut off from any source of emotional, academic or social support. She studied alone and *never* conversed with any of her teachers or school staff. She couldn't tell her family because she thought it would destroy them. In short, *no one knew what I knew* about this discrepancy between preparation and performance! She felt shame, embarrassment and a profound sense of failure in letting herself and her family down. There were a handful of Black women and men and a few more white women in her class. She didn't feel she could confide in any of them, and whenever anyone in her class asked how she was doing, she always responded, "OK."

I saw Ms. B. for a little over a year. I was able to connect with her around her profound isolation and guilt-laden feelings by helping her to better see *her role and that of significant others* in hiding important parts of herself from people all around her. Basic to this was her inner feeling of not being accepted as a legitimate member of her school environment. This inner feeling caused intense anxiety and somatic symptoms. She fostered a perception of not "belonging" or "being valued" which, as it turned out, *was* shared by a few at the school, but not by everyone. She did have to leave the school for a term; however, she is now re-enrolled there. This time, she has identified and sought out mentors, study groups, an active Black organization, and a greater sense of "entitlement" to study there as a Black woman. I'm happy to say that this activity is also reflected in her grades. She has learned to use a number of stress reduction techniques to move past the anxiety blocks and to relax more. She also knows now that her family loves and respects her, no matter what happens, because she freed herself up to share some of the pressure she felt about being the first woman in her family to achieve professional status. This pressure was tied in with her internal fears about losing her place with them, and in a sense "leaving them behind." On an affective level, this fear contributed to her depressed feelings, while on a cognitive level she wanted to believe that they would still love her as they always had. Because she felt vulnerable to a "perceived loss," her academic pursuits had been conflicted and inhibited.

This woman offers a prime example of the experiences I have seen in a large number of Black women clients and associates in predominantly white academic and/or work environments. Most of them are very successful in their external achievements but feel diminished, devalued, unappreciated, and mainly "unknown" in a full sense by those around them. They sometimes also fear being distrusted or not fully included anymore in primary family and ethnic relationships since they feel more distanced from them because of their academic pursuits or jobs.

Many of these women report being treated at work and at school as though they are "invisible" until someone wants or needs something they can provide. This is further complicated by internal and external "perceived losses" when prior significant relationships either accommodate to or change due to the women's achievements. The women's reactions range from complete compliance to "expected majority norms" to uncontrollable rage because they can't be their complete selves and don't feel they are vital, welcome additions to the school or organization. If they let these feelings build up inside them too long before expressing them, they are seen as inappropriate, "bad fits," trouble makers, complainers, "bad team players," and the like. It is vital that we all provide safe, nonjudgmental environments for these feelings to be aired. They then can complement these women's skills, effectiveness and achievements. We also have to try harder to listen and respond in a way that will help empower these women to express a wide range of feelings and behaviors to significant others. This will, in turn, lead to pro-active engagement and healthier connections rather than more isolation and reactive disengagement. They deserve the opportunity to bring all the meaningful parts of their experiences into processes where they can flourish and be fully accepted for who and what they are as human beings. This is not only good for the women and the clinicians, but also good for the schools and organizations of which they are a part. It's the difference between working collaboratively for mutual goals and working alone with separate goals.

The accompanying issue for many Black women (and men) is the reality of "leaving others behind" and not being meaningfully connected. A struggle ensues to do well, meet new people, move more comfortably into the majority world while deciding if and how one will give "something back" to the Black community and also maintain cherished ties there.

A STRONG RECOMMENDATION FOR
CROSS-CULTURAL TRAINING

If a clinician has never received any cross-cultural training, and decides to treat a racially diverse clientele, training is a *must*! I rely quite heavily on strategies developed by other Black clinicians as adjuncts and tools to help implement the "self-in-relation" theoretical approach. Knowledge of cross-cultural counseling techniques is vitally important in working with this population as well as with women from other cultural backgrounds. Elaine Pinderhughes, a Black woman professor of social work at the Boston College Graduate School of Social Work, has written extensively about the cross-cultural interface between ethnicity, race, and power, as well as providing guidelines for teaching empathy (1982). Pinderhughes (1984) states that "knowing how power and powerlessness operate in human systems is a key to effective intervention." She has developed strategies for constructively managing powerlessness on individual, familial

and social systems levels to benefit client and worker. I urge all to become familiar with her guidance in providing treatment.

Further, clinicians can use a technique called "ethnotherapy," developed by Price Cobbs, a Black male psychiatrist based in San Francisco, to sensitize and raise their levels of consciousness (1982). This
plan involves meeting in groups with others who are like you as well
as not like you racially and ethnically to process feelings about your
own and others' ethnicity. If we can all learn to appreciate, value and
like ourselves with our similarities and differences, we come that
much closer to being receptive in mutually empowering ways to others who are not like ourselves.

SUMMARY

In conclusion, I'd like to say that the Stone Center "self-in-relation"
clinical approach is very useful in working with Black women as they
develop and differentiate themselves in a relational, systemic context
within two cultures. This model is a fluid one which sees maximum
health as inclusive of *all* the experiences these women have without labeling their cultural uniqueness as deficient, pathological or deviant.
The process involves seeing development in Black women in the context of relationships which emphasize being understood, as well as
understanding the other(s), in a mutually interactive model. This kind
of interaction, in turn, leads to becoming empowered as well as being
able to empower others. This dynamic has to occur in the therapeutic
alliance if the client is to benefit in her life outside the alliance. It involves attending to this process together with mutual goal setting, caring, listening, validating, sharing observations as well as risk-taking in
expressing a variety of feelings. The process is active, supportive, educational, and systemic. Psychosocial networking is highly encouraged,
and support systems (including those which are bicultural) are utilized as healthy, desirable adjuncts to this type of therapy as they foster more connection to others.

I hope that this chapter has provided some "evolving" food for
thought and for action in our important clinical work with minority
women.

DISCUSSION SUMMARY

*After each colloquium lecture, a discussion session was held so that students
and visitors could exchange ideas with each other and with the speaker. Por-*

tions of the discussion are edited and presented here to expand and clarify the speaker's ideas. In this session Drs. Jean Baker Miller and Carolyn Swift of the Stone Center and Myra Rodrigues, M.S.W, of the Massachusetts Institute of Technology Health Services joined Ms. Turner in leading the discussion.

Comment: I think the Black churches always have been a major source of the connections you're talking about for Black women. They've given the kind of connections which contain a sense of valuing Black women.

Rodrigues: I certainly agree. Black churches have been, and are today, of great importance. Black women find both a sense of very personal connection and also connection to a larger community and tradition that has great meaning; and there is also a spiritual connection which deepens the meaning.

Comment: Unfortunately, as a Black female minister, I am witnessing a disturbing phenomenon. Some of my fellow female ministers are excluding the nurturing and relating roles as they take on more traditional male models of working with their congregations. I think we have to re-work our roles to address the disconnections we have fostered in our churches which mimic those that exist in our other institutions.

Rodrigues: I see this "re-working" already beginning to occur. There is a resurgence of many young Black professional women attending the Black church to counteract a sense of isolation and devaluation. The church is one of the natural sources of help which intersect with various life-cycle events, such as births, christenings, marriage, death, and illness, whether one is a member of a church or not. There is a great need for clinicians and ministers to connect with each other as valuable resources in systemically working with the disconnections women are trying to address. This can serve more fully to reconnect women in a whole sense to achieve a stronger, healthier re-affirmation of self.

Comment: It was very moving in your first example when the mother and daughter talked and cried together when they were able to speak about a very deep issue which had affected them both. It was a striking illustration of how daughters sometimes really can empower mothers. It's really an illustration of the mutual empowerment we talk about.

Turner: Yes, it was a very important time for them both. I want to stress that it illustrates how that can happen for many daughters and mothers, and also that for this woman it happened because she began to examine this essential part of her identity as a Black woman. If therapy hadn't opened that exploration, she wouldn't have gotten to that—and she wouldn't have been able to turn to her mother about it.

Comment: I was thinking about what you said about Black women fearing that they will lose their connections with their families and community if they move into careers or jobs that are more in the "white world." These days many people talk about many women feeling conflicts if they are achieving in the world far more than their mothers were able to. Do you think that Black women, too, have a fear of losing their ties to their mothers, in particular?

Turner: For Black women, I think that there is a fear of losing ties to a whole community, and this is different from white women. However, there may be similar kinds of conflicts for people from other ethnic groups or who rise from lower socio-economic groups. On top of this, there can be specific features around fear of disruption of the woman's relationship with her mother. It is normal for many Black women to feel conflicted around integrating ethnic and majority identities in ways which help them to feel more "whole" and not so fragmented.

Miller: It seems to me that many younger women today have to deal with the feelings involved in letting themselves really have more than their mothers had. They may have some real conflicts and criticisms of their mothers, but they often also have a deep sadness about their mothers' deprivation or suffering; and they have to deal with that in order to not deprive themselves.

Turner: I think similar feelings exist for Black women, but there are also differences on this point too. I spoke about these in describing how much Black mothers work to try to build strength in their daughters just because of the dangers and obstacles they know their daughters will face in the world. I don't think white mothers have so consciously "worked with" their daughters in this way. This can give Black daughters a different feeling about what will make their mothers feel fulfilled or happy. If these daughters can avoid the emotional pitfalls of devaluing their mothers' way of uplifting them, they can feel they are carrying out what their mothers wished so much for them in mutually empathic ways.

Comment: In the second example you gave, you did such a beautiful job of showing how the whole surrounding environment gave the Black woman the kind of messages that made her feel isolated and not wanted. And then the woman herself gets deeper and deeper into isolation and down on herself without really identifying what's happening. I think this occurs without anyone consciously saying, "Let's make this Black woman feel isolated and not valued," don't you? It happens just by carrying on "business as usual" in our usual institutions. Are you suggesting that this can happen so long as educational and work settings don't take specific steps to recognize that this is a high probability, and don't create relational contexts that will be welcoming and congenial for Black women, and other women of color?

Turner: Yes, I would say so. I would say, too, that people like us can help to make all women of color aware of this probability, so that women, themselves, can act on it even before institutions make all of the changes that they should. The women can recognize how important it is that they seek out other people to create the kind of relationships they need. I think that this probably applies to other women of color and other minority groups, too.

Miller: By extension, we could say that educational and work institutions probably don't provide the kind of environments that are based on a good understanding of what women need and that help women to flourish to the fullest. Many women have felt isolated and not valued in the institutions as they exist, but this situation is compounded for Black women. Would you say so?

Turner: Yes, I would. That relates to the main point of my presentation. The sense of being a part of relationships is central for all women's sense of self, and most institutions do not provide the *kind* of relationships which speak to women's needs *and* experience. However, the Black woman may come from a history of having many ties to her Black community; then she often encounters an even greater lack of connection when she enters schools or workplaces in the larger culture which doubly devalue her because she is both Black and female. By becoming aware of the societal, emotional and institutional pressures which feed these disconnections, we can all be in a better position to address them.

REFERENCES

Cobbs, P. (1972). Ethnotherapy in groups. In L. Soloman & B. Berzon (Eds.), *New perspectives on encounter groups*. San Francisco: Jossey-Bass.

Jordan, J. (1984). *Empathy and self boundaries*. (Work in Progress No. 16.) Wellesley, MA: Stone Center Working Paper Series.

Jordan, J., Surrey, J., & Kaplan, A. G. (1982). *Women and empathy*. (Work in Progress No. 2.) Wellesley, MA: Stone Center Working Paper Series.

Kaplan, A. (1984). *Self-in-relation: Implications for depression in women*. (Work in Progress No. 14.) Wellesley, MA: Stone Center Working Paper Series.

Miller, J. B. (1984). *The development of women's sense of self*. (Work in Progress No. 12.) Wellesley, MA: Stone Center Working Paper Series.

Pinderhughes, E. (1982). Empowerment for our clients and for ourselves. Social Casework: *Journal of Contemporary Social Work*, June, 331–338.

Pinderhughes, E. (1984). Teaching empathy: Ethnicity, race and power at the cross-cultural treatment interface. Paper presented at the Annual Meeting of the American Psychiatric Association, Toronto, Ontario, Canada, May 1982. *American Journal of Social Psychiatry, 4*(1), 5–12.

Surrey, J. (1984). Self-in-relation: A theory of women's development. (Work in Progress No. 13.) Wellesley, MA: Stone Center Working Paper Series.

Turner, C. (1984) *Psychosocial barriers to Black women's career development.* (Work in Progress No. 15.) Wellesley, MA: Stone Center Working Paper Series. (Reprinted as Chapter 8, this volume)

This chapter was presented at a Stone Center Colloquium in February 1987. © 1987 Clevonne W. Turner.

5

Racial Identity Development and Relational Theory: The Case of Black Women in White Communities

BEVERLY DANIEL TATUM

The Stone Center Theory Group challenged themselves in the introduction to their book, *Women's Growth In Connection* (Jordan, Kaplan, Miller, Stiver, & Surrey, 1991) to take on the task of better understanding the specifics of women's experience based on class, race, age, ethnicity, and gender. This chapter is presented in the spirit of adding more specific understanding by providing information about a particular group of women—Black, middle-class, college-educated women—and their racial identity development, framed in relational terms.

Though we each have multiple identities based on our membership in various social groups, as Vicki Spelman, author of *Inessential Woman* (1988), has pointed out, these identities cannot be separated like pop beads. For instance, we Black women cannot isolate our Blackness from our femaleness. We are always both simultaneously. Yet little research is being done on the combination. There are, of course, some exceptions, among them the work of Wellesley College professor Alice Brown-Collins (1991). Such exceptions not withstanding, racial identity development theorists have done little to address gender. Relational theory has done little to address issues of race.

In this chapter I want to talk about the connection between racial identity development theory (which essentially describes a process of moving from internalized racism to a position of empowerment based on a positively affirmed sense of racial identity) and relational theory. Specifically, it is an attempt to look at the points of intersection between the two theoretical perspectives in understanding the experiences of young Black women growing up in white communities. The examples I will use throughout the course of this discussion come from interviews I have done with young African American women who grew up in predominantly white communities.

If, as Stone Center theorists suggest, connectedness is the goal of development, and those connections which are growth-enhancing are mutually empathic and mutually empowering, how do Black women in white communities develop these growth-enhancing connections as they move outside the boundaries of their families? With whom? What role does racism play in this process?

If we understand racism to be a pervasive system of advantage based on race (Wellman, 1977), which has personal, cultural, and institutional implications for our daily lives, then we must acknowledge its daily impact on interpersonal relationships. If mutual empathy requires the interest and motivation to know the other, then everyday racism often, if not always, represents the failure of mutual empathy. As Judith Jordan writes, "in order to empathize one must have a well-differentiated sense of self *in addition to an appreciation of and sensitivity to the differentness as well as the sameness of another person* (Jordan, Surrey, & Kaplan, 1991, p. 29, italics mine). Yet when a person discriminates or intentionally or unintentionally acts on perceptions based on racial stereotypes, the appreciation of sameness is violated. On the other hand, when a white friend denies the impact of racism in the friend of color's life, the recognition of difference in experience is denied. As Wendy Rosen (1992) pointed out in her discussion of heterosexism, so too in the case of racism, our culture almost guarantees empathic failures, experiences of disconnection. Given this context, what are the implications for young Black women in predominantly white communities? How does their growth in connection take place?

A MODEL OF RACIAL IDENTITY DEVELOPMENT

Because many of you may not be familiar with racial identity development as conceptualized by Cross (1991), Helms (1990), and others, a brief overview may be helpful. Racial identity and racial identity development theory are defined by Helms (1990, p. 3) as:

. . . a sense of group or collective identity based on one's *perception* that he or she shares a common racial heritage with a particular racial group. . . . [R]acial identity development theory concerns the psychological implications of racial-group membership, that is, belief systems that evolve in reaction to perceived differential group membership.

It is assumed that in a society where racial group membership is emphasized, the development of a racial identity will occur in some form in everyone. Given the dominant/subordinate relationship of whites and people of color in this society, however, it is not surprising that this developmental process will unfold in different ways for the different racial groups. Because of our time limitations, my discussion will be limited to Cross's (1971, 1978, 1991) model of Black identity development. While the identity development of other people of color (Asian, Latino/a, Native American) is not included in this particular theoretical formulation, there is evidence to suggest that the process for these oppressed groups is similar to that described for African Americans (Highlen, et al., 1988; Phinney, 1989).* In each case it is assumed that a positive sense of oneself as a member of one's group (which is not based on any assumed superiority) is important for psychological health.

According to Cross's (1971, 1978, 1991) model of Black racial identity development, there are five stages in the process, identified as Preencounter, Encounter, Immersion/Emersion, Internalization, and Internalization/Commitment. In the first stage of Preencounter, the African American has absorbed many of the beliefs and values of the dominant white culture, including the notion that "white is right" and "Black is wrong." Though the internalization of negative Black stereotypes may be outside her conscious awareness, the individual seeks to assimilate and be accepted by whites and may actively or passively distance herself from other Blacks.

In order to maintain psychological comfort at this stage of development,

. . . the person must maintain the fiction that race and racial indoctrination have nothing to do with how he or she lives life. It is probably the case that the Preencounter person is bombarded on a regular basis with

---

* While other similar models of racial identity development exist, Cross and Helms are referenced here because they are among the most frequently cited writers on black racial identity development and white racial identity development, respectively. For a discussion of the commonalities between these and other identity development models, see Phinney (1989) and Helms (1990).

information that he or she cannot really be a member of the "in" racial group, but relies on denial to selectively screen such information from awareness. (Helms, 1990, p. 23)

Movement into the Encounter phase is typically precipitated by an event or series of events that force the individual to acknowledge the impact of racism in one's life. For example, instances of social rejection by white friends or colleagues may lead the individual to the conclusion that many whites will not view her as an equal. Faced with the reality that she cannot truly be white, the individual is forced to focus on her identity as a member of a group targeted by racism.

The Immersion/Emersion stage is characterized by the simultaneous desire to surround oneself with visible symbols of one's racial identity and an active avoidance of symbols of whiteness. As Parham (1989, p. 190) describes, "At this stage, everything of value in life must be Black or relevant to Blackness. This stage is also characterized by a tendency to denigrate white people, simultaneously glorifying Black people. . . ."

As individuals enter the Immersion stage, they actively seek out opportunities to explore aspects of their own history and culture with the support of peers from their own racial backgrounds. Typically white-focused anger dissipates during this phase because so much of the person's energy is directed towards her own group- and self-exploration. The result of this exploration is an emerging security in a newly defined and affirmed sense of self.

The emergence from this stage marks the beginning of Internalization. In general, "pro-Black attitudes become more expansive, open, and less defensive" (Cross, 1971, p. 24). While still maintaining his or her connections with Black peers, the internalized individual is willing to establish meaningful relationships with whites who acknowledge and are respectful of her self-definition. The individual is also ready to build coalitions with members of other oppressed groups.

Cross suggests that there are few psychological differences between the fourth stage, Internalization, and the fifth stage, Internalization-Commitment. However, those at the fifth stage have found ways to translate their "personal sense of Blackness into a plan of action or a general sense of commitment" to the concerns of Blacks as a group, which is sustained over time (Cross, 1991, p. 220). Whether at the fourth or fifth stage, the process of Internalization allows the individual, anchored in a positive sense of racial identity, to both proactively perceive and transcend race. Blackness becomes "the point of departure for discovering the universe of ideas, cultures, and experiences beyond Blackness in place of mistaking Blackness as the universe itself" (Cross, Parham, and Helms, 1991, p. 330).

Though the process of racial identity development has been presented here in linear form, in fact it is probably more accurate to think
of it in a spiral form. Often a person may move from one stage to the
next only to revisit an earlier stage as the result of new Encounter experiences (Parham, 1989), though the experience of the stage may be
different than it was the first time. The image that I find helpful in understanding this concept of recycling through the stages is that of a
spiral staircase. As a person ascends a spiral staircase, she may stop
and look down at a spot below. When she reaches the next level, she
may look down and see the same spot, but the vantage point is not exactly the same.

A RELATIONAL PERSPECTIVE ON
RACIAL IDENTITY DEVELOPMENT

Though this process is not discussed explicitly in relational terms, in
fact, movement through these stages does occur in emotional connection with others. In the context of the experiences of Black women
growing up in white communities, the identification with the dominant society occurs in relationship with white friends and teachers.
For example, one young woman I interviewed described the love she
felt for her kindergarten teacher and her childhood wish that her
mother could also be white. Most of my interviewees felt connected to
their communities in elementary school and had mostly white friends.
Jean Baker Miller, in her paper "The Development of Women's Sense
of Self," (1991) describes girls in childhood as intensely involved in relationships, and there is nothing to suggest that these young Black
women were any different. Though many had experienced instances
of name-calling and had sometimes been aware of lowered teacher expectations, these experiences might be considered what Miller has
called "minor disconnections" (Miller, 1988). I refer to them as minor
not because they were unimportant experiences (years later they were
significant enough to be recalled in an interview with little prompting), rather they are called minor because they were typically balanced
by positive experiences of connection at home and at school.

The kind of social rejection that precipitates movement into the
Encounter stage of racial identity development typically begins to occur in adolescence. During adolescence, Miller (1991) writes that "the
girl picks up the strong message that her own perceptions about her
bodily and sexual feelings are not acceptable" (p. 20). Black girls in
white communities may be getting the even more loaded message that
their actual bodies are not acceptable. For example, one young woman

described an interaction she had with a white girlfriend in junior high school. She said,

> [She] introduced me to somebody and her friend gave her a look like "I can't believe you have a Black friend." And I remember that one friend saying, "She's not really Black, she just went to Florida and got a really dark tan." And that upset me incredibly because it was like, "What? Yes, I am, wait a second here."

A white male friend also began to feel peer pressure in junior high school to deny his connection, to this Black girl. She explains,

> It eventually got very difficult for him to deal. And so it was easier for him to call me a nigger and tell me, "Your lips are too big. I don't want to see you. I won't be your friend anymore." than to say like he used to, "Oh, you're so pretty."

For other young women, the message was less directly communicated but was discerned from the acts of omission which were a part of their experiences, for example, not being asked to dance at parties or not being introduced to the brothers or male friends of their white girlfriends.

Though these might be considered Encounter experiences in the model of racial identity development theory just presented, the withdrawal from the dominant group did not occur in high school. For young Black women to sever ties with their white friends in communities where there are few other choices available would mean certain isolation. Miller (1988) writes:

> When children and adults feel the threat of condemned isolation, they try to make connection with those closest to them in any way that appears possible. . . . In essence, the child or adult tries to construct some kind of an image of herself and others, and of the relationships between herself and others, which will allow her entry into relationships with the people available. This is a complicated process. In order to twist herself into a person acceptable in "unaccepting" relationships, she will have to *move away from and redefine* a large part of her experience—those parts of experience that she has determined are not allowed.

This may mean denying those aspects of herself which are perceived as culturally different from the majority, or denying her own perceptions of racism. When, as quoted earlier, Janet Helms (1990) writes that "the Preencounter person is bombarded on a regular basis with information that he or she cannot really be in a member of the 'in' racial group, but relies on denial to selectively screen such information from awareness," she is describing a process that allows the person of color to remain in connection with those who are conveying the message of exclusion.

Describing this process in her own words, one young Black woman said,

> I really didn't see my Blackness in high school at all. I mean I was aware of how I was treated differently, but for so long my mom was always saying, "You think you're white. You think you're white. You think you're white." [Her reply.] "No Mom, we don't see color here. Everyone is friends and they treat me the same." I couldn't see then what she was trying to point out to me.

The cost of this denial of experience is internalized oppression, blaming oneself for the relational disconnection. This young woman found herself engaged in a process in high school that continued into college. She said,

> I knew my high school experience was just very weird, just by the way the whites treated me. But my self-esteem has gone down the toilet since I've been here. . . . Being made to feel that you're never quite good enough, never quite pretty enough, never quite smart enough, or even if you're all of those things, just being made to feel that you're different, something's not quite right.

Now approaching her college graduation, this young woman has decided to go to graduate school at an historically Black institution. Her desire to enter a predominantly Black community is part of what has been described in terms of racial identity development as the Immersion stage. In relational terms, we can also see this decision as an attempt to disengage from destructive nonmutual relationships and to find an environment which may be more conducive to the development of mutually empathic and empowering relationships.

Though the young woman just described had to deny aspects of her experience to remain in connection, is it possible for young Black women in predominantly white communities to maintain relational authenticity (an empowered stance) in response to other's lack of empathy (i.e., their racism)? The answer is yes, but it seems encouraged by the availability of mutually empowering relationships in other settings. For example, one young woman described an interaction she had with white friends in high school which she found offensive. She said,

> When it was time to apply to schools, people were like, "Oh, you don't have to worry; you're a minority. Everyone needs minorities." You're

like, "Wait. I've been going to school with you for the past seven years. I've been going to class like you have. I don't think I've been sitting in my room everyday going, 'Oh when it's time to apply to college, it's not going to matter anyway. I'll go whether I can read or can't read, whether I can add or can't add.'" I was very pissed off . . . I told them how pissed off I was at them.

In this instance she was able to express her anger authentically rather than internalize self-doubts about her academic qualifications. The fact that she had a supportive network of family and friends outside of school probably contributed to her ability to challenge her classmates' comments without fear of "condemned isolation."

THE HEALING POWER OF MUTUAL RELATIONSHIPS

The opportunity to connect with peers from one's own racial group during the Immersion stage of racial identity development is a corrective relational experience for many young Black women. The validation of one's own experience by others who have shared aspects of that experience is empowering and contributes to the positive redefinition of racial identity that is occurring at the Immersion stage. For many Black women growing up in predominantly white communities, the opportunities to develop such relationships with other Black women are extremely limited. Though parents can play a role in actively working to construct such opportunities by intentionally building Black social networks for their children (attending a Black church, for example), not all Black parents have acknowledged this developmental need (Tatum, 1987). Most of the young women I have interviewed did not move into the Immersion stage until they went away to college.

One young woman who struggled with a lot of internalized oppression as a result of her growing-up experiences described the impact of meeting an African American woman in college who was obviously proud of her own racial identity:

One of my best friends on this campus is Black and she's very aware of her Black identity. And it's been a great help for me because it makes me look at it and be just as proud as she is of my Black heritage, of my Black identity, and be vocal about it. Whereas I was never vocal, but now I can be.

Though her friend was not from a predominantly white community herself, she shared the common experience of being devalued as an African American woman in U.S. society. Yet her friend had been able to resist the internalization of that oppression and was able to model another way of being Black and female. The exchange of information and survival strategies that occurs at the Immersion stage occurs in the context of mutual relationships in which one feels heard, seen, and understood.

Must this process take place in the context of same-race relationships? While it is possible for a white person to support and encourage this process (e.g., a white teacher could encourage a Black student to get involved in a Black student organization), the impact of racism on interracial relationships makes the required mutuality more difficult to achieve. In her paper, "The Meaning of Mutuality," Judith Jordan describes how one is positively affected by mutual interaction but also describes the potential threat of mutual interaction. She writes, "Growth occurs because as I stretch to match or understand your experience, something new is acknowledged or grows in me" (Jordan, 1991a, p. 89). However if in stretching to understand a Black woman's experience, a white woman learns something new about herself and doesn't like that new thing (e.g., I have white privilege, or racism has affected me in ways I didn't expect), is she tempted to not understand, to keep out that information? My own experience teaching white students about the psychology of racism suggests that the temptation to keep out race-related information is often great (Tatum, 1992). If a white person is unable or unwilling to hear and try to understand the experience of a Black woman, mutuality is not possible.

Jordan (1991b) writes in her paper, "The Movement of Mutuality and Power," that real safety and growth in relationships for adults depend on the ability to engage in mutually empathic and mutually empowering relationships as well as on the ability to recognize nonmutual relationships and to disengage from them. It is ironic then that the attempts of Black women to seek each other out for mutually empowering connections, particularly in the context of predominantly white settings, are often seen as problematic by whites. "Why are they sitting together in the dining hall?" is the often-asked question on campuses around the country. We might ask the question differently. Why is the fact that they are sitting together so often seen as threatening by white students and administrators? Why is it not seen as a healthy response to frequently experienced nonmutuality? In fact, the opportunity for same-race relationships which are growth-enhancing ultimately leads to the Internalization stage of racial identity development.

As African American women in predominantly white settings move toward the empowerment that comes with internalization of a positive sense of racial identity, the question posed by Miller (1991, p.

24) becomes very salient: "How to be the kind of self she wants to be, a being-in-relationship, now able to value the very valuable parts of herself, along with her own perceptions and desires—and to find others who will be with her in that way." For the young woman in the Internalization stage, the range of relationship choices may widen beyond her own racial group. However, her choice of relationships will be predicated upon her perception that those with whom she is interacting are respectful of her self-definition and the range of her experiences.

Those of us who would work with young Black women in a mutually empathic relational mode must ask ourselves if we are prepared to hear, see, and understand their authentically told experience. Unless the answer is "yes," we will not be able to help facilitate the empowerment of these young women as they move through the process of racial identity development.

DISCUSSION SUMMARY

After each colloquium presentation a discussion was held. Selected portions are summarized here. At this session, Drs. Alice Brown-Collins and Robin Cook-Nobles joined Dr. Tatum in leading the discussion.

Question: Do you ever find Black women who have stopped at the first or second stage of racial identity, or is it generally a continuous thing?

Tatum: It is possible to get stuck. I think there's a lot that concerned adults—therapists, counselors, teachers—who have an understanding of racial identity development can do to help people move along. If we assume that this is a process of healthy growth and development, there are ways to facilitate it.

For example, I think it's very common for adolescents to be in the Encounter stage, which is often a stage of feeling very angry about the race-related experiences that you're having. Often it's a very anti-white stage because you're expressing that anger at whites. But it's also a stage at which your own sense of identity has been largely shaped by stereotypes. You have not been provided the information you need to really redefine your identity in more positive, more empowering ways. One of the things that happens for young women, and men too, when they come to college, if in fact they get to college, is that they have the opportunity to take African American Studies courses. It's often access to that and similar new information that helps move people along into the next stage of really redefining their identity in positive terms. The problem is, of course, that many African American students don't get to college and, therefore, don't have access to those African American Studies courses. But, in fact, there's no reason why that information couldn't be communicated at the high-school level. Those who are able to take those college courses often ask, "How come nobody told me about this before?" That question comes up a lot in my interviews. I think we really need to look at the ways in which the very Eurocentric, exclusionary curriculum that is the experience of many high-school students acts to keep people stuck in the Encounter stage rather than facilitating their development in this way.

Question: What is the role of anger in this process? Are you only angry at the Encounter stage or, as you develop, do you leave anger behind? And is the anger that Black women are expressing toward white women within the women's movement a function of their stage of identity development?

Tatum: I would like to say that you get to be angry at any stage. Certainly anger is a very important aspect of the Encounter stage of development. If you are having Encounter experiences, you are angry about that. At the same time, that doesn't mean that once you've worked through and redefined your identity, you never get angry again. One of the differences may be that at the Internalization stage you are better able to deal with your anger in more constructive ways. For example, many people are experiencing the Encounter stage in adolescence, their anger is often expressed in an antiwhite attitude which can be somewhat counterproductive. For example, a Black student might say, okay, before I was trying to identify with the dominant group, and now I'm getting the message that this is not possible for me. So then what I need to do is really assert my identity, and part of that assertion of identity is not be anything that I think is associated with "whiteness." That might include not doing well in school, because academic achievement is seen as "white" behavior. That's problematic.

The question that I always ask is, "Well, how did academic achievement get identified as exclusively white behavior?" We have to really look at the curriculum. This attitude is something that tends to emerge in 7th, 8th, 9th grades, and into high school. What was happening in 1st, 2nd, 3rd, 4th, 5th, 6th grades in terms of what was being presented as models of academic achievement? But I think this is where an understanding of the stages can be helpful because, if I am the teacher and I have a student who seems to be in this angry Encounter stage, I might introduce the student to some personally relevant information about their own cultural experience that may help them redefine that experience. For example, a number of people I've interviewed have mentioned reading *The Autobiography of Malcolm X* as a pivotal experience in moving them from one stage to the next. Or, for example, young Black women who are in this isolated situation might be interested in reading Lorene Cary's book, *Black Ice*, which is about the experiences of a young Black woman at a predominantly white prep school. So there are ways in which that information can be shared.

The young woman I described in the chapter, whose friends were saying that she didn't need to worry about college because "everybody needs minorities," was very irritated by that statement. But rather than internalize her anger, I think her response was an empowered response characteristic of the Internalization stage. She challenged their remarks very directly. Her friends might have heard her response as sounding angry, and she was! But that is legitimate anger, and you can find that at any stage.

Question: I'm wondering if you could talk about bridging the gap between theory and practice in terms of racial relationships. I don't see white women practicing what they preach.

Tatum: I think a lot of it has to do with coming to terms with your own identity as a white person and that is a process that develops over time. Janet Helms (1990) describes a model of white racial identity that parallels in some ways the stages of racial identity for people of color. As whites move through the stages, there is an increasing awareness of the ways in which you've been affected by your own racism, or by racism in the society, the way you've breathed it in like people in Los Angeles breathe in smog. I use the analogy of people in Los Angeles breathing smog because when we talk about racism a lot of white people get very nervous. They're afraid you are going to say that they are racist, and that's part of the "condemned isolation" Black women may experience in white communities.

If I as a Black woman am experiencing racism, and I'm trying to explain it to my white friends, and they are concerned that they may be implicated in this discussion, then there's a way in which they don't want to acknowledge the experience as racism. They may say, "Oh, she didn't mean it, she's a really nice person. You might have misunderstood. That couldn't have been it." But because racism is so pervasive in our society, people do breathe it in, and it does influence their everyday interactions. (Probably, if you went to California nobody would like to be called a "smog breather," but it's so pervasive that that's what people are!) So, one of the things that I find in my teaching about racism is that, white students, as time goes by, become increasingly aware of their own racism. In some ways this awareness leads them to act less, because they don't want to expose their racism. People can get stuck there. But if they're able to be in environments where they're continually being pushed to look at and think about racism, and think about what they can do about it, then it's been my experience that these people start to move. They start to reach out, and not in a condescending or patronizing way, but in an authentic way. But again, I think this movement has a lot to do with stages of racial identity development.

I feel somewhat limited by time here to go into this aspect of women's development at greater length, but I would refer you to my article, "Talking about Race; Learning about Racism," in which I talk about the stages of racial identity development for both whites and people of color, and the ways in which those developmental processes may collide, and what we can do educationally to facilitate development on both sides.

Question: I want to follow up on the question about relationships between Black and white women. When an African American person is going through the developmental stage of expressing anger, and then reconnecting, how can we best support the reconnection?

Cook-Nobles: How to reconnect, how to have mutual friendships—relationships across ethnic and racial boundaries? First you have to deal with the anger and the guilt. And you have to be so motivated to deal with those intense feelings that you think it will be worth the expenditure of energy. Other factors impact the individuals in their lives, and people have to choose where to expend their energy. So those in supporting roles have to look at the social forces impacting on the individual and where they can invest their energy, because racism will wear a person out!

Brown-Collins: I think that part of bridging the gap is for white women to begin to acknowledge their racism. There will be no true bridging of the gap without acknowledging racism. Now you may say, "I don't know *what* this means. Due to what happened in the past, I am now inheriting the legacy of racism. I mean I didn't formulate it, I didn't set it up, but I've inherited it. So, what is the acknowledgment of racism?" It is connecting with other white women to work on your own racism. African American women are typically very sensitive to and willing to connect when people begin to do this. Here at Wellesley there is a group of white women who come together to work on their own racism. Part of the anger here at Wellesley is that whites are expecting us (African American women) always to give, give, give, give, give. white women can take an Africana Studies course, you too can read Malcolm X, you too can do all these things. We think that you have to begin at some point to not only acknowledge but to find a way that you can work on racism because it is not only destroying us as African Americans, but is certainly destroying all human beings.

Cook-Nobles: We can use the male–female analogy and talk about making the connection across gender. The fear is that, when you address the issues, you will lose connection, that there will be a disconnection, that someone will lose. But the reality is that everybody is brought up to another level. People have to be committed to going through the process of going up to that other level. And I like the analogy of smog, because who wants smog in our systems? We want to get it out, and therefore this analogy helps us to see that it is not just an individual problem, but a societal problem in which we *all* play a role. Similarly, if we're going to get rid of it, we *all* have a role to play.

Tatum: I would like to add to that. I didn't describe all the stages for whites, but one of the stages is when someone has started to recognize her own racism and is trying to figure out what to do about it. Often at this stage she will look for the help of a person of color to educate her. "Okay, I see that there's a problem. I want to do something about it. You, person of color, tell me what to do." If the person of color at that point is in the Encounter stage, that person is not interested in playing that role. And, in fact, as Alice was saying, there's no need for a person of color to do that. There are other ways to be educated.

But there is a stage that Janet Helms calls the Immersion stage, like Cross's stage of Immersion, in which white people seek to redefine whiteness. One of the things that happens as somebody becomes aware of the racism in this society and the way in which they have been affected by it, is that they become alienated from the present definition of whiteness. They see whiteness as a dominating, oppressive category, and they don't want to be a part of that. So the question becomes, "How can I be white and not be a part of that category?" Well sometimes the person will try to not be white, to try to hang out at the Black student union or to take on a different identity and say "I'm not like them, I'm distancing myself." But ultimately that kind of separation doesn't work because it's not real, and the person is then forced to acknowledge, "I am in fact white,"—"I am in fact a white woman," in this case. So the question is, "how can I redefine whiteness in a way that makes me feel good?" There are ways to do it. There's more than one way of being white. You can define yourself as a white ally for example. You can define yourself as an agent for change or an antiracist activist.

One of the things that disturbs me about our educational system, beyond what I said about the experiences of African American students, is that if I were to ask each of you to name a nationally known racist, you could all do it. You could think of David Duke or Jesse Helms or George Wallace—somebody would come to mind. If I were to ask you to name a nationally-known white antiracist, my experience is that many groups struggle a long time before they can think of one person. The names of Anne Braden and Morris Dees of the Southern Poverty Law Center sometimes come up—there are people you could name. However, the point is that if you can't think of any antiracists, then it's hard to imagine yourself being one. So that one of the things that happens in the Immersion stage for whites is a real desire to find examples of other people who think the same way.

If I am a white person who is working against racism, who doesn't want to be involved in this process of smog breathing that we have been talking about, then is there a way for me to do that without a life of "condemned isolation"? I need to find other white people who are engaged in a similar process, and that's the role of white allies groups. Sometimes people get really nervous when you say, "Okay, white women should go off and meet together." Well, the Black women have already done it. I mean they are doing that in the Immersion stage, but it's after white women, or white people in general, have done the same work that they can become better able to do their part of the bridging-so it's not just a one-way bridge.

REFERENCES

Brown-Collins, A. (1991). An empirical investigation of the African American woman self inventory. Paper presented at the Fifteenth National Conference of the National Council for Black Studies, Atlanta, GA, March, 1991.

Cross, W. E., Jr. (1971). The Negro to Black conversion experience: Toward a psychology of Black liberation. *Black World, 20*(9), 13–27.

Cross, W. E., Jr. (1978). The Cross and Thomas models of psychological nigrescence. *Journal of Black Psychology, 5*(1), 13–19.

Cross, W. E., Jr. (1991). *Shades of Black: Diversity in African American identity.* Philadelphia: Temple University Press.

Cross, W. E., Jr., Parham, T. A., & Helms, J. E. (1991). The stages of Black identity development: Nigrescence models. In R. Jones (Ed.). *Black psychology (3rd ed.),* 319–338. San Francisco: Cobb & Henry.

Helms, J. E. (Ed.). (1990). *Black and White racial identity: Theory, research and practice.* Westport, CT: Greenwood Press.

Highlen, P. S., Reynolds, A. L., Adams, E. H., Hanley, T. C., Myers, L. J., Cox, C., & Speight, S. (1988). Self-identity development model of oppressed people: Inclusive model for all? Paper presented at the American Psychological Association Convention, August 13, 1988, Atlanta, GA.

Jordan, J. (1991a). The meaning of mutuality. In J. Jordan et al. *Women's growth in connection: Writings from the Stone Center.* New York: Guilford Press.

Jordan, J. (1991b). *The movement of mutuality and power.* (Work in Progress No. 53.) Wellesley, MA: Stone Center Working Paper Series.

Jordan, J. V., Kaplan, A. C., Miller, J. B., Stiver, I. P., & Surrey, J. L. (1991). *Women's growth in connection: Writings from the Stone Center.* New York: Guilford Press.

Jordan, J. V., Surrey, J. L., & Kaplan, A. G. (1991) Women and empathy: Implications for psychological development and psychotherapy. In J. Jordan et al. *Women's growth in connection: Writings from the Stone Center.* New York: Guilford Press.

Miller, J. B. (1988). *Connections, disconnections, and violations.* (Work in Progress No. 33.) Wellesley, MA: Stone Center Working Paper Series.

Miller, J. B. (1991). The development of women's sense of self. In J. Jordan et al. *Women's growth in connection: Writings from the Stone Center.* New York: Guilford Press.

Parham, T. A. (1989). Cycles of psychological nigrescence. *The Counseling Psychologist, 17*(2), 187–226.

Phinney, J. (1989). Stages of ethnic identity in minority group adolescents. *Journal of Early Adolescence, 9,* 34–49.

Rosen, W. (1992) *On the integration of sexuality: Lesbian daughters and their mothers.* (Work in Progress No. 56.) Wellesley, MA: Stone Center Working Papers Series. (Reprinted as Chapter 12, this volume)

Spelman, E. V. (1988). *Inessential woman: Problems of exclusion in feminist thought.* Boston: Beacon Press.

Tatum, B. D. (1987). *Assimilation blues: Black families in a White community.* Northampton, MA: Hazel-Maxwell Publishing. (Originally published by Greenwood Press.)

Tatum, B. D. (1992). Talking about race, learning about racism: An application of racial identity development theory in the classroom. *Harvard Educational Review, 62*(1), 1–24.

Wellman, D. (1977). *Portraits of white racism.* New York: Cambridge University Press.

This chapter was presented at a Stone Center Colloquium on December 2, 1992. © 1992 Beverly Daniel Tatum.

6

The Conundrum of Mutuality:
A Lesbian Dialogue

NATALIE S. ELDRIDGE
JULIE MENCHER
SUZANNE SLATER

Over the past decade, the Stone Center theory group has created a rich theoretical perspective on women's growth through connection, establishing that mutuality is a central hallmark of healthy relationships for women. Judith Jordan has developed and elaborated on the concept of mutuality and pointed to its importance in psychotherapy (1986, 1991b). In 1989, lesbian feminist liberation theologian Carter Heyward took an additional step to alert feminist therapists to the dangers of nonmutuality in most therapies (1989a). She challenged us to explain and correct the fundamental contradiction between the feminists' definition of what constitutes a healthy relationship and the reality of what characterizes a typical therapy relationship. We of the Lesbian Theory Group believe that it is no coincidence that a lesbian pressed this challenge, since lesbian relationships outside of therapy fundamentally challenge traditional arrangements of power and connection, and since lesbians historically have articulated the radical edge of the feminist critique.

The Stone Center theory group has featured mutuality in psychotherapy as a major topic in virtually all of its work over the past four years on psychotherapy relationships. In such papers and presentations as Jordan's "The Movement of Mutuality and Power" (1991a),

Heyward and Jordan's "Mutuality in Therapy: Ethics, Power, and Psychology" (1992), Heyward's and Surrey's workshops and trainings on mutuality, Miller and Stiver's "A Relational Reframing of Therapy" (1991), and the Stone Center's Cape Cod summer seminars, these theorists have questioned the traditional models. They have challenged the notion of the therapist as expert within a rigid, hierarchical structure of power over the client. Instead, they have struggled to define mutuality in therapy and have clearly endorsed the necessity of mutuality within the relational perspective's definition of what constitutes good therapy.

Other theoretical communities and groups of scholars and practitioners have been examining this issue as well. In the pages of *Psychoanalytic Dialogues: A Journal of Relational Perspectives*, a (mostly male) community of contemporary psychoanalysts has been debating various challenges to traditional theory and practice. This community has been alternately referred to as "relational," "interpersonal," or "relational-perspectivitist" psychoanalysis. These discussions—such as Mitchell's (1988) and Aron's (1991) work on intersubjectivity in the analytic relationship, Modell's (1991) examination of the interplay of reality and transference, Burke's (1992) exploration of the use of countertransference disclosure, and Hoffman's (1992) and Tansey's (1992) questioning of the nature of psychoanalytic expertise—represent an exciting challenge to some of the most basic principles of analytic thought, an exploration that runs parallel to and often intersects with our own feminist debate here at the Stone Center.

The work of other feminist thinkers, such as Rogers' "A Feminist Poetics of Psychotherapy" (1991) and Bograd's "The Duel Over Dual Relationships (1992), has also enriched our exploration of mutuality in psychotherapy. Recent conferences on such topics as intimacy between therapist and client, boundaries in psychotherapy, and love in the therapy relationship indicate that many others in our field are thoughtfully considering the various issues related to mutuality in psychotherapy.

At this point, we in the Lesbian Theory Group have felt the need for the discussion to move forward, from advocating the importance of mutuality in therapy, to examining more closely how to incorporate mutuality effectively in treatment. We must turn our attention now to the various complexities that emerge from a more mutual psychotherapy. As we move from establishing the importance of mutuality to discussing how it is manifested in therapy, it is critical to include the many voices of therapists and clients—women of various ethnic, racial, and cultural backgrounds, women of various sexual identities, and women from various professional disciplines.

In this chapter, we will be introducing the voices of lesbians—to be precise, three white lesbian feminist therapists. We do so not merely for the sake of enhancing diversity or broadening the discussion, but also because we believe that lesbian therapists have always been required to wrestle with questions related to mutuality. We hope that our particular experiences will, therefore, not only broaden but also deepen our collective re-visioning of mutuality.

Once we agree that mutuality has an important place in relational therapy, many complicated questions emerge:

- What is mutuality in psychotherapy?
- Are there essential structural elements of therapy that determine whether and how mutuality is possible in psychotherapy?
- How can the treatment relationship maintain its unique and precious qualities while incorporating mutuality?
- Can mutuality exist without authenticity? What is authenticity for a therapist? What are the limits on authenticity and mutuality for the lesbian therapist who is not out to her clients? Is it possible to hold to traditional notions of termination and also believe in the importance of mutuality?
- What exactly are the clinical applications of mutuality in therapy?

First, a few comments about our process as a group: In meeting after meeting over the past nine months, we struggled with these questions, often wondering if we were getting anywhere. Every time we tried to grab hold of some meaty specifics about what mutuality actually is, our thinking turned to mush. We came to little more than an agreement that mutuality should be a goal of psychotherapy, with only vague generalizations about what that meant.

Our discussion of the boundary questions in more mutual therapy relationships edged us closer to genuine engagement. Disagreements surfaced among us as we discussed the use of self-disclosure, both as it relates to revealing personal information about the therapist and also concerning the therapist's expression of spontaneous feelings to her client. The group debated the optimal parameters for managing the inevitable entry of the therapist's needs into the therapy, and we discussed whether we can draw a line between the "real" relationship and the transference relationship. In some of our most lively meetings, we challenged each other's thinking on post-termination relationships, and we argued openly about when boundaries honor the client and when they allow a therapist to hide.

By the time we needed to put pen to paper, we had come to recognize that this is not a topic that lends itself to clear questions and concrete answers. However, we realized that we had reached a more complex understanding of the range of factors that must be considered each time we set out to move a therapy relationship toward mutuality. Our group had learned how to move beyond the facile generalizations, how to think complexly about mutuality, and how to make choices in a myriad of distinct situations.

Our discussions, and particularly our debates, have led us to the conflicts that pulled us deeper into relationship with each other and into our investigation of our topic.

Our chapter consists of three sections, written individually, with input and critique from the other members. Except for this introduction and a brief conclusion, each of us will present our own thoughts and perspectives as we examine and develop a different facet of our ongoing dialogue about mutuality in psychotherapy. There are both overlaps and disagreements in the content of our sections. The combined elements of agreement and conflict reflect the success of our process, in which we have moved beyond the simplistic, to a deeper engagement with the conundrum of mutuality in psychotherapy.

Structural Possibilities and Constraints of Mutuality in Psychotherapy

JULIE MENCHER

Just as the Stone Center's relational perspective first affected me a decade ago, these recent discussions of mutuality have provoked in me an exciting and restful sensation of coming home. As I have listened to and participated in these discussions, I have heard the formal articulation and celebration of what I've found to be most healing in psychotherapy. I have gained a sense of the therapist as a real person, truly engaged and participating actively in the rhythms of discussion and silence, willing to talk about the relational process on both sides, acknowledging the real-life factors and circumstances of therapist, client, therapy, and community which both intrude on and enrich the treatment relationship. This is the person I aspired to be as a therapist, and this is the therapist who I tried to find as a client. (I will be using the word *client*, deliberately avoiding the use of the word *patient* because of its association to the hierarchies and power dynamics of the doctor/patient relationship.)

There were moments in recent discussions of innovations toward mutuality in treatment, when I had that 'of course' feeling and wondered, "Haven't we all been working this more mutual way for years?" While many clinicians have been engaged in a silent rebellion against nonmutual traditional methods behind the closed doors of our therapy offices, I, for one, have really felt the urge to come out from the therapy office closet—not merely to proclaim my own authenticity as a more mutual therapist, but also to formally describe, delineate, and honor a more mutual approach—so that future therapists won't have to hide behind closed doors.

Until now, my more mutual treatment approach has consisted only of a catalogue of mental snapshots, images of moments where my client and I have led each other off (what I have known to be) the beaten path of psychotherapy and into exquisite moments of intensity.

MUTUALITY IN THERAPY—SOME ANECDOTES

• A client complained that in the previous session I had seemed uncharacteristically preoccupied and far away. I thought back to the day of our last session and remembered that there was a lot going on for me at that time. I said, "Thinking back on it, I realize that you're right, that I was preoccupied that day. I'm very sorry—it was a mistake for me to let what was going on for me intrude on our time together." She thanked me for the apology and my candor with her. We moved on to another topic, but I still felt a loose thread of strain between us. I asked her if she felt there was more to discuss about my preoccupied state in the previous session, and she said yes but couldn't identify what exactly. I asked her if she wanted to know what was so engrossing to me that it took me away from her that day. She said yes, and I revealed that at the time I'd just learned of my cousin's sudden death in a car accident. She responded that she felt incredibly moved and close to me because I shared my loss with her, because I was willing to be so vulnerable, and that I treated her "like an equal." Without rushing in to take care of me or abandon her own feelings, she expressed her condolences and inquired if I was O.K. In hindsight, I understand how important it was that I validated the client's perceptions of me, explained my affective state, and revealed my own vulnerability to pain.

• When a client woodenly and mechanically described a horrific incident of being brutally raped by her father, I started to cry. Suddenly concerned, she said, "You look so sad and scared!" I agreed that sadness and terror were indeed what I felt, and we went on to try to recover her lost affect about the incest. Although (or perhaps because) this was a completely spontaneous reaction for me, my client experienced my nonverbal expression of affect, and I was unconsciously connecting with her most deeply repressed pain.

• A client I'd been seeing for several years came in one day and began to discuss an acquaintance of hers who is also an acquaintance of mine. Toward the end of our conversation, I flippantly made a remark warning my client about this other woman's untrustworthiness. Visibly stung, my client said, "Actually, I kind of like her." Immediately recognizing my error, I apologized for my offhanded remark and acknowledged that while my protectiveness toward her had an important place in our relationship, my judgments of people we both knew clearly did not. My client persisted, saying, "You *never* do stuff like that—why do you think you did that?" Because I felt as if I had initiated this role reversal, and as a result she had a perfect right to continue it to its conclusion, I agreed to take a moment to think about her question. I said, "The only reason I can come up with right now is that I'm feeling nervous today because I have my own agenda—something I'd like to bring up with you, based on my own need, not yours—something I know from our past experience that it's hard for us to talk about." We went on to discuss the issue of whether I could include case material from our therapy in this presentation, a question she'd had complicated feelings about before. Later on in the session, after she'd agreed to be included in my chapter, she said, "I don't want to tell you what to do, but I think you should use *this*—our talk today—in your mutuality chapter." In this session, the only relationally responsible response I could have had to my stumbling was to be willing to examine my own process as it was located in our particular treatment relationship, and to reveal it to her. In addition, the issue of my occasionally bringing my own needs to our relationship became explicit and available for discussion.

The imprecision and artistry of the therapeutic process often demands that we take risks in the moment that we only fully comprehend much later. With enormous reverence for the particularly powerful process of connection in the psychotherapy relationship, I think that much of how we grow through therapy is mysterious, unknown, or indescribable. I believe it is the unique qualities of the therapy relationship that create a context in which the mystery can work its magic, in profound and life-changing ways.

THE STRUCTURAL ELEMENTS OF
THE TREATMENT RELATIONSHIP

The following essential structural elements of the treatment relationship provide the basic context for its uniqueness.

- It is a time-limited relationship with a formal beginning and ending.
- The relationship is primarily and explicitly dedicated to the growth of the client, based on agreed-upon goals.
- There is a contract about when, where, how often, and how long to meet, but the therapist differentially wields power in determining this contract—usually the therapist determines time slots, usually in the therapist's office, usually by conventions of the profession, 50 minutes weekly.
- The client comes to the therapist because she/he is experiencing difficulty and asks for the therapist's help, based on clinical training, expertise, and experience.
- For the individual client, therapy is usually the only current therapy relationship; for the therapist, this particular therapy relationship is one of many current treatment relationships (Slater, personal communication, 1992).
- The client shares much more information about his or her life than the therapist shares about his or her life.
- The therapist agrees to keep the relationship confidential, and the client is free to reveal it to others at will.
- The client pays and the therapist is paid.
- The therapist's communications to the client are supposed to be purposeful and are intended to further the treatment relationship; the client's communications to the therapist are virtually unconstrained.
- The therapist has the responsibility and the power to make recommendations to the client; the client has the ability and power to respond.
- The therapist operates within a broad professional context (including training, professional affiliation, ethics, and legal and licensing requirements), of which the client may or may not be aware.

- It is primarily the therapist's job to monitor and maintain the structural elements of each treatment relationship.

These characteristic elements of the therapeutic relationship are not incidental details; rather, they are essential factors which make this particular connection sometimes quite odd but always unique. I believe that these essential elements are what we have to work with, and work within—not get beyond.

ASYMMETRY AND MUTUALITY

We cannot ignore that these elements predetermine an inherent *asymmetry* in the therapy relationship. When we attempt mutuality within the context of asymmetry, we face the enormous challenge of traveling in two seemingly opposite directions simultaneously.

But maybe asymmetry and mutuality are not entirely mutually exclusive. In an attempt to delineate a relational approach to psychoanalysis, contemporary analyst Aron (1992) defines asymmetry as the dissimilar and unequal division of responsibility, roles, and functions within the treatment relationship. In contrast, mutuality (as he defines it) involves "how reciprocal the interaction and the experience of interaction are; that is, do the two participants mutually and reciprocally influence each other" (Aron, 1992, p. 482). Aron also states,

> The fact that the influence between patient and analyst is not equal does not mean that it is not mutual. Mutual influence does not imply equal influence, and the analytic relationship may be mutual without being symmetrical. (Aron, 1991, p. 33).

Burke (1992) wrestles with the question of how to implement this contemporary analytic goal, concluding that the therapist must constantly negotiate "a central dynamic tension between the mutual influence of the participants and the asymmetry inherent in a relationship that emphasizes understanding the motivations of only one participant" (p. 241).

While the concept of a dynamic tension between asymmetry and mutuality is extremely helpful in understanding how to incorporate mutuality into psychotherapy, I find that these contemporary psychoanalytic discussions are critically flawed in their lack of attention to the issue of power. These analysts' ability to conceive of mutuality within asymmetry depends on ignoring the power dynamics of the treatment relationship. The dimensions of asymmetry and mutuality do not merely represent drastically different directions in *technique*; fundamentally, they represent stark dichotomies of power, with asymmetry implying power differential and mutuality implying shared power. When we include an analysis of power in the psychotherapy relationship, I conclude that extreme allegiance to the asymmetry principle is disrespectful of clients, ineffective, and probably at the heart of most forms of therapist/client abuse; *and* I conclude that true mutuality is impossible within a treatment relationship that is intrinsically constrained by power imbalances and differentials. When we, as feminists, expose the structural, institutionalized power differential of the therapy relationship, our negotiation of that central tension between asymmetry and mutuality becomes ever more complex and challenging.

I believe that in psychotherapy *movement* towards mutuality is both possible and desirable, but that the actual achievement of mutuality is impossible within the asymmetry of power of the therapy relationship. When we acknowledge exactly what prevents true mutuality, we facilitate the relationship's movement toward mutuality. Only if we acknowledge the existence of the power differential, the hierarchies and the boundaries, will the client feel we understand and experience each of our positions in the therapy relationship.

MOVEMENT TOWARDS MUTUALITY

Our recognition of therapy as a relational context of unequal investment and unequal vulnerability lays the groundwork for movement toward mutuality. In traditional approaches, the hierarchy and rigidity of the roles of therapist and client are infrequently acknowledged and even less frequently challenged. Only at termination does the therapist share more of her or himself as a real person, in order to break down the hierarchy and move towards equality.

Within a more relational treatment approach, from its beginning the growth of the therapy relationship fundamentally involves movement towards mutuality. Movement towards mutuality involves fashioning the treatment not solely from theoretical constructs or clinical experiences; rather, we allow both ourselves and our clients to consider that the client may have the most expertise on her or his problems— and her or his solutions. We allow and encourage unequal but reciprocal impact and the expression of mutual influence.

The movement towards mutuality may be achieved by various means. The therapist's disclosure of personal information about her life is only one method—one I have found to be too easy to do and too difficult to use effectively. It doesn't involve much creativity on my part to impart information about my life; but the usefulness of that information is often doubtful. However, there are several other movements towards mutuality at our disposal.

- The therapist can be open to being affected and changed by the treatment relationship (Jordan, 1991).
- The therapist can express affect about the client. The therapist can disclose opinions about the client.
- The therapist can admit uncertainty or error, including fumbling and indecision; the therapist can propose tentative hypotheses, instead of delivering sure interpretations.
- The therapist can accept and validate the client's expressions of caring and concern for the therapist.
- The therapist can validate the client's accurate perceptions about the therapist.
- The therapist can tell the client what she (the therapist) has learned from the client.
- The therapist can refuse to take precautions to prevent the client from seeing the therapist as "a real person."

Movement toward mutuality, of course, requires attunement to the client's needs; the therapist must use these techniques selectively, as their impact will vary from one treatment relationship to another, as well as from one point in time to another with each client.

PARAMETERS AND BOUNDARIES

As we've opened the door to reconsidering some of our basic notions about psychotherapy, I've found that our discussion sometimes makes me quite uncomfortable, and I chafe at some of the more extreme challenges to the traditional structures of treatment. I find myself concerned that in the spirit of critique and movement toward mutuality, we are overturning some of the cornerstones that make the therapy relationship uniquely valuable. Sometimes, our discussion of mutuality feels as if we were on a slippery slope, where we end up sliding into making the therapy relationship just like all others. For example, I've heard such questions as:

- "If the therapist's expression of her feelings towards the client is helpful, why limit it to only certain feelings—what about jealousy, competition, sexual attraction—why not share those feelings with clients as well?"

- "If we aim towards mutuality, then why can't we convert the intense connection of the therapy relationship into a friendship after termination?"
- "If mutual responsiveness and impact is a measure of movement towards mutuality, then doesn't it mean that something is awry in the treatment relationship if the therapist *isn't* growing from it?"
- "Isn't the whole concept of boundaries outmoded in a more mutual treatment approach?"

While I agree that we must ask such questions in order to determine the outer limits of the treatment innovations we're considering, I personally do not answer them in the affirmative. I believe that the bizarre, distinctive features of the therapy relationship are what allow for a kind of freedom for the client to grow, in ways that other relationships do not. If this was a relationship just like any other, clients wouldn't be paying for it. The movement towards mutuality depends on *acknowledgment* of a power differential, a role differential, and certain hierarchies—it does not depend on the eradication of these asymmetries. Once those parameters are established, mutually understood, and their limitations confronted, the client can use the treatment relationship in ways that she or he has not been able to engage in other relationships.

Further, I believe that boundaries remain important in psychotherapy. I agree that the hypervigilant guarding of ego boundaries has been used to protect the therapist, sometimes at the expense of the client, and to frighten therapists away from their own authenticity and creativity. I conceptualize the *useful* boundary in psychotherapy more relationally, as a boundary around the relationship that provides a container which protects the relationship, allows much freedom within it, and contributes to making the treatment relationship uniquely valuable. The relational boundary involves time boundaries, space boundaries, and psychological boundaries.

Likewise, I view termination within a relational frame: I do not view termination as a final ending, beyond which I will permit no contact. I believe that the connection lives on beyond the ending, either through internalization, or through the clients overt desire to touch base with me from time to time, or for me to remain available for further therapy. As Herman, Gartrell, Olarte, Feldstein, & Localio (1987) write, "neither transference nor the real inequality in the power relationship ends with the termination of therapy." Likewise, Hall (1984) recognizes the difficulties in post-termination relationships because of the "half-life of transference exceeding that of plutonium." Although in my termination grieving I am often tempted by my own wish to continue our connection, I believe I am always more valuable to my client as her therapist than as her friend.

MUTUALITY IN LESBIAN THERAPIST/LESBIAN CLIENT RELATIONSHIPS

Now, how does being a *lesbian* therapist affect issues of mutuality? I think things become considerably more complicated in the lesbian therapist/lesbian client relationship. Dillon (1992) has commented that mutuality in treatment is especially critical with lesbian clients because lesbians experience great mutuality in their nontherapy relationships and therefore require nothing less in their relationships with us. In a cultural context where lesbians are largely isolated, invisible, and cut off from peer or ancestral role models, lesbian clients may look to lesbian therapists to fill this gap. As with any oppressed population, a therapist's adherence to traditional edicts about neutrality can be dangerously interpreted by the lesbian client: silent neutrality within a context of oppression may be interpreted as the therapist's collusion with the status quo of homophobia—"no comment is a comment" within a climate of oppression.

While these factors would argue for the need for increasing attention to mutuality in treatment with lesbians, there are additional elements which complicate the lesbian therapist/lesbian client relationship. In order for the therapist to be more mutual, she must be willing to express herself with authenticity. However, Natalie, Suzanne, and myself are among the fortunate few who are able to be authentic with our clients if it is clinically useful. But many lesbian therapists work in agencies or communities where they must guard the secret of their sexual identity from their clients, and this secrecy fundamentally and powerfully constrains authenticity and, therefore, mutuality.

In addition, working as a lesbian therapist with lesbian clients means that you live and work in a small-town atmosphere, even if that small town is the New York City lesbian community. Dual forms of contact with my clients is the rule, not the exception. The lesbian client who is talking with me about her deepest pain at four is likely to be dancing next to me at a lesbian bar at ten, or working out next to me at the gym on Saturday morning, or marching next to me at a political rally next week. My response to the inevitability of dual contact with my lesbian clients is to become more vigilant in protecting the relational boundary and preventing *dual contact* from turning into a *dual relationship*. This distinction often brings up complicated, mixed feelings about the limitations and unique qualities of our therapy relationship-and we work together in each treatment relationship to use our confrontations with the particular realities of therapy within the context of the therapeutic connection.

Contributions of the Lesbian Experience to Mutuality in Therapy Relationships

SUZANNE SLATER

"I got your name from the lesbian referral service at the women's center," began my brand new client. "I told them I wanted to find a lesbian therapist who could work with me individually and who does long term therapy." With this beginning, the frame for our new therapy relationship is already forming, based on the acknowledgment that we are two lesbian women coming together to create a one-to-one, potentially close relationship with each other. Many of my lesbian clients know I am a lesbian before they come to see me. As members of an oppressed group, it is adaptive and often necessary for them to elicit this information about potential therapists before they risk inviting a therapist into their most private emotional worlds.

The first information exchanged between us pertains, then, to me, not to the client, and it is personal knowledge about me, relevant to my own relational and sexual life with women. Over time, whatever meanings this particular client will attach to my lesbian identity or to this commonality between us will emerge as we proceed and will differ from those of other clients. However, my client's knowledge of such personal information about me moves the connection beyond the bounds set forth in traditional constructions of therapeutic relationships and establishes that we are creating something outside of that restricted model of relationship. While heterosexual women therapists and clients may also discover their shared heterosexual identity, the all-female therapy relationship does not recall for them the same reminiscences of their lover relationships, and, in fact, specifically distinguishes the therapy relationship from the heterosexual lover relationships they form in their personal lives.

Even prior to therapy, lesbians gather experience in creating their relationships with no models of how *healthy* lesbian relationships should look. All lesbian relationships reflect a choice to move beyond social restrictions and invite both women to venture into clearly forbidden territory. Lesbian friendships, lesbian family relationships, collegial partnerships, and other lesbian-to-lesbian ties all demonstrate this independence, with the women looking to their own needs, desires, and individual priorities to shape their resulting bonds. Each relationship takes on the quality of an unfolding and unpredictable intimacy where the full emergence of the connection is jointly developed.

I will focus here on the parallels between lesbian love relationships and the therapy relationships formed between lesbian therapists and lesbian clients. I will suggest that the therapy relationship is intangibly influenced by both clients' and therapists' associations with each woman's experiences in her lesbian love relationships. This underlying nuance—or reminiscence—may be wholly or partially unconscious and ties the primary elements of the lover bond to some aspects of the structure of the therapy relationship. Parallels can be observed in the way lesbians frequently prioritize high levels of emotional closeness, in the way they create unique relational boundaries around the couple or therapy dyad, and in the contact some lesbians maintain with one another after the therapy or lover relationship ends. While much of the carry-over is specifically outside the sexual realm, I will recognize the potential presence of sexual attraction within this reminiscence, as well.

LESBIAN IDENTITY AND MUTUALITY

All lesbians reach a critical crossroad. When two women find that fully entering into their closeness includes sexual and romantic feelings, women must choose between authenticity and conformity. Either the women can act on their authentic sexual attraction to each other *or* conform to powerful social injunctions against unrestricted intimacy between women—not both. By definition, lesbians are women who have faced this decision and have chosen to deepen their bond and go beyond the point at which society orders them to stop. Lesbian identity is achieved by prioritizing this desire for full and forbidden connection over complying with the imposed structure for the relationship.

Studies done by Loulan (1988), by Blumstein and Schwartz (1983), Peplau, Padesky, and Hamilton (1982), Eldridge and Gilbert (1990), Mencher (1984), and others have examined the relational features most central to lesbian couple relationships and have found that lesbian couples prioritize exactly those interpersonal elements which are most essential to the development of mutuality—empathic identification, a focus on emotional closeness, high expectations of self disclosure, and emphasis on relational equality. Partners commonly work to hone their abilities to negotiate both getting their own needs met and meeting the needs of another within the context of an all-female relationship. The couple continually balances identifying with each other as women, and as lesbians, while still differentiating between each woman's unique identity.

These components are especially conducive to developing a mutual relationship in therapy as well, where therapist and client share crucial personal commonalities despite their clearly distinct identities and roles. While in therapy, the focus is, and should be, disproportionately placed on meeting the client's needs; movement towards mutuality is nonetheless enhanced and complicated by reminiscences of lesbian love relationships present in both women's lives. Client and therapist alike may be prepared to view each therapy relationship as an especially unique and uncharted exchange, looking to themselves to shape the complexities and boundaries of their developing relationship as a result of their experiences in constructing without models their own personal lesbian relationships outside of therapy.

Movement towards mutuality between client and therapist requires a rejection of traditional, nonmutual, male-defined models of relationship that bear partial similarity to the nonconformity required of lesbian women. As is true for lesbian lovers, the client and therapist reach a crucial turning point that can also be characterized as a choice between authenticity and social conformity Either they can comply with the restrictions imposed in traditional models of therapy or venture into the still-controversial realm of collaboratively constructed therapy relationships. This choice serves as the clear point of departure from social convention. While lesbians are not the only women who value exclusively woman-to-woman relationships, lesbians have given these connections particular prominence in their lives, and have done so at tremendous social cost. Each lesbian brings to the therapy relationship a special seriousness about her connections with women and a desire to form genuine intimacy without the socially required participation of men. Therein, these lesbians demonstrate a commitment to the relational process at the expense of traditional social or professional approval. The two relational experiences, of being lesbian lovers and of being a lesbian client and therapist partnership, contain crucial parallels that can inform and shape the development of the therapy relationship. In therapy, these parallels may be manifested in a variety of ways, including a high level examination of the real (in addition to the transference-based) therapy relationship typical of some lesbian therapy dyads, a particular and mutual openness to negotiating how the therapist will and will not use self-disclosure in a relationship that began with a revelation of personal information about the therapist, and possibly also in a testing of boundaries on the part of some lesbian clients. In these and other ways, lesbian clients may be less likely to conform passively to a provided model for the therapy relationship and may expect to have input into the relationship's character and parameters.

Both lesbian lovers and lesbian therapy dyads striving for mutuality come up against a similar ambiguity when they opt for the uncleared path toward a more obscured but promising relational journey. Without maps to indicate how lesbian love or more mutual therapy relationships should look, both couples and therapy dyads are simultaneously burdened and freed up to construct their relationships virtually from scratch. While lesbians forming *therapy* relationships are guided by clearly different goals than are lesbians creating *couple* bonds, both invite the inevitable ambiguity that emerges when women allow their bonds to develop in their own unique way. Heyward (1989b) captures the essence of this relational unfolding in her statement, "Mutuality, like equality, signals relational growth and change and constitutes an invitation into shaping the future together" (p. 34). She continues, ". . . both people should be growing and changing in the relationship, mutually empowered to become more fully themselves with one another" (p. 35).

Lesbian couples must invest continual effort in this creative process—constructing their relationships according to their own needs and choices and monitoring their progress vigilantly. Frequently, lesbians are world-class processors, able to analyze at length (and occasionally ad nauseam) the most intangible of interpersonal dynamics. As Dillon (1992) has pointed out, lesbians are familiar with and open to relational complexity. Lesbians often view getting in there and working on their relational process as a source of closeness in and of itself. They may come to therapy equally prepared to examine the dyadic process emerging between client and therapist.

CONSTRUCTING BOUNDARIES

In both therapy and couple relationships, lesbians must discover what boundaries are needed between the two women and also between the relationship and the outside world. Lesbians commonly respect the utility of relational boundaries, and they expend much energy in creating and preserving selected boundaries. Lesbians commonly cultivate lesbian-to-lesbian friendships that are highly mutual and also clearly nonsexual. Many lesbians skillfully navigate the particular complexities of forming nonsexual intimacy with one another.

Likewise, more mutual therapy relationships also demand particular boundaries. While movement toward mutuality does involve transcending *traditional* conceptions of therapy relationships, these more mutual therapy dyads are not formless relationships where all boundaries are automatically discarded. Lesbian clients may come to therapy specially equipped to help select useful relational boundaries. However, unlike the situation in couple relationships, establishing and preserving those boundaries in therapy is a mutual but unequal exchange. The therapist assumes ultimate responsibility for boundary maintenance, frequently collaborating with her clients but not capitulating in disputes over needed relational limits.

In addition, societal homophobia imposes a continual need for lesbians to present their most intimate and private relationships either as nonexistent or as superficial to the surrounding mainstream community. Lesbian couples face pressures to hide the true nature of their relationships due to the very real dangers associated with coming out. Similarly, therapists deliberately keep the treatment relationship secret, resulting in the powerful duality of great intimacy behind closed doors and little or no acknowledgment that any such attachment exists in front of others. Lesbians in therapy may recognize this contrived but necessary pattern of interaction from their experiences in lover relationships. Because lesbian therapists and clients share what are usually small lesbian social communities, there is a strong likelihood that they will travel in overlapping social circles. They may, therefore, frequently be confronted with the need to enact a duplicitous exchange, where minimal head nods suffice as recognition of actually intimate, private bonds. The similarity to their lover relationships may be at times quite conscious for one or both as this familiar dance is repeated.

> Terry and Andrea didn't often go to plays in Springfield. It was one thing to be out together as a recognizable couple in Northampton, but neither felt the same safety being identified as lesbians in Springfield. Throughout the evening, they avoided touching and watched the crowd more vigilantly than felt comfortable. Part way through intermission, Terry spotted her therapist sitting in a nearby section of the theater. Clearly aware of each other, the therapist nodded to Terry in an acknowledging but understated way. Privately, Terry felt vaguely amused that two of the most important women in her life were here, and no observer would ever be able to tell.

BEYOND TERMINATION

Lesbians' experiences in couple relationships also color their therapy relationships after termination. While heterosexual couples more frequently end contact with each other after they have broken up, lesbians frequently work to maintain connection after they are no longer a couple. This effort is based on the belief that relational bonds extend beyond the two women's roles as lovers. The basis for relationship is less wholly dependent on their lover status than is true for other kinds of couplings. Likewise, lesbians in therapy may challenge traditional conceptions of termination, where clients and therapists relinquish all contact with each other and avoid future connection of any sort. Lesbians' normative efforts to create post-break-up relationships with ex-lovers may inform their responses to the traditional prohibition against post-termination contact between clients and therapists. Hence, the lesbian therapy dyads may exhibit a wider range of post-termination arrangements between clients and therapists. Also, as Julie has mentioned, because the lesbian community is small in most areas, unplanned contact between lesbian clients and therapists after therapy has ended is quite likely, whether or not either considers this interaction desirable. This may actually limit the options for clients and therapists, as in practice a choice to have no further contact may be difficult to accomplish.

> "I can't believe I won't be back after seeing you every week for four years," my client commented tearfully. "I'll miss seeing you and being able to connect with you." My client and I knew we would be running into one another this very weekend, since both of us were invited to a small memorial service for a mutual friend. We both acknowledged the paradox of working to bring closure to our relationship knowing we'd be seeing each other again right away. It was too soon after this final session for us to have contact, and yet, neither would agree to forego the weekend's important event. How could I help my client fully experience this ending, when we both knew we'd repeatedly cross paths before any time had passed at all?

SEXUAL TENSIONS

Finally, it cannot be ignored that the commonality shared by lesbian therapists and clients is a sexual as well as a relational one. Within the intimacy and privacy of the therapy relationship, lesbian clients and therapists develop relational features which bear similarity to their love relationships. Specifically, client and therapist renounce overly confining relational boundaries, increase their collaboration in shaping their relationship, and prioritize the development of their authentic connection. Each woman knows that in their private lives outside of therapy this process has included sexual feelings. Heyward (1989b) has bravely articulated the sexual nuance in the development of mutuality in her statement, "Our sexualities are our embodied yearning to express a relational mutuality in which the tensions are sustained, not broken. . . . There is remarkable erotic power in these tensions" (p. 33–34). Within a therapy relationship there is potential for this sexual tension at moments of relational breakthrough.

> For many weeks I could feel we were nearing a profound secret. My client's eyes studied me constantly, clearly looking for clues as to whether or not I would be able to handle the truth she was considering sharing with me. Finally, she found her moment and took the risk. "My best friend and I were secret lovers for twelve years," she said. "We would meet every night after our husbands went to work for the 11 to 7 shift, and we would stay together until they were soon due home. We'd set a clock to be sure to be back in our beds before they arrived home." The content of her secret surprised me only slightly and was not difficult to hold. The look in her eyes, however, gave me pause, as we sat silently in her moment of greatest exposure. My client shifted anxiously, uncomfortable in the silence that followed her disclosure. She knew she was suddenly more exposed, revealing a sexual truth about herself that filled her with both fear and shy excitement. The resulting tension between us felt distinctly sexual and I, too, was uncomfortable as I recognized that my own feelings had become sexually charged as well. At exactly this moment of revelation that she, too, is sexually involved with women, our own connection was being tested. We were both women for whom moments of great intimacy with another woman had in our lives become sexual. Neither of us could escape the unspoken fact that vestiges of that same blending of close and sexual feelings which were so welcome in our personal lives had subtly found their way into the therapy relationship as well.

In conclusion, while lesbian love relationships and lesbian therapy relationships contain critical and fundamental differences, lesbian client and therapist dyads engaged in working towards mutual (though unequal) therapy relationships do so in the presence of an underlying reminiscence to each one's experience in forming lesbian love relationships. The association between these two central forms of lesbian-to-lesbian connection occurs at varying levels of conscious awareness and is certainly not universal for all lesbians. However, lesbians bring unique experience to the tasks of redefining the boundaries between client and therapist, of welcoming relational ambiguity, and of making their connections with women primary at particular social cost. In addition, lesbian experience also informs clients' and therapists' approaches to managing the dichotomy of sharing great closeness behind closed doors yet hiding the relationship from others, of juggling complex realities related to their therapist-client contact after termination, and of recognizing the potential for sexual feeling inherent in the developing emotional connection. While nonlesbian therapy dyads may also achieve these relationship qualities, the association between lesbian experience and the tasks of developing genuine client-therapist mutuality offers a particular contribution to the wider discussion of therapeutic mutuality between women.

Mutuality, Psychotherapy, and Ethics

NATALIE S. ELDRIDGE

Why is ethics a key element in our discussion of the movement toward mutuality in psychotherapy? In our discussions, we found ourselves stumbling over the limitations of our more traditional conceptions of ethical standards of practice. At the same time, it became increasingly necessary to make a clear link between a defined ethical framework and our own movement toward mutuality in our practices. It is by this domain of ethics and professional identity that we can distinguish between psychotherapy relationships and all other relationships in which we engage.

My thoughts on mutuality, psychotherapy, and ethics have been nourished by many people: Carol Gilligan (1982) and her colleagues' work on moral development, the work of both Laura Brown (1989, 1991) and the Feminist Therapy Institute (1987) on feminist ethics, Carter Heyward's (1989a) moving challenges in her papers here at the Stone Center, and the pioneering work of Melba Vasquez (1992) in voicing the importance of gender and ethnic diversity in training clinicians to practice ethically. I have been further stimulated and challenged by my involvement with the Stone Center Lesbian Theory Group.

From this rich context of feminist theory I want, first, to suggest a way for therapists to view ethics from a relational model. Next, I'll give an example of how this relational view can be useful in understanding the movement toward mutuality in psychotherapy. Finally, I will offer some cautionary suggestions for considering ethics in psychotherapy to those of us traveling in the uncharted territory between traditional views and not-yet-clearly formulated alternative frameworks.

ETHICS FROM A RELATIONAL FRAME

> "Thou shalt not have sex with your client. . . ."
> "Thou shalt not have dual relationships with your clients. . . ."
> "Thou shalt not use therapy relationships for personal gain. . . ."

Regardless of how the ethical codes are worded, most of us have been trained to conceptualize the ethics of our practice as a list of commandments, or rules. If the rules are broken, the result could be a compromised treatment for our client, negative judgments by our colleagues, and/or a legal suit brought against us. Some of the most agreed upon rules have been reified by becoming laws dealing with confidentiality, the duty to warn, and, in some states, sexual contact between client and therapist. Those "ethical practices" that have become laws are the most clearly understood and discussed in professional circles, because of the threat and enormous cost of legal liability. An orientation around rules is what Gilligan (1982) has defined as a morality of rights, where justice and fairness prevail—an orientation most pronounced in the moral reasoning of men. It is on this frame of morality that our legal system, and much of Judeo-Christian culture, is based. Gilligan (1982) compares the morality of rights with a morality of responsibility, where an ethic of care and relational considerations prevails—an orientation she discovered as she listened to women struggle with both hypothetical and real decisions. In a morality of responsibility, reasoning is based on weighing conflicting responsibilities to the various relationships in which a person is engaged.

The work of psychotherapy is certainly about care, and our ethical standards and codes do reflect underlying principles of care, such as our responsibility to do no harm to our clients (Kitchener, 1984, 1988). Yet the emphasis in our ethics training seems to be on what we should avoid, rather than what we can do, to ensure an ethical stance of doing no harm. We learn to avoid certain behaviors, but are not always provided with a theoretical frame that describes what it is about that behavior that makes it unethical or that helps us respond to the less defined, more subtle situations which can arise in our practices.

I am suggesting that while the effective practice of psychotherapy relies heavily on a morality of responsibility and care, our professional standards and codes of ethics are communicated to us largely within a morality of rights and justice, with the implication that fairness and universality should prevail. Although there are ethical imperatives which should be applied universally, I believe that some areas of ethical deliberation need a more complex and flexible kind of reasoning. It is the ethic of care, most pronounced as we listen to how women reason, that we need to understand more fully in order to apply an appropriate ethical frame to a relational therapeutic model.

A relational context in psychotherapy, and in our ethical thinking, allows for greater variability and diversity in our practices which, in turn, can reflect the needs of our increasingly diverse clientele. However, variability runs counter to a basic tenet of our training. We are taught to develop *universal* rules and standards of practice and to apply them with no variation to all clients. Indeed, if we vary our practice from one client to another, aren't we taught that we are risking a potential ethical violation through our own countertransference reaction? I have found this question arising often with colleagues and supervisees. My response is that we should indeed observe, and recognize, any variations in our practice from client to client. The goal, however, is not to ban all variation, but to question why there is variation and if it is therapeutic. Where traditional thinking and a "fairness and consistency" model of ethics prevail, such a variation is suspect by its very existence. I suggest that we must take the next step and ask the relationally therapeutic questions of what is appropriate care for the particular client, for the particular therapeutic relationship, and for the given therapist? Could a particular response (such as silence and a neutral affect) be therapeutic with one client and abandoning with another? I think the answer is a resounding yes. Could a therapist's response (such as tears) be unthinkable (a clinical error) with one client and therapeutic with another? Absolutely. For example, I have found it therapeutic to sometimes share my tears with a client who is discussing a significant loss. With terminally ill clients, I have been moved to tears by the prospect of the loss of my client through death. Yet the client who is facing her own death, and finds everyone in her life dissolving into tears when she tries to discuss how she feels about dying, may need a different response from her therapist if she is to experience her process in a fuller way. It is a consideration of the relational context of each dyad, at each stage of the relationship, that guides the therapist about this ethic of care.

As we take a step deeper in negotiating mutuality in psychotherapy, we move beyond discrete behaviors, such as showing an emotional response or sharing a piece of personal information. At the base we find the psychotherapeutic frame and our responsibility as therapists to construct and preserve that frame.

Yet how clear are we about what that frame is? How do we each, personally and professionally, understand and experience the process of constructing and preserving this frame? In considering this question, I came up with a working definition for myself: The therapeutic frame is both an internal image and a set of concrete behaviors, held and acted on by the therapist and communicated, over time, to the client. Within the parameters of this frame, both therapist and client engage in a negotiation of intimacy and power that will maintain safety and a therapeutic climate for the healing and growth of the client. Various therapeutic orientations and cultural experiences affect how we, as therapists, might envision this frame. I believe the Lesbian Theory Group's particular views of the therapeutic frame, though not absolutely congruent among those in our group, are still informed in some common ways by our experience as lesbians, personally and professionally.

On a personal level, certain cultural factors emerge which have been discussed by both Julie and Suzanne. As lesbians, we are likely to have been relatively unconstrained by the heterosexual "frame" for couple relationships; instead we have negotiated normative lesbian paradigms of high-intimacy, shared-power relationships (Eldridge & Gilbert, 1990; Blumstein & Schwartz, 1983; Peplau, Padesky, & Hamilton, 1982).

On a professional level, unless we refuse to work with lesbian clients, or unless we deprive ourselves of lesbian community involvement and support, our social and political community is comprised of us and our clients. Therefore, we are challenged to find therapeutic and ethical ways to maintain a therapy frame that will neither deny the other contacts that may occur, nor be destroyed by them. I will use this dilemma of working within a small community to illustrate some principles of ethical thinking from a relational orientation.

EXAMPLES OF RELATIONAL ETHICS

Dual roles between therapist and client are specifically taboo in the professional codes of ethics, one of what Brown (1989) calls "the thou shalt nots." Since the traditional ethical stance of complete separation between personal and professional contacts is impossible for many lesbian therapists treating lesbians, the first step is to reframe and name our common experience. Berman (1985) has suggested the term "overlapping relationships" to describe those aspects of therapists' and clients' lives that will intersect within a small community, even when the therapist exerts great effort to avoid dual roles. If we begin with the premise that some overlap is unavoidable, we must go on to explore ways to delineate and maintain clear boundaries around the therapeutic frame in this more mutual therapeutic context. How can we embrace the predictable reality of overlapping relationships and yet avoid what is dangerous and harmful in the broader concept of "dual relationships"?

I would like to suggest several guidelines. First, we can recognize and validate the existence of overlapping relationships, to ourselves, our colleagues, and to our clients. Otherwise our own shame or denial of the existence of these "breaks in the traditional frame" will get in the way of conscious and thoughtful decision-making about how to maintain a useful frame in this particular system. Jordan (1989) has written eloquently on the power of shame to destroy connection.

Second, we can be active in preplanning the ethical management of anticipated overlapping relationships. We can predict potential overlaps with clients at the outset and collaboratively set up norms with the client that will contain both boundaries and connectedness in such outside encounters. The Feminist Therapy Code of Ethics (1987) developed by the Feminist Therapy Institute is unique in addressing the concept of unavoidable overlapping relationships, and offers the following as one of its guidelines: "A feminist therapist recognizes the complexity and conflicting priorities inherent in multiple or overlapping relationships. The therapist accepts responsibility for monitoring such relationships to prevent potential abuse of or harm to the client" (p. 2). This suggests that we don't need to flee from the possibility of role overlap, but rather we are to take responsibility for making the first step toward boundary management.

Third, we can develop a more complex concept of the therapeutic frame than the traditional one. The traditional frame is what Brown (1991) has called an "abstinent frame," and is conceptualized as invariable from client to client, with any variations seen as breaks in the frame, and, thus, as opportunities for boundary violation. For example, within an abstinent frame, self-disclosure of certain personal information or emotional responses would be seen as a boundary violation regardless of the relational context of the particular situation. Similarly, within a different frame, a therapist who views self-disclosure as always valuable, holding it as a kind of ideal, may also fail to recognize the circumstances in which self-disclosure is clearly contraindicated. Mutuality must begin with a very clear focus on the particular cultural and therapeutic context of each therapy relationship.

As an example, all lesbian therapists must deal with the question of whether, when, and how to come out to clients. From an "abstinent frame," the therapist might choose never to directly come out to clients. But even if the therapist espouses a norm of never disclosing her sexual identity to clients, the client may uncover this information and may bring it to therapy. How does the therapist hold the therapeutic frame and deal with this intrusion of information? How does the therapist deal with this authentically? What harm could come from the therapist's failure to acknowledge her sexual identity? On the other hand, if a therapist holds a norm of always coming out to her clients, what happens if a client doesn't want to know? There are some clients who are simply not ready to hear this information and effectively defend against it by denying it, and there are those who, to their detriment, will hear it and feel bombarded by such a disclosure. The therapist who makes this decision on a clinical basis, case by case, must deal with the complexities of reviewing her therapeutic frame within the context of each therapeutic relationship. It is often more comfortable to stay in an abstinent frame than to deal with the demanding process of negotiating these complexities.

Fourth, the application of a feminist analysis of power in therapy can help us to clarify and set appropriate boundaries for the therapeutic frame. We can include the client's expertise in determining appropriate boundaries by providing options for discussion. At the same time, we must acknowledge that our power is not equal and not capitulate to the desires of our client when they differ from our own clinical judgment. I think my clinical judgment must be based on what the client wants, on what I think is best for the client, *and* on what I am comfortable with as a therapist and a person. Still, some boundary violations can be avoided simply by asking the client what will work best for her rather than making a priori assumptions from an expert position.

Finally, weaving an ethical framework into our training and practice rather than treating it as something we add on later will help us to develop a more integrated orientation to our ethical and theoretical understanding. Each of us has to begin by developing our own ethical code, in consultation with others and in a way that is congruent with the existing codes to which we have already agreed to abide. An example of how one lesbian therapist has woven an ethical code for herself is offered by Gartrell (1992) in her recent article on "Boundaries in Lesbian Therapy Relationships." Although others, including myself, would not necessarily come to the same decisions about our practices,

Gartrell's clear delineation of her stance on boundaries provides a good example of the development of one therapist's relationally-responsible code of ethics.

PRACTICAL SUGGESTIONS FOR AN ETHICAL USE OF MUTUALITY IN PSYCHOTHERAPY

1. Acknowledge and own the power we have as therapists and the inevitable power differential between therapist and client that forms the frame of psychotherapy. Denial of our power is dangerous.

2. In reviewing our own practice and ethical standards, go beyond concrete do's and don'ts to ask ourselves "why" or "why not" about each behavior. This questioning practice can help to keep our ethical framework more conscious and aligned more closely to our theoretical orientation. It is easy to violate the spirit of an ethical code or standard without violating the letter of the code.

3. Therapist self-care is an ethical imperative. If we are not fairly consistent in caring for our changing personal needs, it will be very difficult (if not impossible) to prevent us from meeting those needs in our therapeutic relationships. A part of this self-care is recognizing the limits to our flexibility as we work with our clients. For those of us with large practices in a small community, there are very real repercussions if we vary certain boundaries with one client and not with another. Our clients talk to one another about their experience of therapy and what they know about us—a normal response for an oppressed group checking out levels of safety and struggling to create mutual models of relationships, including therapeutic relationships, that reflect their unique needs. The therapist would be wise to consider this broader context for her practice and assert the boundaries she needs in order to provide adequate privacy and consistency. This kind of self-care is particularly critical when the therapist is a member of the same extended community.

4. The last, and probably most essential suggestion, is to make ethics a relational process: consulting, questioning, discussing, disagreeing, clarifying . . . these relational processes help to heighten our awareness and capacity to create a living ethics for relational psychotherapy.

I leave you with more questions than answers about mutuality, psychotherapy, and ethics. I have suggested the complexities involved by highlighting a few of the interlocking pieces. We need to grapple with the combination of the need for some universal ethical imperatives and the importance of aspects that must be handled on a case-by-case basis. We must be careful not to replace traditional edicts with "relational edicts," not to substitute one set of "thou shalt nots" for another.

I believe that by integrating more of the voice of responsibility and care into our understanding of ethics, along with the voice of the "thou shalt nots," we can enrich our practices and weave an ethical framework more congruent with a relational model of psychotherapy.

CONCLUSION

In conclusion, once we, as therapists, have relinquished the security of an allegiance to asymmetry (at the expense of mutuality) or to mutuality (ignoring asymmetry), we find ourselves in the more complicated territory of engaging in the tension between these two seemingly opposed elements of psychotherapy (Burke, 1992). In this chapter we have examined the challenges of engaging in this tension in each therapy relationship, in each session. Furthermore, the process of incorporating mutuality into psychotherapy involves always being mindful that each individual therapy relationship is firmly rooted in a tradition and structure of power, as well as being embedded within a broader context of culture and community. Raising questions rather than giving answers, we have tried to build a frame around which to negotiate a very complex topic and to add our voices to what we hope will be a continuing dialogue on the conundrum of mutuality in psychotherapy.

DISCUSSION SUMMARY

After each colloquium lecture, a discussion was held. Selected portions are summarized here. Drs. Judith Jordan and Irene Stiver joined in the discussion.

Question: I want to thank you for taking risks and addressing some difficult issues. To address one of Julie's examples: When a client picks up accurately that we are preoccupied in a session, how far do we go with that? Do we give her her money back?

Mencher: No, I don't think that we have to go that far. I think that interaction becomes part of the fabric of the therapy relationship. It's the reality of relationships of all kinds that attentiveness and attunement are not perfect. I think there's something to be gained in a client seeing that we are not perfect, and in using that in the therapy. I often say to clients, "Let's look at how it feels to you to learn that I'm not perfect." For some clients, it feels like an assault; for other clients, it feels like a welcome relief. It has to be negotiated in each particular relationship.

Jordan: I'd like to add that the client may get double her money's worth in the session—where the discussion of the "failure" can be incredibly empowering and validating.

Slater: We need to distinguish between different kinds of preoccupation. When there is an event in the therapist's own life that makes it understandable that the therapist will feel called away, that's one thing. A different situation is when I find that with a *particular* client, I'm more likely to feel preoccupied than with others. In those cases, we need to examine what is going on in the client, or in that particular treatment relationship that is causing that reaction.

Stiver: We expect that there will be rhythms of connection and disconnection in the therapy relationship. It is the ethical responsibility of the therapist to examine her part in these rhythms and work on them with the client.

Question: I also want to thank you for the risk-taking. I'm concerned, though, about some of the assumptions I heard in Suzanne's section and also in the beginning of Natalie's—that lesbians bring to therapy great previous knowledge of mutual and intimate relationships. We need to remember that all lesbians are women first. That means that many of our lesbian clients are survivors of abuse, are substance abusers, and have grown up in a violent world. I don't think that we can generalize that they'd have experience with selective boundary-making and with knowing about mutual and intimate relationships. Every client is unique.

Also, can you, Suzanne, discuss how you handled the situation of experiencing sexual tension with your client?

Slater: I really agree with the first part of your comment. I am not attempting to say that lesbians do it best. But because lesbians form relationships with no models whatsoever, because we really have to start from scratch, we come to relationships with more experience of having to work on the process. It does not necessarily mean we've all done a spectacular job or that some lesbians don't bring impediments to that process.

About the clinical example: The presence of sexual tension is one of the most difficult things to handle in therapy. For many people, it comes up infrequently. I certainly don't mean to suggest that this happens all the time between lesbians. In many situations, I would choose not to talk about my sexual feelings, because of the risk of reenacting a frequent situation in female experience, i.e., the imposing of other people's sexual feelings on women. I think you have to be very clear that the revealing of your sexual feelings is in the client's best interests and not a way of coping with your own discomfort. I wouldn't say *never,* but I'd have to have some very clear reasons for it, and if I didn't I'd err on the side of not discussing it openly.

Mencher: I *would* say *never*. I would never reveal to a client that I have sexual feelings for her that come from anything outside of a response to her feelings for me. I think this is because the therapy relationship exists within a culture in which sex is *so* burdened, so laden with baggage, that I think that my saying to a client, "I'm attracted to you" cannot be surely therapeutic within that cultural context. The issue of erotic transference and countertransference is extremely complex, and our training is very inadequate. I think that it's often important to bring these questions about particular cases to a consultant or supervisor, while also realizing that our consultants may not feel solidly expert on this issue either. This is clearly a topic that we could explore much further.

Question: I want to raise a dilemma that my colleagues and myself encounter a lot—how to manage participating in a 12-step program, being lesbian-identified, working with lesbian clients, and going to lesbian meetings. I've tried many different ways of dealing with this. I talk to clients about what meetings I go to, and which meetings I'd like them not to attend because I speak there and they are my home meetings. There's quite a lot to that. It pushes against the culture of 12-step programs, that they are open to everyone. It also has implications for anonymity; if I'm at a meeting and I hear a client speak, and I hear something that concerns me, then how do I deal with that piece? It's another issue I'd like us to consider.

Mencher: I think your comment is very important, both within a 12-step context and for therapists and therapy clients as well, e.g., therapists participating in group therapy. You raise the question, how does the therapist communicate and delimit her own authentic needs? At what point do I say to my clients, "I need something from you." "I need you not to go to that meeting." "We need to figure this out." I think it's important that the therapist take the step to say, "We need to figure this out together."

Eldridge: I think that, in your comment, you really delineated your own ethical frame and struggled with how you're going to balance your own needs within that—that's what we need to do more of, proactively and in consultation and collaboration with our colleagues.

REFERENCES

Aron, L. (1991). The patient's experience of the analyst's subjectivity. *Psychoanalytic Dialogues, 1*, 29–51.

Aron, L. (1992). Interpretation as expression of the analyst's subjectivity. *Psychoanalytic Dialogues, 2,* 475–507.

Berman, J. S. (1985). Ethical feminist perspectives on dual relationships with clients. In L. B. Rosewater & L. E. A. Walker (Eds.), *Handbook of feminist therapy: Women's issues in psychotherapy* (pp. 287–296). New York: Springer.

Blumstein, P., & Schwartz, P. (1983). *American couples.* New York: William Morrow.

Bograd, M. (1992). The duel over dual relationships. *Family Therapy Networker, 16*(6), 33–37.

Brown, L. S. (1989). Beyond thou shalt not: Thinking about ethics in the lesbian therapy community. *Women and Therapy, 8,* 13–25.

Brown, L. S. (1991). Ethical issues in feminist therapy. *Psychology of Women Quarterly, 15,* 323–336.

Burke, W. F. (1992). Countertransference disclosure and the asymmetry/mutuality dilemma. *Psychoanalytic Dialogues, 2,* 241–271.

Dillon, C. (1992). *Bringing theory alive with lesbians.* Paper presented at the Harvard University/Cambridge Hospital Conference on Women and Therapy, Boston, MA.

Eldridge, N. S., & Gilbert, L. A. (1990). Correlates of relationship satisfaction in lesbian couples. *Psychology of Women Quarterly, 14,* 43–62.

Feminist Therapy Institute (1987). *Feminist therapy ethical code.* Denver, CO: Feminist Therapy Institute.

Gartrell, N. K. (1992). Boundaries in lesbian therapy relationships. *Women & Therapy, 12,* 29–50.

Gilligan, C. (1982). *In a different voice.* Cambridge, MA: Harvard University Press.

Hall, M. (1984). *Client/counselor sex and feminist therapy: A new look at an old taboo.* Paper presented at the Third Advanced Feminist Therapy Institute, Oakland, CA.

Herman, J., Gartrell, N., Olarte, S., Feldstein, M., & Localio, R. (1987). Psychiatrist-patient sexual contact: Results of a national survey. *American Journal of Psychiatry, 144*(2), 164–169.

Heyward, C. (1989a). *Coming out and relational empowerment: A lesbian feminist theological perspective.* (Work in Progress No. 38.) Wellesley, MA: Stone Center Working Paper Series.

Heyward, C. (1989b). *Touching our strength: The erotic as power and the love of God.* San Francisco, CA: Harper.

Heyward, C., & Jordan, J. (1992). Mutuality in therapy: Ethics, power, and psychology. Stone Center Audiotape, No. A7.

Hoffman, I. Z. (1992). Some practical implications of a social-contructivist view of the psychoanalytic situation. *Psychoanalytic Dialogues, 2,* 287–304.

Jordan, J. V. (1986). *The meaning of mutuality.* (Work in Progress No. 23.) Wellesley, MA: Stone Center Working Paper Series.

Jordan, J. V. (1989). *Relational development: Therapeutic implications of empathy and shame.* (Work in Progress No. 39). Wellesley, MA: Stone Center Working Papers Series.

Jordan, J. V. (1991a). *The movement of mutuality and power.* (Work in Progress No. 53.) Wellesley, MA: Stone Center Working Paper Series.

Jordan, J. V. (1991b). Empathy, mutuality, and therapeutic change: Clinical implications of a relational model. In Jordan, J., Kaplan, A., Miller, J. B., Stiver, I., & Surrey, J., *Women's Growth in Connection* (pp. 283–289). New York: Guilford Press. (Originally presented in 1986).

Kitchener, K. S. (1984). Intuition, critical evaluation and ethical principles: The foundation for ethical decisions in counseling psychology. *The Counseling Psychologist, 12,* 43–55.

Kitchener, K. S. (1988). Dual role relationships: What makes them so problematic? *Journal of Counseling and Development, 67,* 217–221.

Loulan, J. (1988). Research on the sex practices of 1566 lesbians and the clinical applications. *Women and Therapy, 7,* 221–234.

Mencher, J. (1984). Changing the lens on female personality development: A challenge to the notion of fusion in lesbian relationships. Unpublished master's thesis, Smith College School for Social Work, Northampton, MA.

Miller, J. B., & Stiver, 1. (1991). *A relational refraining of therapy.* (Work in Progress No. 52.) Wellesley, MA: Stone Center Working Paper Series.

Mitchell, S. A. (1988). *Relational concepts in psychoanalysis: An integration.* Cambridge, MA: Harvard University Press.

Modell, A. H. (1991). The therapeutic relationship as a paradoxical experience. *Psychoanalytic Dialogues, 1,* 13–28.

Peplau, L. A., Padesky, C., & Hamilton, M. (1982). Satisfaction in lesbian relationships. *Journal of Homosexuality, 8*(2), 23–35.

Rogers, A. G. (1991). A feminist poetics of psychotherapy. In C. Gilligan, A. G. Rogers, & D. L. Tolman (Eds.), *Women, girls and psychotherapy: Reframing resistance* (pp. 33–53). New York: Harrington Park.

Tansey, M. J. (1992). Psychoanalytic expertise. *Psychoanalytic Dialogues, 2,* 305–316.

Vasquez, M. J. T. (1992). Psychologist as clinical supervisor: Promoting ethical practice. *Professional Psychology: Research and Practice, 23,* 196–202.

This chapter was presented at a Stone Center Colloquium on April 7, 1993. © 1993 Natalie S. Eldridge, Julie Mencher, and Suzanne Slater.

7

Relational Development: Therapeutic Implications of Empathy and Shame

JUDITH V. JORDAN

Western science, including psychology, rests on the assumption of a primary reality composed of separate objects that secondarily come into relationship with one another. As Helen Lynd notes, "The separation having been intially assumed, the problems of relation and integration are posed" (1958, p. 81). Moving from Aristotelian logic and Newtonian physics to quantum physics, we begin to see reality defined by relationships, continuities, and probabilities rather than by discrete objects and dualities. Traditional psychological theories view "the self" as the basic unit of study and emphasize its independence, security, and separation from other selves. In the existing paradigm of "self-development" the task is to internalize resources of love in order to create an ever more unique, self-sufficient, and separate structure: the self. Control, boundedness, and ownership of action have been essential to psychology's view of the individual (Jordan, 1988).

In the image of a separate self, boundaries are construed as necessary protections, giving shape and strength to the inner person who is threatened from without. Viewing development from a *relational* rather than a *self* perspective, boundaries could be understood as processes of contact and exchange, moments of knowing, and movement and growth. Thus, we evolve from a metaphor of a bounded self whose task it is to "master" reality, to a relational self "meeting" reality and growing with others.

The Stone Center relational perspective on human experience posits that, optimally:

1. We grow in, through, and towards relationship.
2. For women, especially, connection with others is central to psychological well-being.
3. Movement towards relational mutuality can occur throughout life, through mutual empathy, responsiveness, and contribution to the growth of each individual and to the relationship (Jordan, 1983; Kaplan, 1983; Miller, 1984, 1986, Stiver, 1984; Surrey, 1985).

Moving away from the primacy of the "intrapsychic self" in no way suggests that there is not a real inner life characterized by organization, a sense of personal history, feelings, expectations, and internal representations of self and other. From a relational perspective the movement of relating, of mutual initiative and responsiveness, is the ongoing central dynamic in people's lives. A psychology of relationship goes beyond the dualities of intrapsychic versus interpersonal, selflessness versus selfishness, altruism versus egoism (Jordan, 1988).

Our perspective emphasizes that in growth-enhancing relationships people take mutual responsibility for relationships and provide the means for each other's development. One client summarized the importance of both people caring for the relationship: "There is Len, me, and the relationship. When I feel that he is paying attention to the relationship, it feels so much better. Usually, I carry that by myself." Another woman, in the middle of a fight with her husband in which both were escalating hurtful remarks and in which she was feeling victimized, suddenly stopped and said, "Wait a minute, who's the *real* victim here?" and found to her surprise that her transforming answer was, "the relationship." When both people share a respect for and desire to nurture the relationship, mutuality is created.

Piaget's theory of adaptation, comprised of accommodation and assimilation, provides one model of the dynamic of realationship (1952). Our internal images, expectations, and organizations of experience change to accommodate newness in our surroundings, and we later change what we take in during the process of assimilating it. Ideally, growth occurs through mutual initiative and responsiveness in relationship, what we might call mutual accommodation and assimilation. Responsiveness to other individuals, as well as having an impact on them, leads to our own growth.

As therapists, we stress the development of relational awareness and an interest in the movement of relationship, not just attention to self and other. With a real appreciation of the "ongoingness" of a need for connection, we cease infantilizing needs for intimacy, tenderness, nurturance, and deep involvement in relationship. The shift from pathologizing the powerful motivation for connectedness to honoring it, produces a marked change in the way we undertake therapy. It would be like taking all the popular books about women, like, *Women Who Love Too Much*, or *Men Who Hate Women and the Women Who Love Them* and retitling them: *The Courage to Care, The Power of Taking Responsibility for Relationship*, or *Women Who Care Enough About Relationships to Buy Thousands of Books on the Subject*.

WHAT IS RELATIONAL THERAPY?

Writing about Dora, Freud suggested that in therapy, "I set myself the task of bringing to light what human beings keep hidden within them" (1905/1959). This is another way of saying that one attempts to make the unconscious conscious or, "Where id was there shall ego be." In the Freudian model of therapy, there should be a decrease in intrapsychic conflict, with a subsequent increase in exercise of will and autonomy. There is also an increasing internalization of function and structuralization leading to greater interpersonal independence. The interpretative activity of the analyst should cause a lifting of repressions, bringing the unconscious to light. In object relations theory if a "good enough" holding environment is provided, the "real self" will emerge (Winnicott, 1971). In Kohut's unidirectional model the empathic therapist, used as a self-object, provides a function for the derailed narcissistic development of the individual, ultimately leading to increased internal capacity for self-esteem regulation (1984). In all these models the transference is honored and observed, but the actual engagement in the therapeutic relationship is paradoxically aloof and counterrelational.

I would like to suggest that the most obvious and overlooked event in therapy is that when one brings oneself more fully and clearly into relationship, one enhances self, other, and the relationship. One increases one's capacity to be more whole, real, and integrated in all relationships; split-off energy begins to flow back into connection. Here I include relationships with people, nature, material objects, and work. In the following discussion I will not focus on matters of technique so much as a change in attitudes and understanding. These guide the practice of therapy so that the perspective shifts from one of control and self-sufficiency to one of relatedness and mutuality (an interplay of initiative and responsiveness) and increased capacity to grow in connection and to contribute to the growing connection.

At the heart of relational therapy is the relationship between therapist and client. A return to the pain of the past becomes possible and healing because in this journey the client is not alone. Empathically present, the therapist joins in the experience. One sexually abused client beautifully expressed her dilemma in therapy, showing her empathy for the therapist as well as an understanding of the task at hand, when she said to her therapist: "I hate to bring you back with me into all this pain. I shouldn't be so specific about all this abuse . . . it's too terrible. But I need someone to help me to be with it." It is by the very specific and, in this case, extremely painful detailing and reliving of the abuse situation, that the client creates real, emotional resonance with the therapist. The therapist, while feeling the pain, is not overwhelmed by it. The message is, "We can bear this together." The client and therapist begin to appreciate the meaning systems that have grown around the pain and how it has shaped the person's life and understanding. And the relational images that have formed as a result of these experiences become more obvious and available for change. The therapist is committed to trying to understand; the failures in empathy are valuable places for the therapist and client to work together towards a clearer understanding.

I would like to address several key issues in relational therapy: authenticity, mutuality, trust, and empathy. I will then explore narcissism and shame as they shed light on this perspective.

WHERE AND HOW DO WE EXPERIENCE ALIVENESS, A SENSE OF BEING REAL?

Movement towards congruence between inner and outer experience is a goal often sought in psychotherapy, as is the goal of personal knowledge. We develop a sense of personal authenticity largely in relationship and, paradoxically, as we move into relationship, coming to know the other more fully, we also greatly expand our knowledge of ourselves.

Sometimes the old spatial metaphor of the "real me," buried deep inside the body makes it seem that the "real self" is only impinged upon and damaged by relationship. The "real self" can take on a reified quality, something inside the child that is unfolding in some coherent and predetermined direction, which then becomes distorted by interactions with others. This leads to conceiving of boundaries as walls protecting vulnerable intrapsychic reality from external influence. In contrast, from a relational perspective, "vulnerability" can become an opportunity for growth rather than an invitation to possible danger. And safety resides in connectedness, not separation and power. Rather than the "emergence" of a reified "real self," we speak of the development of clarity through connection, a kind of co-creation. That is, there is not a "real self" which can "emerge" fully formed, but the possibility of the co-creation of an increasingly authentic self.

If there is a consistent imbalance so that one person is always altering her experience to fit the other person's needs or, alternately, demanding that the other person be a certain way in order to stay in connection, there will be serious distortions in self-and other-expression. The sense of aliveness in the relationship will suffer. As one of the women I work with said, "If I distort myself to be loved, is it real? Is it worth it? What, who gets loved?"

Often in dealing with a sense of lack of personal authenticity (which usually coexists with a lack of relational vitality), people mention striving to "speak their truth" or to find their voice. Carol Gilligan's book, *In a Different Voice*, brings this into clear focus (1982). Being able to say what you see, think, feel, and need is tremendously important. I am reminded of a quote by Adrienne Rich: "Listen to the small, soft voices, often courageously trying to speak up, voices of women taught early that tones of confidence, challenge, anger, or assertiveness, are strident and unfeminine. Listen to the voices of the women and the voices of the men; observe . . . the male assumption that people will listen, even when the majority of the group is female" (1978, p. 243).

Both the voice as reality and the voice as metaphor are to be taken seriously. Voice, like the notion of "real self," rather than being something that emerges fully formed from within, is contextual (Jordan, 1988). Thus the "audience" to whom we speak greatly affects the way we speak and the content of our utterances. In real dialogue both speaker and listener create a liveliness together and come into a truth together. Dialogue involves both initiative and responsiveness, at least two active and receptive individuals. In speaking to groups about our perspective on the psychology of women, we have felt the flow of life and confidence coming back to us from groups of women clinicians as they find the freedom to utter their truths regarding clinical practice, sometimes for the first time in public.

TRUST AND MUTUALITY

Therapy occurs in a context of trust; both therapist and client must develop trust for each other and for the relationship developing between them. Many clients come to us experiencing difficulty trusting others; but many also feel untrustworthy, a powerful experience for those suffering with shame (which I will discuss later). It may be just as important that therapists learn to trust clients, that the trust created be mutual. Therapy involves growth in trust of the other which— again, seemingly paradoxically—leads to growing confidence in our own view of reality, a process of gaining a sense of our own voice or truth.

Mutuality does not mean "sameness." It involves openness to change and healing on both sides. Therapy requires mutual trust, respect, and growth. It is not just two people getting together to talk about their lives; in the therapy relation, the two individuals join in the intention to assist the client. While the therapist exercises certain kinds of authority and the client moves into a place of vulnerability, the attitude is one of empowerment rather than "power over." The client's position of vulnerability is at all times respected and protected; the therapist is there to serve the client's needs. Helen Lynd notes, "Relating to another person in terms of superiority and inferiority, aggression and submission can only interfere with mutual discovery and love" (1958, p. 155). The therapy relationship should never include an attitude of superiority; both members of the interaction must be open to influence by the other. Both must risk change and the uncertainty which accompanies growth. This does not imply that both grow in the same way, or that there is no difference between therapist and client. But mutuality in therapy does rest on the assumption that real growth of an individual can occur only in the context of a real, mutually responsive relationship.

Clearly, this model values relatedness, although it in no way undermines the capacity to experience joy and nourishment in solitude. Though alone in solitude, one can relate fully to nature, books, animals, or one's internal images, and one can expect to return to the human community. By contrast, in isolation, one feels cut off from others, wishing for reconnection but unable to achieve it.

Furthermore, this perspective in no way negates the importance of initiative and responsibility, features that have often been connected with "autonomy." Rather than talk about "autonomy" which carries with it connotations of freedom *from* relational consequences, I prefer to speak about the capacity for

1. initiative, creativity, and responsiveness;
2. clarity of perception and desire;
3. capacity to act with intentionality;
4. the capacity to effect change.

All of these capacities are expressed in a relational context where we feel active concern about the consequences of our actions for others. This concern should also include an openness to others' impact on us. Perhaps we could call this "responsive initiative." This is the dwelling place of morality, which Carol Gilligan explores, and it is at the vital core of human caring (1982).

Goals of therapy do not include the attainment of some conflict-free state of harmony and happiness, but the development of an increased openness to learning and growth and more capacity to tolerate tension and conflict so that movement into isolation and, hence, fragmentation does not occur. Suffering is recognized as inevitable and the common lot of human beings. As such, suffering becomes a cause for joining others in alleviating pain and developing compassion. This is very different from experiencing suffering as a personal injury which reveals personal insufficiency. Relational competence, reaching out to others *for help* and *to help* are ultimate human responses, acknowledging the ongoing interdependence of all people. Instead of a therapy that supports the myth of attainable self-sufficiency and individual perfectibility (self as intrapsychic island), we recognize the necessity of mutuality in the face of inevitable uncertainty and suffering. We are not "bad" and therefore guilty if we cannot control and shape our lives in some ultimate way; we are simply subject to the inevitable human limitations which create the humility upon which our interdependence and humanity is predicated.

EMPATHY AND THERAPY

Empathy allows an understanding of each other's subjective world; it involves a direct movement from subject-object relating to subject-subject relating. Here is another person I can understand, in some ways different from me, but also like me, like all people. Poets have suggested that in moving more fully into the particular, we can experience the universal. It is the paradox of empathy that we appreciate the unique, differentiated characteristics of this particular other person, and we move past the particular to join in a place of commonality.

Translation of the original German word for empathy, *Einfuhlung*, stresses the capacity to "feel into" another's experience. Another possible way to think about this word is "to feel at one with." The *joining* aspect of empathy, the mutuality involved, and the increased sense of relatedness is not of primary interest in most models of development that address empathy, including Kohut's (1984). There, the therapist's resonance with the other is seen as important because it leads to the therapist's better understanding of the other. In fact, in addition to increasing their understanding, *both* people draw nearer each other in the empathic moment in a way which expands their sense of human community. Kohut talks about the "recognition of the self in the other" as the central dynamic in empathy (1978). But there occurs an equally important experience of recognizing the other in the self.

Similarly, in the process of self-empathy, one also develops an empathy for that which is human in oneself, often for very real and inevitable human failures or losses. Where expression of feelings has been curtailed or the premium on control has led to a suppression of spontaneous affect, the capacity to experience empathic resonance with others or to develop empathy towards one's own feelings suffers.

We all struggle with the need to recognize our unique experience; yet we also wish to be with others in some identifiable commonality or sameness. Because much of boys' gender socialization is based on making them *not like girls or women*, the wish for joining in commonality or likeness may become a source of conflict or anxiety for boys and men. Identity for men is importantly shaped by "differentness." The great emphasis on boundaries as forming protection and securing separation also evolves in this context. Hence, any movement towards sameness may be viewed with alarm; I suggest it is this fear that is mirrored in psychology's overconcern about movement towards "regressive merging" or experience of sameness. Connecting around difference is exciting, expanding, and challenging, but the capacity to move into a place of resonance is equally growth producing.

Emphasis on the autonomous self, or the "real self" unfolding, can culminate in the creation of a pathologically isolated individual struggling to maintain the illusion of self-sufficiency and boundaries: the narcissistic solution of the 20th century Western man. The wish for connection and the inevitable vulnerability to shame that accompanies this wish are largely disavowed aspects of the human condition which women often carry, as Jean Baker Miller notes (1976). This imbalance is most clearly expressed through gender and leads to male disconnection and overreliance on "power over" others; in women pathological shame develops. Both men and women suffer in such a system. Mutuality, the movement towards integration of initiative and responsiveness, where both the individual's and the relationship's well-being are honored, becomes severely curtailed.

THE NEED TO BE CONNECTED AND THE NEED
TO FEEL SPECIAL: EMPATHY AND NARCISSISM

I suggest that the need for connection and emotional joining is our primary need; empathy serves this need. The need to feel *special* becomes paramount when the need for relatedness is not met. The failure of connection and the resulting need for admiration can often take the form of needing to be "better than." Kohut's understanding of narcissistic development posits that failures of admiring self-objects lead to an internal deficit in the capacity for regulation of self-esteem (1978, 1984); there is then an ongoing narcissistic need to be "mirrored" and an unconscious anxiety about the resulting dependence on others to provide this function.

It is not their difficulty with self-esteem regulation which, I think, is most damaging for narcissistic people, but their difficulty in letting others really have an impact on them, their difficulty being responsive to others. This difficulty leads to encapsulation, a failure of connectedness, and a disruption of the sense of well-being which comes from relationship. The search for adulation and admiration is a futile attempt to restore a sense of connection; there is an illusion of safety and control in being highly esteemed by others. The need to feel *special* defensively replaces the desire for connection.

The capacity to take joy in the growth of another is utterly absent where narcissistic issues predominate; the other's existence is but a reflection of the self, to be used by the self to buttress self-esteem. Real responsiveness, mutuality, and the creation of something new and spontaneous together are not possible. The other person cannot be allowed to be genuinely responsive because the response may not contribute to one's image, and one cannot respond freely because that admits the possibility of being affected by the other. Dominance and control become an essential strategy in narcissistically distorted relationships, and vitality is drained from the connection, contributing to the inevitable interpersonal boredom and the quest for newness and excitement. Using the metaphor of voice, the dialogue has become imbalanced, with little energy devoted to real listening.

SHAME: WISHING FOR CONNECTION,
FEELING UNWORTHY

Thus, with narcissistic problems there is often increased effort towards invulnerability and diminished responsiveness to the reality of the other; interpersonal injuries lead to narcissistic rage. In shame we experience a heightened sense of vulnerability and our sense of initiative falters; in interpersonal failures we attribute personal responsibility and unworthiness to ourselves. Many of the problems we deal with in therapy reflect the pervasive pain created by shame: addictions, sexual abuse, eating problems, many depressions, impulse problems, and post traumatic stress disorders.

Shame is often seen as the opposite of narcissistic pride, the loss of self-respect or self-esteem (There may be sex differences in the experience of shame; what I am about to describe may be more characteristic of shame in women.) I would like to suggest that shame is most importantly a felt sense of unworthiness to be in connection, a deep sense of unlovability, with the ongoing awareness of how very much one wants to connect with others. While shame involves extreme self-consciousness, it also signals powerful relational longings and awareness of the other's response. There is a loss of the sense of *empathic possibility*, others are not experienced as empathic, and the capacity for self-empathy is lost. One feels unworthy of love, not because of some discrete action which would be the cause for guilt, but because one is defective or flawed in some essential way.

In the moment of shame, one feels exposed, looked at; the characteristic response is to blush, pull away, avert the gaze. Nathanson comments, "During mutual gaze we feel attached. In the moment of shame, we feel shorn not just from the other but from all possible others" (1987, p. 9). One feels separate, outside the pale; Jean Baker Miller has spoken of "condemned isolation" or "being locked out of the possibility of human connection" (1988), a feeling state which I think is central to much of our work in therapy. Tomkins places shame as one of the original negative affects (1987). Helen Block Lewis notes, "In this affective tie the self does not feel autonomous or independent, but dependent and vulnerable to rejection. Shame is a vicarious experience of the significant other's scorn" (1971, p. 42).

Shame can occur in response to many different events. Common precipitants involve some exposure in which one is made to feel defective, weak, out of control, "foolish," babyish, dirty, stupid, awkward, betrayed, or, in a love relationship, more involved or vulnerable than the other. Loss of a sense of containment or of being in control figures importantly in most of these feelings and reflects our cultural preoccupation with control. Sometimes merely being "different" becomes a source of shame. But all of these imply some interpersonal situation in which one no longer can feel valued or worthy of connection. The effect of shame is global and immobilizing. One does not feel capable of making the situation better. So we move into hiding and secrecy; in this case the opportunity for a reparative interaction with another is lessened. It is as if we lose the ability to reach out. The helplessness of the situation leads to further shame. It is the very tendency to pull away from relationship to protect oneself that, in fact, most locks one into the shame. In the extreme, shame contributes to dissociation and inner fragmentation as the person struggles to be free of the experience of personal defectiveness. Guilt is about identifiable acts and transgressions; reparation is generally possible. Amends can be made. Shame is about *being* and feels less easily modified, at least in our culture.

Mild shame may actually be a healthy signal that one must bring awareness to one's relating, balancing initiative and responsiveness. But in an unequal power situation or where mutual empathy is absent, shaming others becomes a means to control them. And this can produce pathological shame. Socialization of children is very shame-based. Children are shamed out of babyhood, away from being helpless, needy, readily expressive of feelings, vulnerable, and dependent. Gender socialization is also laden with shaming, both in the home and in the world. Boys are shamed if they act or feel too dependent, scared, out of control, "weak," tearful; anything that is categorized (stereotypically) as feminine is to be avoided at all costs. Girls are shamed for being uncaring, angry, competitive, unloving, "selfish." Much adult gender-determined behavior is burdened with shame; if we cross the line of what is considered gender-appropriate, we often feel intense shame, unworthiness, a wish to hide.

WOMEN'S SENSE OF SHAME

Male standards of psychological maturity and adult functioning have consistently judged women's way of knowing and being as less "good" than the male way (Broverman et al., 1970). A debilitating response to these societal standards has led women to feel defective or inadequate about who they are. Helen Block Lewis notes women are far more susceptible to shame than men (1987). 1 think there are three major reasons for this:

1. Patriarchy is actively invested in shaming and in silencing women's reality.
2. Because women are especially open to their desire for connection, they are especially vulnerable to its threatened loss, which occurs with shame.
3. If we care how we are, with, and for, other people in relationship, we will experience shame when we feel we have let oth-

ers down or when our being impinges on or hurts them in some way. This I would call healthy shame.

As a result of prevailing male standards and the silencing of women's reality, for women there is a broad and widespread sense of "being" wrong; that is, one's *being* is wrong. One's reality is not right, one looks for the wrong things in life, one's cognitive capacities are not developed in the right direction. Such a pervasive sense of deviance and inferiority leads to a profound disempowerment, and one loses the ability to represent one's own reality, ultimately, to even know one's truth (Miller, 1988). Shame becomes a way of *being* and a way of being disempowered; in shame we lose our ability to speak, initiate, and expect respect. In shame we feel painfully disconnected, longing to repair the rupture but unable to move in that direction. Thus, shame is a powerful factor in women's lives. A characteristic lament from one woman was, "Bob doesn't listen to me; then, when I 'up' the volume, he calls me a screamer." (Or, in the field of psychology, we are called hysterics, manipulators, borderlines, masochists, dependent personalities).

Another path to disempowerment and the paralyzing experience of shame, is to be treated as if one is invisible and inaudible. William James noted, "No more fiendish punishment could be devised, were such a thing physically possible, than that one should be turned loose in society and remain absolutely unnoticed by all the members thereof. If none turned around when we entered, answered when we spoke, or minded what we did, but if every person we met 'cut us dead,' and acted as if we were nonexisting things, a kind of rage and impotent despair would ere long well up in us" (1890/1968, p. 42). What James describes fits well, I think, with the experience of shame, wanting to be acknowledged and connected and feeling hopelessly cut off from that connection, "cut dead," as he notes. An intrapsychic, self-psychology rendering of this might suggest the person needs to be adored, acknowledged, admired; a relational perspective views the essential injury here to a sense of connection and, hence, to vitality.

THE SILENCE THAT SHAME CREATES

A powerful social function of shaming people is to silence them. This is an insidious, pervasive mode of oppression, in many ways more effective than physical oppression. In a supposedly egalitarian society, shaming becomes a potent, indirect exercise of dominance to subdue certain expressions of truth. By creating silence, doubt, isolation, and hence immobilization, i.e., shame, the dominant social group (in this case white, middle class, heterosexual males) assures that its reality becomes *the reality*. This dynamic has dictated the social experience of most marginalized groups, be they women, Blacks, lesbians, gays, Hispanics, or the physically challenged, whose voices have for too long been unheeded and whose reality has thus been denied.

When people are shamed and silenced by their shame, they cease trusting their own perceptions and sense of reality. Their sense of injury and violation of trust in themselves and the world is often profound (Lynd, 1958). Isolation enlarges the sense of self-doubt, uncertainty, and "wrongness." This renders them more vulnerable to other people's reality claims, self-distortion, and hence to further victimization. This may account for some of the revictimization that occurs for survivors of sexual abuse and contributes to the difficulty for many in leaving an abusive situation. In recent years, sexual abuse survivors have begun to help each other speak out. This courageous capacity for utterance is also developing among clients abused by therapists, doctors, and other caregivers. The 12-step programs have already discovered the power that comes from joining in the admission of a need for help and thereby loosening the grip of shame and secrecy. There is also the empowering experience of giving to others. This is a profoundly balancing and relational program.

People who are "shame prone" are used to taking responsibility or "the blame" for relational failures; in an interpersonal situation where there is an injury, there are several possible responses. One can get angry and blame the other (perhaps the narcissistic solution); one can take personal responsibility, sometimes inappropriately (the place of shame). Another response, suggested by a relational model, is to take both people into account and move towards understanding the relational patterns that led to the failure, assuming a kind of relational responsibility. Creating this kind of "relational empathy," similar to Kaplan's notion of "process empathy" (1988), may be at the heart of growth-enhancing relationships. Therapy offers an invaluable opportunity to heal the long-range wounds of shame. We are finally heard. Our reality is acknowledged. We are trusted and become trusting. We have an opportunity to create a relationship in which we can more fully represent our experience and find acceptance. In an empathic milieu we can look at shameful experiences freshly, with a view to understanding how they came to be, rather than with a view towards judgment. Very importantly, the therapist acknowledges and respects the client's experience, something that might be called empathic respect. In affirming the client's experience, the therapist conveys the recognition that the client's feelings and behavior make sense in the context of her or his situation.

S. is a woman I worked with who dealt with multiple issues of shame. At age 12 she was hospitalized with severe anorexia; her prognosis was guarded. She felt deeply ashamed of her body, but it was not until five years later when she began treatment with me that she could share the shame of sexual abuse by her stepfather from the time she was nine until age 13. Added to this was her sense of self-blame and shame at not having been able to protect herself; over and over she anguished, "Why didn't I tell anyone? Why didn't I stop it?" She felt profoundly immobilized and had great difficulty moving from this position of withdrawn self-hatred. Her desire to reach out and to be accepted was blocked by her absolute conviction that she was bad, unlovable, and not to be trusted. Her self-hate and despair were often painful for me to experience with her, although sharing the pain was valuable for both of us. Then, in the course of treatment, she was revictimized in a grueling rape. Again, her sense of shame increased, as she wondered why she hadn't perceived the danger and averted it. This idea was fueled by her reading of popular psychology which suggests that at all costs we must see ourselves as being in control; hence, victims too are to blame. The initial violation in which her vulnerability as a child made her prey to a destructive parental figure left her feeling shame, cut off, beyond understanding. What then ensued is characteristic of the cycle of shame; more and more isolated and silenced, she became increasingly fragmented and suffered with an intense sense of unworthiness. Only very slowly, by learning to trust and finding herself trustworthy in treatment, through our building a reliable, safe, and growth-enhancing relationship together in therapy, could she begin to bring these silenced aspects of her experience back into relationship. The beauty of her growth from isolation and shame into self-empathy and real relatedness has been deeply moving.

SHAME IN THERAPY

Therapy often challenges us to be with the most extraordinarily painful experiences. Much suffering arises in the context of shame, and often therapists may have the impulse to avert our gaze as well, to move out of the pain of the empathic moment. But we are committed to trying to see and listen and understand. Therapy, by its very nature, addresses shame; we ask people to talk with us about those things that they feel most uncomfortable about in themselves, things they might not be able to speak about with anyone else, things we may feel uncomfortable about in ourselves . . . helplessness, rage, lust. Therapists, too, can create feelings of shame by interpreting only the regressive or infantile aspects of an individual. Infantilizing clients and seeing their needs for connection as pathological is powerfully shaming.

Therapists sometimes further shame clients by assuming a position of power through knowledge which suggests, "I know better than you." The way some therapists interpret unconscious material, or resistance and the like, also may carry shaming implications. The therapist's silence itself may be experienced as scornful. And therapists often shame with their attitudes of judgment and condescension, as typified by the pejorative use of such concepts as masochism, borderline personality, and manipulation (Stiver, 1985). Nothing could be more countertherapeutic and damaging than these attitudes of disrespect, whether subtle or blatant.

A relational therapy also works towards releasing the shame which so frequently arises in this culture about not being an autonomous, self-sufficient person, in control of one's life. In a way, the shame experience often pushes one back into an almost preverbal mode. Others often withdraw from people experiencing shame in this way, leaving them alone in their silence. In therapy which emphasizes empathic attunement, the therapist will note these moments and will, through empathic listening, provide the client a response that does not rely solely on the client's capacity to verbalize the experience. This, then, slowly allows the experience to be brought into the verbal, communicable domain. One client, commented, "When I can't articulate things so you understand them, I feel abashed and embarrassed." An exploration of our mutual responsibility for achieving clarity diminished her sense of embarrassment and shame.

Often work on shame must precede work on sadness or grief; in clear sadness or grief, one is usually reaching out, believing in the possibility of reparative connection (Stiver & Miller, 1988). In more complicated grief reactions and depressions, shame may prevent the person from feeling the connection necessary for expressing sadness, or a person may feel ashamed of negative feelings, embarrassed about being out of control or about some undesirable reaction to the pain (i.e., seeming selfish). Often there is shame about caring so much about relationships in a culture which values them so little. Sadness also places one in a more vulnerable position, thus more open to shaming.

Healing pathological shame is not about increasing the narcissistic self-sufficiency or self-esteem of the individual or building some intrapsychic structure. Healing shame essentially involves enhancing empathy for self and other and bringing the person back into connection in which empathic possibility exists. This point highlights one of the major differences between a therapy guided by a theory of self-development versus one occurring within a relational perspective.

THE THERAPIST'S SHAME

Therapy cannot be a mechanistic enterprise but must take the therapist as well as the client to deep places of vulnerability and possible shame. Unlike many professions that count on definable skills or taking particular roles, psychotherapy calls upon the presence of the whole person of the therapist. How we *do* therapy is a lot about who we *are* as people. Therapy is importantly about *being*. It does not depend on a clear and easily mastered set of skills. We, too, must struggle to stay in connection in the face of vulnerability. There is, then, much room for the experience of shame in the therapist, particularly the beginning therapist. Therapy happens behind closed doors, with little direct validation of what we do. Because the work is difficult and often not immediately rewarding, there is much room for self-doubt or possibly shame, a secret belief that someone else would be better at this. The rendering of the process in textbooks often contributes to a feeling that the books do it right, and we do it wrong; there, highly rationalized interventions and emphasis on the successful moments give a very skewed and unrepresentative picture of the process. (If there is one plea I can make to anyone writing about therapy, it is to please say what is actually happening in the therapy relationship, not what theory prescribes or what sounds smart or clever or theoretically informed.)

Much supervision is carried on in an atmosphere of shaming. Supervisors with clear theories of what should happen, particularly in terms of neutrality, nongratification, and nondisclosure can also be very critical of supervisees who have a different notion of the therapeutic process. A young therapist came to me after one of my presentations about the importance of mutuality in the therapy process and shared the following experience: She had been with a client who was experiencing terrible grief about her mother's death. The therapist herself began to cry as she listened to this pain, and her quiet tears were noted by the client, in a appreciative way. When she reported this to her supervisor, however, he exploded: "You just raped that patient. Why did you inflict your feelings on her? Where were your boundaries?" With a sense that what she did was humanly compassionate, therapeutically useful, and certainly not destructive or hurful, this young therapist felt assaulted by her supervisor but not ashamed. She had a clear sense of the importance of relationship and of allowing herself to be affected by clients. Had she been more uncertain she would have felt devastated rather than appropriately critical of her supervisor's rigidity. Another beginning therapist commented that a supervisor had criticized her "lack of boundaries" when she stood up and passed a box of Kleenex to a sobbing client.

A psychiatric resident commented that one of the most important things she had learned in her residency was how to lie to supervisors. She was told she was "too relational" by her male supervisors, so this young woman stopped telling her supervisors how she was responding with patients. As a result she felt lonely and vulnerable. One often feels this way even when supported by a supervisor, but her loneliness and sense of risk were even greater.

Old theory dictates that we remain impassive, "neutral," nongratifying. Many beginning therapists have been shamed by supervisors for being too responsive or too transparent. While different responsibilities are assumed in the therapy relationship, the relationship develops between two real people. The therapist must be real as well, and this authenticity is informed by an ever-present sense of responsibility to and, initially, for the relationship and the client. As the therapy progresses, the client will, in fact, assume more responsibility for the relationship.

C. is a woman I had seen for two years in treatment who appeared very disconnected from herself and others and who had recurring dreams of being made of brittle metal, unable to bend or feel. She had never cried or expressed any spontaneous feeling with me or with her two former therapists. Following the death of my mother, which she knew about, I was in deep grief. On one occasion tears came to my eyes in response to something she said about her grandmother, a person to whom she had felt close and who had died the previous year. She stopped and said, "You're sad about your mother right now, aren't you?" I said I was. She too began to cry and said, "I've felt so bad for you. I'm so sorry about what you've been through." I thanked her and let her know how much I appreciated her responsiveness. All of my training would suggest that I had committed the error of burdening my client with my personal concerns, or that I had made the mistake of allowing her to help me. In effect, this was a moving, alive moment in our work together that dramatically altered the quality of our relationship and subsequent therapy.

Such responsiveness can pose problems. If one has a rule *never to respond in a personal way*, the decisions are arbitrary, clearer (although I get less and less sure about how one actually does this). When we choose to be more real and revealing in therapy, we must make more difficult judgments about what will be in the service of the client and the relationship. This intentionality is at the core. Each relationship will shape different decisions. It is the particularity of the relationship that must be honored.

In summary, our model of development influences our practice of therapy. Evelyn Keller has pointed to the difference between the Platonic knower who "seeks to approach and unite" with the essential nature of things and the Baconian scientist who equates knowledge with power and dominion over things (1985, p. 95). Therapy at its best represents an effort to understand through empathic joining not through exercising "power over." In the empathic listening of therapy, we must be more open, and capable of uncertainty than is ordinarily comfortable in a society that stresses control and predictability. Until recently, our scientific model has pushed us in the direction of answers, certainty, theory. The more I practice therapy, the less theoretical and certain it becomes. Each therapy is radically different, as each relationship has a texture, shape, and pattern of its own. We must *listen,* not *impose;* we must *follow* as well as *lead.* Each person's voice is valuable; each person's capacity to listen is important. The tension of creating a dialogue can be difficult; it can be wonderful. We must be mutually responsive and initiating in order to grow. Jean Baker Miller (1986) has suggested that in order for a relationship to be enhancing for one person, it must encourage growth in both participants. In therapy, we move, not in the realm of control and prediction, but together we create connection and understanding. The therapeutic dialogue is between two real people, each experiencing more aliveness in connection, with a shared primary goal to enhance the client's wholeness, well-being and capacity for relationship. Perhaps more useful than any "scientific," clinical guidelines for doing therapy is Rilke's advice in his letters to a young poet:

> Be patient towards all that is unsolved in your heart and try to love the questions themselves. . . . Do not seek the answers which cannot be given you because you would not be able to live them. And the point is to live everything. Live the questions now. Perhaps you will gradually, without noticing it, live along some distant day into the answer. (1934, p. 35)

DISCUSSION SUMMARY

After each colloquium presentation, a discussion was held. Selected portions are summarized here. At this session, Irene Stiver of McLean Hospital and

Jean Baker Miller and Alexandra Kaplan of the Stone Center joined Judith Jordan in leading the discussion.

Question: I wanted to make a comment about shame as it's related to humiliation. I had an experience in couple's therapy where I felt my husband and the therapist ganged up on me. My feeling was one of extreme humiliation. I left very upset. I could no longer work with them. I couldn't understand my reaction at the time, but now, listening to what you're saying, I think that humiliation is connected to rage that cannot be expressed in the situation. I was powerless.

Jordan: I think there is a connection. If the anger at being hurt or exposed can't be expressed either because of power imbalances or because you're concerned about hurting the person to whom the anger is directed, then you may pull away sometimes to protect the other person as well as yourself. You are in a no-win position. You feel powerless, and that in itself can feel shameful. In that moment you feel that there's no empathic possibility.

In your case, the other two people were not able to be there for you in a way that you needed them to be, so your response was to do what people do when shamed: to pull away and withdraw from the situation. Another factor with anger, in particular, is that for women there are a lot of "shoulds" about anger; in other words, we are not supposed to "be" angry. We are definitely not supposed to show it. If we feel ashamed of certain emotional reactions, which is what happens when we feel something that we think we shouldn't feel (involuntary and involving our whole being), the feeling can become laden with shame. I think that in the case of anger and shame, this can lead to a kind of silent fury which then makes us feel even more ashamed since it seems so out of proportion with the original instigating event.

Stiver: In listening to your question and in response to Judy's paper, it seems that in couple's work we could do a lot of reframing in terms of looking at what we can do to help the relationship. Couple's work often focuses on one or the other in the couple as if one is to blame. Judy's paper suggests a shift from an individual to a relational perspective. I think this is important because I think there is a lot of blaming in couple's therapy.

Jordan: One of the common examples I've seen in couples' work with men and women is when the relationship is very difficult, and one person, typically the woman, has been putting a lot of energy into trying to make it better, she may be blamed by mental health professionals for "loving too much" or be labelled as masochistic. This is often the burden of the one who takes primary relational responsibility: to be seen as "trying too hard" or as "self-sacrificing." A better way to think about this would be to look at the real imbalance in the couple about who is taking responsibility for the relationship and try to work on that. Mutual responsibility-taking for the welfare of the relationship would be the goal.

Question: When you distinguished between guilt and shame, you said that guilt was about actions that could possibly be amended and that shame was about *being*. Can you elaborate on what you mean by *being*?

Jordan: I think one of the distinctions between guilt and shame has to do with the difference between voluntary and involuntary action. Guilt is about an action that one sees as voluntary and that one sees oneself as having some control over, some moral responsibility for, if you will. Shame is experienced often as about something that happens involuntarily to one or about some failure to live up to some ideal about how one should be; it involves the entire sense of self. I meant by *being* that it involves the whole person, our whole being. Guilt is about particular transgressions and violations of standards.

Miller: When people experience shame, it's about everything they are. You feel less than human when you're made to feel ashamed. As Judy said, you feel you are outside the possibility of human connection because of this awful "thing" that you are. Guilt seems to be about a more discrete act and not about your total existence as a person.

Comment: Part of a research study done at the University of Michigan found that when they asked depressed women to talk about their guilt and embarrassment, that embarrassment was experienced very frequently by the women; whereas guilt, which is normally associated with depression, really wasn't noted that often. I could never make sense of that finding until tonight; so, thank you.

Comment: I wanted to comment on dealing with shame, with being shamed in a relationship. My husband uses shame to control. He uses nonresponse when I ask him something he doesn't like. He acts as if I don't exist. One of the things that helps me reject being shamed is the realization that if he needs to control me, he is dependent on me. He is dependent on my cooperating with him. That frees me to perceive his dependency in that situation. He is operating out of fear and a need to control, and I don't have to buy into his fear.

Comment: It seems to me there's a great deal of implicit criticism in what you say of the way psychiatrists and psychologists are being trained. I wonder what sort of changes you might make in training.

Jordan: First, since the most important training in therapy occurs in supervision, it is very important that supervisors become sensitive to the issue of shaming the trainee. With so much uncertainty and sense of personal exposure on the part of the trainee, it is terribly easy to be shamed by a critical or judging attitude on the part of the supervisor. Similarly, the supervisor should explore with the trainee how easily clients are shamed in the therapy setting. It is terribly important to help a beginning therapist develop sensitivity to the client's sense of exposure and feelings of being cut off from empathic possibility. Openness to uncertainty and exploration, rather than defining and labeling, are central to therapy. Therapists are there to understand, not to shame or judge.

Question: When you talked about the potential for the therapist to shame the client, I thought you were pointing to the fact that the end does not justify the means. I struggle with how to help people who are engaged in very self-destructive behavior without shaming them, how to help them give up the behaviors without attacking the self.

Jordan: One of the places where that happens is when people are in relationships that are destructive. If the therapist takes a relational perspective and looks at the relational imbalances, that is very freeing for people. It removes a sense of self-blame, and together you can really try to understand the destructive relationship. Also, when the therapist becomes more sensitive to the possible shaming implications of certain interventions, that is quite helpful. It also helps to be clear that while you are upset with the self-destructive actions, you can appreciate that the person often is trying to do something constructive through these behaviors, often trying to understand or communicate something. Ironically, the person is frequently working to establish a better sense of connectedness. It's important for us as therapists to appreciate that person's "ends" as well as to work on shifting the sometimes self-destructive "means." *Respect* for the client's *efforts to connect* and to make sense of experience is terribly important always, but especially when shame is involved.

Comment: I was glad, Judy, that you mentioned minority women and lesbian women in your talk. I was thinking how for lesbian women there is such a large part of us that we need to keep hidden when we're not in safe situations, particularly professionally. I was also thinking about how my gay male clients share that experience of shame, and they have that empathic ability. It leads me to wonder about the experience of shame and the connection of that experience with the ability to be empathic.

Kaplan: That opens up a huge area for all of us. We all carry our own shame as therapists in our work. In some cases we know where our shame is, and in some cases we don't. It is an important task to know where our shame is and how that affects our clients. If we know it, it can help us to be more empathic.

Question: With guilt, we make the distinction between neurotic guilt and appropriate guilt. Is that distinction meaningful where shame is concerned? Or is it always deleterious?

Jordan: I think there is a mild shame which might be thought of as appropriate humility. Appropriate guilt is about doing something wrong, realizing it, and feeling remorse about it. Similarly, for instance, in mild shame or humility, I realize in an interpersonal situation that I am not perfect, my *being* is imperfect in certain ways. I become aware of a wish to be more worthy of relationship, to be more lovable and loving. It brings my attention to the desire for connection in a healthy way. Humility, if you will, is at the heart of the relational self; I think it represents a balance of awareness of the other person and of oneself. Compassion comes alive here . . . for self and other.

Comment: I'd like to elaborate on something you said which I think is relevant to the treatment of sexual abuse. An important acknowledgment is not just that violence was done to the victim, but that violence was also done to the relationship. From what you've said, we could see that part of the anger at the perpetrator is about his failure to take responsibility for the relationship and for the damage done to the relationship as well as to the abused individual.

Jordan: Yes, both the abused person and the relationship are betrayed and violated in such situations. And one of the outcomes is that the victim learns not just that this particular perpetrator is destructive or dangerous, but also comes to fear that all close relationships can be similarly hurtful. Building relationships marked by mutual responsibility for the relationship becomes very important and can be an important focus for the treatment.

REFERENCES

Belenky, M., Clinchy, B., Goldberger, N., & Tarule, J. (1986). *Women's ways of knowing: The development of self, voice, and mind.* New York: Basic Books.

Broverman, I., Broverman, D., Clarkson, F., Rosenkrantz, P., & Vogel, S. (1970). Sex role stereotypes and clinical judgements of mental health. *Journal of Consulting and Counseling Psychology, 43,* 1–7.

Freud, S. (1959). Fragments of an analysis of a case of hysteria. In E. Jones (Ed.), *Sigmund Freud Collected Papers* (Vol. 3). The International Psychoanalytic Library, No. 9. New York: Basic Books. (Original work published 1905)

Gilligan, C. (1982). *In a different voice.* Cambridge, MA: Harvard University Press.

James, W. (1890). The self. In C. Gordon & K. Gergen (Eds.), *The self in social interaction.* New York: Wiley.

Jordan, J. (1984). *Empathy and self-boundaries.* (Work in Progress No. 16.) Wellesley, MA: Stone Center Working Paper Series.

Jordan, J. (1986). *The meaning of mutuality.* (Work in Progress No. 23.) Wellesley, MA: Stone Center Working Paper Series.

Jordan, J. (1987). *Clarity in connection: Empathic knowing, desire and sexuality* (Work in Progress No. 29). Wellesley, MA: Stone Center Working Paper Series. (Reprinted as Chapter 3, this volume)

Kaplan, A. (1982). *Women and empathy.* (Work in Progress No. 2.) Wellesley, MA: Stone Center Working Paper Series.

Kaplan, A. (1988). *Dichotomous thought and relational processes in therapy.* (Work in Progress No. 35.) Wellesley, MA: Stone Center Working Paper Series.

Keller, E. (1985). *Reflections on gender and science.* New Haven: Yale University Press.

Kohut, H. (1978). The psychoanalyst in the community of scholars. In P. Ornstein (Ed.), *The search for the self: Selected writings of Heinz Kohut, 1950–1978* (Vol. 2). New York: International Universities Press.

Kohut, H. (1984). *How does analysis cure?* Chicago, IL: University of Chicago Press.

Lewis, H. (1971). *Shame and guilt in neurosis.* New York: International Universities Press.

Lewis, H. (1987). *The role of shame in symptom formation.* Hillsdale, NJ:. Erlbaum.

Lynd, H. (1958). *On shame and the search for identity.* New York: Wiley.

Miller, J.B. (1987). *Toward a new psychology of women* (2nd ed.). Boston: Beacon Press.

Miller, J.B. (1984). *The development of women's sense of self.* (Work in Progress No. 12.) Wellesley, MA: Stone Center Working Paper Series.

Miller, J.B. (1986). *What do we mean by relationships?* (Work in Progress No. 22.) Wellesley, MA: Stone Center Working Paper Series.

Miller, J.B. (1988). *Connections, disconnections, and violations.* (Work in Progress No. 33.) Wellesley, MA: Stone Center Working Paper Series.

Nathanson, D. (1987). *The many faces of shame.* New York: Guilford Press.

Piaget, J. (1952). *The origins of intelligence in children.* New York. W.W. Norton.

Rich, A. (1978). Taking women students seriously. In *On lies, secrets and science.* New York: Norton.

Rilke, R. (1934). *Letters to a young poet.* M. D. Herter (Trans.). New York: W.W. Norton.

Stern, D. (1985). *The interpersonal world of the infant.* New York: Basic Books.

Stiver, I. (1984). *The meanings of "dependency" in female-male relationships.* (Work in Progress No. 11.) Wellesley, MA: Stone Center Working Paper Series.

Stiver, I. (1985). *The meaning of care: Reframing treatment models.* (Work in Progress No. 20.) Wellesley, MA: Stone Center Working Paper Series.

Sullivan, H. (1953). *The interpersonal theory of psychiatry.* New York: W.W. Norton.

Surrey, J. (1983). *Women and empathy.* (Work in Progress No. 2.) Wellesley, MA: Stone Center Working Paper Series.

Surrey, J. (1985). *Self-in-relation: A theory of women's development.* (Work in Progress No. 13.) Wellesley, MA: Stone Center Working Paper Series.

Tomkins, S. (1987). Shame. In D. Nathanson (Ed.), *The many faces of shame.* New York: Guilford.

Winnicott, D. (1971). *Playing and reality.* New York: Basic Books.

Wurmser, L. (1981). *The mask of shame.* Baltimore: Johns Hopkins University Press.

This chapter was presented at a Stone Center Colloquium on April 5, 1989. © 1989 Judith Jordan.

8

Psychosocial Barriers to Black Women's Career Development

CLEVONNE W. TURNER

PREFACE

This chapter could not have been written without the collaboration and shared stories of resilient, multitalented, resourceful Black women who *do* survive and *are* successful in their own ways, even when times are hardest. This "learned talent to survive" was passed on to me chiefly from my mother and her network of women friends, relatives, and neighbors in the Black community. They modeled the difficult yet successful integration of working inside and outside the home, preserving relationships, providing community service and maintaining dignity and perseverance that surrounded me during my formative years. My father both complemented and supported this model of growth in me.

I, like the majority of Black women in this society, grew up with the notion of getting as much education as I could, working, marrying and having children as "the norm." Implied in this, and sometimes explicitly said, were two interwoven givens: to make other Black folk proud of me and to uplift the race in some way by making good, myself.

INTRODUCTION

To be Black and female in today's society poses unique and complex issues in thinking about, planning for, and working towards a career. This complexity is due, in great part, to Black women's dual minority status. Work is an indispensable part of life for most people. It serves to integrate them into social, political and economic networks in the society at large. Our society, which values the "Protestant work ethic" as part of its backbone, has insidiously and systematically produced roadblocks of gigantic proportion for Black women, even though they have worked fairly consistently throughout their existence in this country, as well as in their original homelands. They have worked long hours and double shifts providing manual labor to scientific breakthroughs in order to survive, maintain and/or improve certain standards of living.

The psychological burden of living with the many false images and myths imposed by this society, while struggling to live and work in it and maintain a positive sense of identity is now over 350 years old. At times it gets extremely heavy. Black women are for the most part aspiring to be in control of their lives in a basically white, patriarchal society. This chapter is not intended to take away from the blatant racism also directed at Black men or the bitter sexism pervading the treatment of women, both of which Black women share. It will attempt to shed some light on some of the issues and feelings unique to Black women, It is hoped that by including and developing data on this often overlooked population a more total picture of work issues will evolve.

Throughout this chapter, four primary barriers will be interwoven: *racism, sexism, classism* and *ageism*. I will attempt to illustrate how these rampant forms of discrimination bar Black women from full participation in our society. Case examples from work done at the Stone Center as well as with Black women in various walks of life will be included. The Stone Center material is the result of a two-year nonclinical Search-Research group I co-ran with a Black woman, Dean Sylvia Robinson, who had prior experience as a career counselor. The group focused on career and relationship issues of Black college women. In general, however, our findings dovetailed with the experience of many working Black women with whom I've spoken both within and outside of my clinical practice.

COMMON THEMES

To know a Black woman in our society today is certainly not to know all of us. To try to describe our female identity entails looking at a rich, complex, multifaceted person who has not been studied or understood adequately. Primarily we are hidden within the words—Black, female, and often just the word "other." There exists within us much variety in individual as well as in collective identities, behaviors, feelings, styles, personalities, skin tones, religions, philosophies, relationships between ourselves and others, etc. It is very important not to form one description or characteristic way of thinking about Black women. Having said this, there do exist some common themes and threads that most Black women share with each other more than with other women. I have compiled a list of eight to keep in mind:

1.   Black women in this country have a history and tradition of combining the roles of worker, wife and/or mother as the "norm." Paradoxically, this tradition continued despite slavery, as well as in large part because of it.

2.   Black women and Black men have a history together of mutual interdependence around work done outside the home in order to achieve some semblance of financial stability and security, as well as to preserve family and community solidarity. Whether low-income or not, these families are characterized by an egalitarian pattern in which neither spouse dominates but each shares decision making and the performance of expected tasks (Hill, 1971).

3.   Black women historically have shared and/or carried out the role of "breadwinner" because of a complex set of racial circumstances which denied meaningful employment to Black men. This situation has led to such myths as Black men being seen as shiftless and lazy and the women being seen as matriarchal, superstrong and emasculating. Subsequently, for survival many of these women had to care for themselves, children and families. Unlike most women in this predicament, they were systematically degraded and blamed for this plight. This hardship damaged Black male/female relationships and the solidarity of the intact Black family (Beale, 1970; Davis, 1983; McCray, 1980).

4.   Black women are the only women in this country to be categorized as "not being human" along with Black men and children. Slave infants and their mothers were seen as "property of the slave master" and could not look to their men for protection as other women and children have done. Death to the men often resulted if they interfered.

5.   From 1619 to 1863, Southern white men had legal license freely to abuse Black women and then labeled them immoral, loose, and sexually degraded. Myths like these and others have continued from that time up to the present. They attack Black women's morals

and character while also serving to give male teachers, supervisors, or co-workers a more entitled sense to sexually harass them. This continues to wreak havoc. It sometimes distorts Black women's perceptions of themselves and undermines or destroys the relationships they share with Black men. These women have higher rates of separation and divorce than their white female counterparts, and statistics show them less likely to remarry.

6. Developmentally, Black women have integrated traditional male roles of achievement, autonomy and independence with the more traditional female caretaking and nurturing roles as a "norm." At the Stone Center, we are evolving a "self-in-relation" theory looking at how women in general develop a primary emphasis on meeting others' needs before their own, and working on cultural differences within it. This theory seeks to examine women's primary sense of self as relational, that is, embedded in mutual empathy in early mother/daughter relationships. It further looks at establishing and maintaining relationships *within* the developmental process rather than through "separation and individuation" as it has been written about for many years. This theory represents a significant part of the Black woman's developmental experience as she adds on other relationships which start with the mother/daughter one and tend to heighten rather than diminish her sense of self. Black mothers often have a heavier sense of responsibility to their daughters because of racism and sexism, and are working constantly to instill deeper feelings of self-esteem, confidence, resourcefulness, inner strengths, etc. in Black daughters to help them face adversities better and to resist discouragement when roadblocks are placed in their paths. These daughters usually are taught very early in life to *rely on themselves* as well as to *learn how to care for others*. They are culturally different from their white women counterparts in the way they integrate traditional male achievement orientation with the more female identified empathic style of considering others, nurturing and caretaking—especially in the broader sense of staying mutually connected with family and the Black community.

7. Black women affected by the remnants of sexism in the Civil Rights Movement and racism in the Women's Rights movement often feel caught in the middle. They are conflicted about how to resolve these "splits" within themselves. The nurturing relational side wants to heal these splits, while the assertive, achievement side wants to demand equality and support.

8. Most economists, sociologists and statisticians seem to agree that the Black female, despite her long history in the role of worker, financially accrues fewer benefits than white females, Black and white males. This disparity is reflected in the form of lower-paying, low-sta-

tus jobs held by the majority of Black women, with less access to diversity and upward mobility. Professor Phyllis Wallace, a prominent Black female economist at MIT, provides hard statistical data on these points in her book, *Black Women in the Labor Force* (1980). Black teenage women and, parenthetically, older Black women are-the "poorest" group of women in America today.

A CLOSER LOOK AT THE BARRIERS

Because racism and sexism are so closely intertwined, Black women often go through the mental exercise of deciding "which is it this time?" I am referring to the mental gymnastics occurring on a daily basis of decoding which type of discrimination lies behind which interaction, and then deciding whether to respond, how to respond or being too overwhelmed by strong feelings to respond at all. In an academic or work situation, many women report a syndrome involving switching gears and rotating alliances between various groupings of men and women. This is a survival technique which is quite stressful, but necessary. I call this the "chameleon syndrome" because the women literally "fine tune" and "adapt" themselves in trying to negotiate various work environments. These efforts to decrease the effects of discrimination and conflict, to acclimate in a "suitable fashion" and to work more smoothly with others in the work place are deemed essential as ways to add to overall work effectiveness. Many Black women see these as requirements as a way "to keep their jobs." It is not necessarily something one is comfortable doing, but automatically finds oneself doing as an option to being confrontational or hostile all of the time. It involves employing various communication styles, depending on the "norm" of the group, and incorporates what I call a "healthy paranoia" as a survival skill in learning whom to trust, how to read people and how to cushion disappointments.

SURVIVING WITH STRESS: SELECTED CASE HISTORIES

Trying to survive stress sometimes can backfire when a woman doesn't also assume *some* responsibility for having her own needs met. This is illustrated by a forty-five-year-old Black woman administrator working on a predominantly white, co-ed campus, who relates:

> I'm completely done in when I get home every night. I know I'm good at my job, even better than most because I have to be. Everything I do at

work is *so* visible; it's like being in a fishbowl. I'm complimented one day for being such a good listener but no one really listens to me, so I'm cool and distant the next day. I'm forever being told how "strong" I am because I'm a successful single mother of five, but I actually have to argue to take time off from work to attend my kids' parent/teacher conferences. On many levels I feel I am many things to many people: administrator, counselor, committee member, mediator between white men and women in the office, and always "mother confessor," but no one in my office really *knows* me the way I know them. They really seem insensitive to my feelings and needs, but expect *me* always to come through for them.

This theme is echoed in the words of two Black female college students. The first one says,

Women of color often tend to be surrogate mothers to siblings when parents/mothers work outside of the home because of economic necessity. This often is a setup for falling into surrogate mothering roles with other students (both white and of color) who then expect me always to be the strong, giving, nurturing one. Consequently, if I'm not careful, others have a hard time being a support for me.

The second student shares:

Minority women often have to bring to college and to reaffirm continually their own positive sense of self-worth here in order to counteract not always receiving a full complement of positive reinforcement once on campus.

Other times, women expect one type of oppression and are hit with others as incorporated in the words of a successful Black female scientist:

I expected to deal with many difficulties breaking into a mainly white, male-dominated profession which *I accept* as a given. I was not prepared for all of the pettiness and mediating constantly required between my more chauvinistic white male co-workers, competitive white female co-workers and Black male co-workers who resented some of the status I acquired upon arriving—I was the first Black female there! Occasionally I'd accept a dinner invitation with one of the Black males and his wife, but I no longer indulge in this because of the suspiciousness from the wife. She was suspicious because I appeared more identified with her husband than with her. This is not to say that everyone I encounter at work does not care about me as a person or a professional, but the *stress* associated with trying to stay on top of my profession, manage my own personal life and get along with co-workers can be unbearable. I'm beginning to believe that the Black professional woman is the most untrusted and betrayed of all in the work place.

Or consider these poignant words of a seventy-year-old Black female domestic worker who has had to be so concerned with basic survival that it would be ludicrous for her to dwell on her "feelings" or problems in the work place:

> My chillun, thank the Lord, is healthy and gets work most of the time. For me, I reckon things is still pretty much the same and I'll never have very much, but I can't complain. We still believe in God and we always had something to eat.

THE INCLUSION/EXCLUSION PHENOMENON

Other women relate stories about inclusion/exclusion and the prices they have paid for success. Many of them seem to be in a "limbo predicament," caught between two worlds where achieving a measure of success has separated them emotionally, geographically, socioeconomically or symbolically from their families or origin or ethnic roots. Some *do* bridge successfully this gap and manage to integrate the concepts of "success" and "staying in touch with who they are"—usually with a mixture of pain, tolerance, guilt and sometimes with feelings of being tested by the "old ties" to prove that they still can relate and be trusted. This presents a very paradoxical dilemma which has strong emotional, social and political ramifications. Concerning this, a twenty-seven-year-old Black, single businesswoman relates,

> I had never felt as alone or isolated in my life before landing my dream job in a major corporation. I had already relocated myself far from family and friends. However, I soon found that in order to keep my job, I had to conform to company and societal norms while showing the world how successful and fortunate I was by learning quickly to play the corporate game. I became angry, resentful, awkward and uncomfortable with my white co-workers "in their world." At the same time, I became sadly very distant and "out of step" with the few Black co-workers I encountered, none of whom even worked in my division. Initially, I felt that life had played a mean trick on me, and that the tradeoffs went too far. Now, I find I'm becoming that assertive, progressive Black woman of the 80's with a whole new set of problems. These encompass male/female problems, but center mainly on the difficult tensions with my family around communication, lifestyles, my "Blackness" being questioned and our not feeling as positive and accepting of each other.

FEELINGS OF "NOT BELONGING"

Black women's lives, emotional histories and current perceptions of themselves do vary, and sometimes what they feel inside is hidden and not shown on the outside. Take, for example, the words of a thirty-year-old married, Black female sales worker,

> When I was told several years ago that I wasn't hired for a certain department store job, I can still remember and feel the uncaring look on the face, as well as the high and mighty attitude, of a certain white female. She was just about my age but short and dumpy and on the prim side. She told me that *I* wouldn't fit into this job because *I* didn't have the right combination of related work experience. The way she said it made me feel like I was in a different time and place. I was transformed instantly in my mind into the too dark, too tall, ugly, lanky slave girl who wasn't attractive enough or smart enough for "Miss Ann" to use in the house, I should go back into the fields and get dirtier, where I belonged. I became so negative about myself and almost everybody around me after that incident that it was hard for me to feel like I could fit in anywhere. She got to me at a bad time, and I probably disliked myself then more than I imagined she disliked me. I felt angry, but all I said before I left was, "Thank you for your time."

Or the words of a nineteen-year-old, Black female college student in a predominantly white college who shares:

> Every time I'm in Professor X's class and he calls on me I freeze, can't get my words or thoughts together, feel dumb and wish I could just disappear. Funny thing is, I always study more for this class and think I'm prepared until he calls on me with that look that says, "you don't really belong here."

Upon exploration of this syndrome of not belonging, one finds that the pressures of trying to fit in, conform or communicate in the "acceptable" form of the majority culture results in an anxiety that literally interferes with one's natural abilities and modes of expression. On many levels and at all ages the feeling or perception that "you really don't belong" serves to complicate career aspirations in the forms of negative projection on one's self, overcompensation, assimilation, homogenization (trying to be like the one with perceived power), over-aggressiveness, submissiveness, giving up, anger, isolation and even fears of failing or of succeeding. I hasten to add that most Black women I've had contact with *do* believe in themselves, *do* have a positive sense of self, and *do* achieve, as one of them put it, "in spite of my oppression and to show them that I can." Though data on emotional coping skills and self-image of Black women is sparse, the literature bears out my observations (Jones and Welch, 1979; Myers, 1980; Jackson, 1973). To go a step farther, Black women more often feel good about themselves for "who they are," but feel angry at our society which is perceived and experienced as "racist, sick and unequal." Ladner (1972) documented this with data for the young urban Black women she studied. In spite of the difficulties presented by sex typing, the Black female generally has emerged with a positive self-concept, high aspirations and expectations.

ADDITIONAL EMOTIONAL BARRIERS

Single Black working women and single Black female parents who work outside the home face special emotional issues. One centers around nontraditional lifestyles that are often not supported, fully accepted or understood by significant others in ways that are meaningful to the women. If these women do not feel the appreciation and emotional support we all need, career goals often are sabotaged or the women fall short of their full potential—one sometimes can lose hope. Recent mental health statistics show that depression, psychosomatic illness and emotional stress *is* on the rise in Blacks, especially poor, young Black single women with children. The older Black woman is also at more risk if she is poor or unemployed and living alone. Suicide rates are low, but on the rise. Traditional supports from extended families and the Black church are no longer as powerful in offsetting these problems. More women than men, however, still use these supports regardless of socioeconomic position (McAdoo, 1980).

REFUTING THE MYTHS

Various myths and lots of confusion have surfaced about Black women retarding the progress of Black men in their pursuit of self-improvement and economic security. Another myth says that these women are better educated than the men. Several researchers (Jackson, 1973; Jones and Welch, 1979) have provided convincing data that demonstrate the higher incidence of career restriction for Black women who receive a college education and refute these myths. In some instances these women *are* hired more often than males because of the perception that they are less threatening to the dominant power structure. According to Wallace (1980), however, Black women are still relegated to the least access to employment opportunities and positions of real power. These are all ploys in which victims are set against one another rather than allowed to join together to make more meaningful gains. Often when a woman is hired rather than a male, she is paid less, is allowed minimal power, has little upward mobility. Often there is a downgrading of reporting mechanisms in the system prior to her starting. This can play into the inclusion/exclusion phenomenon in which there is access to certain "middle or low" management areas of work, but little or none to top management and policy making decisions. These women are not generally included in the establishment network or institutional hierarchies. Bell-Scott (1979) has written about the necessity for Black women to understand hierarchies and to learn how to function most effectively in them.

FACTS AND REALITIES

It must be noted, according to Wallace (1980), that one out of every three Black families in 1977 was headed by a woman, compared with one out five hispanic families and one out of nine white families. Black women heading these families were younger, more than twice as likely to be single and had more children, lower labor force participation rates, higher unemployment rates, higher rates of poverty and lower educational levels than their white counterparts. It seems a better educated, younger and highly qualified Black middle class is developing at the same time that a larger Black underclass struggles to survive in worsened economic conditions. Although roughly 30% of these low-income women reportedly combine work and welfare intermittently, Wallace predicts that within the next decade only a "token few" will make significant inroads into new occupations and better jobs. *Poverty* represents, then, an "ultimate barrier" to these women. It will continue to undermine work and career development unless new strategies utilizing combined effort from those in all income brackets are created and utilized. This will have to include more widespread support systems from the minority as well as the majority populace. This kind of support is precisely what the Stone Center is working on in another one of its projects, innovative groups for low-income mothers in transition to employment. About 80% of the mothers participating in this program are Black women.

CONCLUSION AND COPING STRATEGIES

I would be remiss to discuss barriers without including a brief look at coping mechanisms. So I'd like to summarize by pointing out a few of the findings from the group at the Stone Center revolving around career and relationship issues facing today's Black woman. They are relevant to the Black female college population as well as to the Black female population at large.

1.   In schools and work places there are not enough "hands on" role models and interested mentors for these women readily to identify with, or who also happen to be Black and female. Those women who are prospects for this role are often put in positions where "mentoring" compromises the work they were hired to do. Or they, themselves, develop "role overload" trying to do both. Some do manage. The only option, however, for many Black women is to seek out Black males, white males and females. As one student put it, "If their advice has your best interest at heart, is sound professionally and includes your world view and will help you get through the system—take it!"

2.   Many Black women rely primarily on themselves or their families as their first resource in "hard times." More traditional counseling and psychotherapy is usually not sought out or accepted unless it is a last resort, or the people in this setting are perceived as "culturally unbiased" and able to help out in a concrete as well as insightful manner.

3.   Many Black women work so hard trying to make it academically and in the world of work that it is hard for them to take time out just for themselves. Mothers of these women usually live in this same pattern. Commonly accepted forms of relaxing were more often communal, e.g., "just getting together with others I feel comfortable with to talk, complain, enjoy a home-cooked meal, play cards, dance and 'just be me' without having to shift gears or be strong for somebody." This points to the next theme.

4.   The importance of forming a personal support system at school and at work was crucial. This involved finding others who were both the same or different color and sex who understood and reaffirmed for the students who they were as women, and could give them moral support professionally. Sometimes these "supportive others" had to be educated and "brought along," as one woman put it, before mutual coalitions and networks could be formed.

5.   Black women need to develop a more *entitled* sense of utilizing whatever resources are at hand or can be added to those already in existence.

In closing, I'd like to say that much more research is needed to define adequately this particular female culture with all of its variations, and to develop a clearer understanding of the Black woman's place in society. As we better understand and reflect each segment of our population, we come closer to doing the same for all of us and to creating a more harmonious world in which to live and work.

DISCUSSION SUMMARY

After each colloquium lecture, a discussion was held. Selected portions are summarized here. In this session, Dr. Alexandra Kaplan, Dr. Jean Baker Miller, and Ms. Sylvia Robinson, Dean of the Class of 1986, joined in leading the discussion.

Question: I have observed among Black women many of the phenomena you illustrated so well in your chapter. I feel, now, that I can better understand and support their struggles for survival and equity. Can other nonBlack women learn from these experiences?

Turner: Most definitely. However, keep in mind that white and Black women start in different places and do not share the same work history. White women have not been seen traditionally as "competing" with men in the workplace, although there are exceptions. Black women are often erroneously seen this way. In reality, both Black men and Black women traditionally have had to work for economic stability. There are struggles Black women historically have faced concerning "who should have the job." These will no doubt surface now for many more white women, especially in the fields which are male-dominated. Tensions and competition with men can surface within relationships, around primary and secondary breadwinner roles. Egos may be bruised and roles will need to be redefined and broadened. Mutual dependency, complementary self-fulfillment in both sexes and a greater sense of working harmoniously together often results, too. Both men and other women can be helped ultimately by participation in diverse, equitable job experiences.

Question: Can you tell us more about how you help Black women overcome, psychologically, some of the barriers to career development?

Turner: In a nutshell, by instilling and nurturing within them a greater sense of entitlement to all of the goodies that living and working should provide. I counsel them to become "better consumers" of what life and work have to offer by shifting their attitude away from viewing themselves solely as victims. I advocate constructive activity rather than helpless passivity. Ego-strengthening exercises and constructive on-the-job experiences are planned and sought after as goals, utilizing whatever resources and supports are possible. Learning to ask for what is due her and feeling OK about doing this is often a first step for many. Learning to document for oneself and others the work one performs and how this is done to benefit one's employer is crucial. Having access to job descriptions is one proven way to attain upward mobility or promotion; enlisting others in the workplace to witness this is also necessary. Adequate training and time to adjust to a job also instill positive self-esteem, security and a feeling of belonging. Educating others about job needs rather than complaining, all go into feeling "entitled" to be in the workplace.

Comment: The Black women of lower socioeconomic class whom we recruit to work in our federally-funded agencies often have difficulty being assertive and many don't last in their positions. Any ideas about what we can do to motivate them?

Turner: Personally, I don't believe one person can solely motivate another. Listen to what the women have to say about where they have been and are now in the work force; what excites and helps them; how they want to be involved in process of motivation and goal direction. Don't assume you are the expert and know what's best for any one of them. Utilize their resourcefulness. For many, your job may be seen as a "quantum" leap away from theirs. They don't see the possibility of obtaining the necessary preparation, training or support.

Kaplan: It is very important, as I've found in the lower-paid, employed Black mothers' group I work with, to find ways to listen to and to validate the experiences they are having. After creating the right conditions, the women regain the sense that these are meaningful and important. Too often, this is overlooked and then you can't connect with their present and future aspirations and/or needs.

Question: Are there things that all of us should attend to earlier in these women's lives, given the complexity of the issues? What can be done to help young Black girls?

Robinson: A strong and sound family background helps tremendously to give young Black girls a sense that they belong and are cared about without considerations based on race. Many families also complement this with early exposure to Black teachers who further instill belief in themselves as positive, self-affirming women who *will* make it in life. Positive Black role models and exposure to Black women doing well in a variety of careers is vital. Once these girls have a solid base, they can extend this further to a larger white and Black network of supports and people who believe in them.

Miller: All of these suggestions are good, but we have to emphasize that we still have to work to make solid opportunities in agencies and companies for Black women. There have to be not only jobs to get into, but places for advancement and growth. Motivation has to be attached to concrete and very real goals. There still are not nearly enough good jobs.

Turner: Yes, it is rare for a Black woman or man, regardless of their talent and skill, to go to the top of a major corporation or to be a college president of a majority institution. It was not until 1955 that a Black woman, Willa P. Playler, became President of Bennett College in Greensboro, North Carolina. She was the first Black woman in the history of America to head a Black women's college. Today, that college again is headed by a man. When more equity exists throughout the work system (from entry level to the top level) Black women can not only just hope for career rewards, but will realize them, too. Ultimately, this benefits all of society.

REFERENCES

Beale, F. Double jeopardy to be Black and female. In Toni Cade (Ed.), *The Black woman, an anthology.* New York: The New American Library. 1970.

Davis, A. Y. *Women, race and class.* First Vintage Books Edition. New York: Random House. 1983 (originally published in 1981).

Hill, R. *The strengths of Black families.* New York: Emerson Hall Publishers, 1971.

Jackson, J. J. Black women in a racist society, In Charles C. Willis et al. (Eds.), *Racism and Mental health,* Pittsburgh, Pennsylvania, University of Pittsburgh Press, 1972.

Jones, J. & Welch, O. The Black professional woman: Psychological consequences of social and educational inequities upon the achievement of high school careers in leadership positions. *Journal of the National Association for Women Deans, Administrators and Counselors,* winter, 1980, 43(2), 29–32.

Ladner, J. A. *Tomorrow's tomorrow: The Black woman.* Garden City, New York, Doubleday, 1971

McAdoo, H. P. Black mothers and the extended family support network. In La Frances Rodgers-Rose (Ed.), *The Black woman.* Beverly Hills, CA, Sage, 1980.

McCray, C. A. The Black woman and family roles. In La Frances Rodgers-Rose (Ed.), *The Black woman.* Beverly Hills, CA: Sage, 1980.

Myers, L. W. *Black women: Do they cope better?* Englewood Cliffs, NJ: Prentice-Hall, 1980.

Scott, P. B. Moving up the institutional hierarchy: Some suggestions for young minority and women professionals from the notebook of a novice. *Journal of the National Association for Women Deans, Administrators and Counselors,* winter, 1980, 43(2), 34–39.

Wallace, P. *Black women in the labor force.* Cambridge MA: Massachusetts Institute of Technology Press, 1986.

This chapter was presented at a Stone Center Colloquium in February 1993. © 1993 Clevonne W. Turner.

9

Building Connection through Diversity

CYNTHIA GARCÍA COLL
ROBIN COOK-NOBLES
JANET L. SURREY

CYNTHIA GARCÍA COLL

During the last six months, Robin Cook-Nobles, Jan Surrey, and I have addressed, in a very personal way, the issues that arise from trying to build connections through diversity. Starting with the microcosm of the evolving relationships among us, we took it upon ourselves to further explore how we could establish a deeper understanding of the ways in which our diverse backgrounds have shaped our worldviews, our attitudes toward ourselves and others, our needs, and our ways of connecting. We have done this as women coming from three very different backgrounds, myself from a colonial, culturally and racially mixed Caribbean island society (Puerto Rico), Robin from the racially segregated South just before the civil rights movement, and Jan from a white, Jewish, middle-class community.

The process has allowed us to acknowledge our similarities as much as our differences, and it has resulted in a deeper connection among the three. Throughout our regular meetings, we have experienced miscommunications and passionate arguments; we have also experienced sadness and exhaustion from sharing very personal, painful experiences. We have become aware of our own misconceptions and prejudices about each other's experiences and have found some commonalities in areas that were quite unexpected. It has been hard work. Going from the personal to the political, the process has also evidenced very clearly to me that the notion that when women acknowledge their differences, the solidarity among them will be lost is a misconception. Actually, I am more convinced now that this process is necessary if a true new world order is to be established and feminism is to become the voice for many voices that feel excluded. If I can speak for the three of us, which I hesitantly do, I would say that the process has not only enhanced our mutual respect and admiration for each other, but also has made us recognize the value and uniqueness of our connection in spite of having some very fundamental differences among us. So . . . what are the challenges? Why is it so hard sometimes to establish connections with persons from different cultures, races, socioeconomic classes, sexual orientations and ethnicities than our own?

Several Stone Center working papers have addressed these issues. Cannon and Heyward (1992) described the ongoing effort to build a friendship, the struggle of creating and sustaining a mutually empowering relationship between a white and a Black woman in spite of society's prevalent racism and other structures of oppression. To quote them: "Can we be different but not alienated? . . . the answer lies in the quality of our relation and whether real dialogue . . . is possible and desired between us and around us, among our sisters, Black and white. The problem with white liberalism is that liberal white men and women do not advocate real relation, not mutual relation, but rather a patronizing relation" (p. 4).

In earlier my working paper on cultural diversity (García Coll, 1992), I raised some similar questions. To quote:

> If we recognize that these groups experience different cultural values, as well as different access to economic and social resources, and that they are subjected to prejudice, racism, classism, sexism, and segregation, we would expect that their world-views, psychic structures, and developmental outcomes would be profoundly impacted.
>
> Where does this reality leave us? How can we collectively (and I would now add individually) recognize how profound these differences are in spite of some basic similarities? (p. 5)

Finally, Tatum (1993) examined why disconnections occur in significant relationships between white male and female friends and Black women, starting during the adolescent years. Black women describe many instances of subtle to overt expressions of racism from white male and white female friends as well. Tatum states, ". . . in the case of racism, our culture almost guarantees empathic failures, experiences of disconnection" (p. 2). Actually, in her framework, these disconnections tend to precipitate movement in the process of racial identity for the Black woman.

In these three Stone Center papers, we all agree that there are some inherent challenges when we attempt to establish connections through cultural diversity. In the present paper we will present, individually, our perspectives on these issues—perspectives that emerge from our personal experiences as well as from our convictions of how connections that recognize, accept, and incorporate diversity can be established and are ultimately necessary in a world which is increasingly interdependent. Each of us will address the following questions:

- What gets in the way of establishing growth-enhancing, mutually empathic relationships across races, classes, cultures, and ethnic groups?
- What works? What can be done to overcome these impasses, these obstacles?
- What is our vision for the future, our ideal of a multicultural, diverse, pluralistic society?

Before I take up these questions, I would like to introduce my personal perspective:

1. My perspective is that of a Puerto Rican, middle-class woman who grew up on the island of Puerto Rico, who was granted U.S. citizenship from birth, and who has experienced Puerto Rico's rapidly evolving colonial relationship with the U.S., which includes tremendous economic, political, cultural, and educational upheavals.

2. My perspective is that of a Puerto Rican woman who migrated to the U.S. at the age of 22 to pursue a graduate education, which, among other things, resulted in a major shift in my experience from being part of the majority to becoming a member of a so-called minority group.

3. My experience in the United States has been mixed.

- I have been granted a lot of privileges as a result of the historical oppression of my own ethnic group, like minority fellowships and special criteria for admission to graduate programs.
- I have experienced, along the way, very subtle to very open forms of prejudice and discrimination.

- I have undergone a process of acculturation that has opened possibilities for economic and social mobility, but that has also created losses, especially the severing of very strong ties to my traditional culture.

4. I am the mother of three tricultural children who are:

   - American by birth and exposure to the dominant culture;
   - Jewish by their father's tradition and heritage;
   - Hispanic by their mother's culture, extended family, and the deliberate creation of a support system that includes their Hispanic nanny and her numerous relatives and friends.

As it is evident, using myself as an example, each of us has a unique perspective that is the product of complex life experiences, past and current. It is hard for me to imagine, even if I strongly identify myself as a Puerto Rican woman, that my perspective can be taken as prototypical. It is hard to believe that any of us will experience the world in the same way. The richness and complexity of all human beings, the acknowledgment, celebration, and incorporation of diversity, also brings about the identification and celebrations of connections.

So, keeping my own perspective in mind, what gets in the way of establishing mutually empathic, growth-enhancing relationships across classes, races, ethnic groups, religions, and/or cultures?

Collective History

I would like to propose that one of the things that impedes the process is our collective histories; by that, I mean the prior and current history of power differentials and conflicts between the groups that the individuals belong to. In my particular case, Puerto Ricans have experienced five hundred years of colonialism, the last hundred under the rule of the United States. Most colonial relationships reflect not only economic oppression and exploitation but also a systematic imposition of cultural and ideological values and a denigration of the existing culture, language, history, values, artistic expression, physical attributes, ways of communicating, relationships, etc. So even if two individuals are interacting and struggling for mutuality, the prior and current historical relationships between the two groups get in the way. This collective history is real, but in most instances it is more a part of the core experience of the oppressed than the oppressor. Among Puerto Ricans, this internal oppression can be overtly expressed with ambivalence, defiance, resistance, passivity, submission, Or a combination of all of these reactions.

In addition, the prior history of each group, independent of the other, can get in the way. By that, I mean that even if historically there have not been power differentials among the groups that the individuals are members of, there are certain internalized assumptions that will be generalized to members of other groups. If you have been colonized/oppressed, you might react to another group as an oppressed individual not expecting mutuality and assuming a power differential between the two, even if there has been no prior power differential with the group that you are interacting with now. It is a perceived power differential, which might be real or not, but is as powerful as if it were real. So, as a Puerto Rican, if I perceive you as an authority figure, I might react to you as if you were one even if you do not so consider or perceive yourself.

Personal History

In addition to the collective history, the individual's personal history can also get in the way. This will include each person's prior experiences with other individuals of the same group, or with other individuals from similar groups. Other aspects of life, such as, specific experiences, socialization processes, attitudes learned in early childhood, and the individual's self-concept, may also be obstructions.

Some individuals may be aware of these sources of influences and be willing to work through them, as did Cannon and Heyward (1992). A lot of the personal work among the three of us has been in gaining awareness of each other by sharing views and perspectives on our personal histories and considering their impact on our evolving connection. In other instances, powerful feelings, generated by the awareness and ownership of the collective and personal history, can interfere with the process. Similarly, strong denial or lack of awareness of either the collective or personal history can also get in the way. As a Puerto Rican woman, I have had to come to terms with my ambivalence about my ethnic identity—the shame and pride of my collective history as well as my personal choices. So, keeping in mind my own perspective, what can be done to surmount these impasses, these sources of possible disconnections and even violations?

Working Through the Impasses

A first step is that we all have to acknowledge and, more importantly, own our collective histories as well as our personal experiences. Acknowledging the collective and personal history can bring about emotional discomfort: guilt for being part of the oppressor group, anger for having been held responsible for your group's historical actions, and shame for realizing your own contribution as a member of either the dominant or the oppressed group. Because of this, individuals might choose not to venture outside their own ethnic or racial group, or might deny that either the collective or personal history has any relevance to the ongoing relationship. This denial, however, fails to validate the other person's experience and thus contributes to further disconnections.

A second important consideration is that both persons have to be willing to take risks. Both have to be willing to listen, to learn, and to adapt to each other and to realize that there may be some losses involved. The challenge of establishing mutuality through diversity may be similar to that of any other relationship, but exacerbated in a cross-racial, cross-ethnic, or cross-class interaction. To quote Jordan: "In order to empathize one must have a well-differentiated sense of self in addition to an appreciation of and sensitivity to the differentness as well as the sameness of another person" (Jordan, Surrey, and Kaplan, 1991, p. 29). "Growth occurs because, as I stretch to match or understand your experience, something new is acknowledged or grows in me" (Jordan, 1991, p. 89). However, Beverly Tatum's own experience teaching white students about the psychology of racism suggests the inherent difficulties in establishing cross-ethnic mutual relationships (Tatum, 1993). To quote her: "However, if in stretching to understand a Black woman's experience, a White woman learns something new about herself and doesn't like that new thing (e.g., I have white privilege, or racism has affected me in ways I didn't expect), she is tempted to not understand, to keep out the information" (p. 5). Tatum's experience is that this discomfort usually gets in the way.

An Ideal Society

So what is my idea of an ideal society? In an ideal society, ethnic, socioeconomic, and racial differences would not be equated with deficits. It is clear that our differences, such as experiences and ways of communication, are going to be influenced by these social variables in some very fundamental ways. However, these differences do not imply deficits. In my ideal society, we would try to create opportunities for establishing connections in diversity as early as possible, so children would learn from early on the pains and gains of building connections through diversity, the necessary work, the necessary growth, the richness, the challenges of these experiences. In my ideal society, there would be structures in place so that working through diversity, both at the personal and collective level, would be part of everyday experiences. In my ideal society, the process that my two friends and colleagues and myself have experienced in the last six months would be more the norm than the exception.

ROBIN COOK-NOBLES

I first want to share a little about who I am. I grew up in Winston-Salem, North Carolina during the times of segregation, when the public water fountains had signs that read, "Colored," and bathrooms at restaurants and filling stations were open only to whites. I lived in an all-Black neighborhood of hard-working, honest families. We were a nuclear family of father, mother, and four children (I am the youngest). We were homeowners, so I guess we would be considered middle class. Most of the families looked like mine. Some held working-class, semi-skilled jobs, some ran small businesses that served solely the Black community, and some were professional. It did not matter what one did, only that one worked and earned an honest living. That alone was respectable, it was enough.

We walked to school and were taught by all Black teachers, some of whom lived in our neighborhoods. They knew us well, had taught our older brothers and sisters, and had gone to school with our parents. We felt safe and secure and lived rather routine, consistent lives. Our Blackness was a nonissue. Our teachers told us we could be anything we desired, even President of the United States, if we tried hard and got a good education. And we were sheltered enough, and naive enough, to believe them.

In retrospect, I think they were over-building up our self-esteem to help us to cope and survive in a cruel, harsh world. Just like a mother may over-clothe her child on a stormy, wintry day, so they over-protected us, hoping that they had put on enough layers of protection to weather the many storms that lay ahead. And there was no warning as to when such storms would occur.

I will share one such story. We were traveling to Charleston, South Carolina to visit my father's relatives. We were so proud of them because they lived on Cook St., which was a short, dead-end street that we, as children, believed was named after our family because they had lived on that street for as long as we could remember. I recall riding for miles and miles, in what appeared to be the dead of night.

Then, I had to go to the bathroom. So I told my parents, and they began to look for a filling station with a restroom where they could stop, get gas, and take a restroom break. What followed was very interesting and new for me. My parents began to discuss tactics of gaining access to a restroom. My mom and dad disagreed on the tactics. My mom's strategy was to approach a filling station that appeared "hospitable," to ask whether we could use the bathroom, and if the answer was yes to buy gas. My father had a different strategy. He wanted to go up to any filling station, be pleasant to the owner, buy gas, and then ask whether we could use the restroom. This resulted in an argument. I heard my mother saying, "Roy, why do you choose this filling station with all those crackers hanging around?" I did not know what in the world my mother was talking about. I looked out of the car on the ground and did not see any crackers. Furthermore, I did not see what saltines had to do with anything anyway. What was the problem? Why was my mother making such a big fuss? (The word "cracker" used in this way, is what Blacks in the south call racist white people. As indicated by my unfamiliarity with this word, my parents did not generally call people names or use such words in their ordinary speech.)

Well, since my father was doing the driving, he got to choose the strategy. After getting a full tank of gas, and paying, and being polite, he asked whether his little girl could use the restroom. The owner, who initially seemed nice, turned with a cold, stony face and said, "We don't have restrooms for niggers." My father did not argue (that would have been too dangerous). He just drove away. He did not say a thing, but I felt his hurt, his humiliation, his feeling of powerlessness in being unable to grant his youngest child, his baby girl, the simple request of using the bathroom in a respectful way. My mother was fuming! Not apparently angry at the white man for his racism and lack of humanity, but at my father for not knowing better. For choosing to negotiate man-to-man with a white man.

They stopped on the side of the road, several miles away from the filling station to assure our safety, and suggested that I go to the toilet outside, in the bushes. It was dark. I was scared. I refused. Instead, I chose to wait until I reached my relatives' home, where I could use the bathroom like a human being with respect, and I would not wet my pants in the car either. I now had a mission. I had to save myself, my own dignity. I had to give my father and mother back some of theirs also.

Now that I have shared a very real and personal part of myself with you, I will address the questions at hand. (1) What gets in the way of establishing growth-enhancing, empathic relationships across races, classes, cultures, and ethnic groups? (2) What works? What can be done to overcome these impasses, these obstacles?

In essence, I feel that racism and classism get in the way. Hidden within racism and classism are more human experiences such as *anger, guilt, politics, inability to manage conflict, a fear of the loss of self, and inability to accept difference*. I will elaborate on each of these issues, and will present possible solutions as each issue is discussed.

ANGER

In Cannon and Heyward's (1992) working paper, Katie asks Carter if she can hold her anger. Katie shares that for the last 10 years she has gotten in touch with her anger, as well as the collective anger of all African American women. Yet Katie goes on to say that being in touch with her anger is not enough. She adds . . . where do I go with my anger?," and states, that ". . . over and over again I hear white women talking about their fear of Black women's anger," and that she has, ". . . watched white women go to any length to repress, suppress, depress, oppress all acknowledgment of Black women's anger" (pp. 7–8). So she asks Carter whether she can hold her anger. In essence she is saying, will you be with me in this process? Will you share this experience with me?

This is no easy task. To hold somebody else's anger involves being able to hear and to listen without being defensive. Since a great deal of Black women's anger is directed at white women, both past and present, this can be very hard for white women to do. Also, given the history of slavery and oppression that Black women carry with them every day, including white women's historical role in it, and the current privileges that white women still have as a result of this historical oppression of Black women, holding the anger is no easy task.

In addition, I think that there are different cultural norms regarding the expression of feelings, particularly anger. To illustrate, take any one of your favorite fairy tales. The white female is typically depicted as passive and submissive, waiting for someone to take care of her or to rescue her. Usually that person is a white male on a white horse. In these tales, there is typically an evil, bad person who gets in the way of the innocent, sweet, white woman being rescued and living happily ever after. That person typically is dark-complected and wears black. She is evil and assertive and powerful; not as powerful as the white male, but she gives him a run for his money. This dark, evil, assertive, powerful person is the stereotypical way that the Black female is portrayed in our culture. She is dangerous and to be feared, especially if she gets angry. She is violent, scary, and can kill you. She is out of control.

Psychologically, these images of the white female being innocent, sweet, virginal, and passive, and the Black female being evil, mean, violent, and scary get incorporated into our unconscious. The expression of anger is one way in which, I think, these images or stereotypes manifest themselves in everyday life. Based on these unconscious stereotypes, African American women have a lot of permission to be angry and to express that anger, while white upper-class women (remember that Sleeping Beauty was a princess, and Cinderella became a princess) are expected to repress their anger and to be polite and to see the raw expression of anger as rude and scary. Thus, when these two groups come together, conflict is inevitable. For at some point during a mutually empathic relationship, anger will present itself. But as Cannon and Heyward (1992) so eloquently express, if the relationship is to progress and move forward, the anger has to be held.

GUILT

One of the reasons why I think it is so hard for white women to hold Black women's anger, is the guilt which many well-meaning, liberal, feminist white women feel over the oppression of Black women and the privileges they have as a result. According to Peggy McIntosh, whites and males need to own their privileged status. To quote (McIntosh 1988):

> As a white person, I realized I had been taught about racism as something which puts others at a disadvantage, but had never been taught to see one of its corollary aspects, white privilege, which puts me at an advantage.
>
> I think whites are carefully taught not to recognize white privilege, as males are taught not to recognize male privilege. (p. 1)

Miller (1986) addresses the issue of difference and states that in most instances of difference there is also a factor of inequality (permanent and temporary). Permanent inequality is defined as unequal due to characteristics that are ascribed at birth such as race, gender, class, nationality, or religion. I, therefore, wonder how one can be engaged in mutually, empathic, genuine relationships when inequality is inherent in the relationship and that status is considered permanent?

Tatum (1992) points out that, "the introduction of these issues of oppression often generates powerful emotional responses ... that range from guilt and shame to anger and despair" (pp. 1–2). Nevertheless, as Alice Brown-Collins stated during Tatum's recent colloquium on "Racial Identity Development and Relational Theory: The Case of Black Women in White Communities," white women have to own their own racism if we are to connect across cultures.

In the Winter 1992 newsletter of the Boston Area Rape Crisis Center, Russo, writes,

> I'm a white, middle-class, Catholic-raised woman. This is not only the position I was born into and raised, but the legacy I carry with me into my life and politics. But it is not a static and unchanging identity, rather something to be reckoned with and challenged on a daily basis.
>
> Unlearning and confronting racism in myself and others must be an active process, because my white privilege allows me to ignore or deny it when I choose. Racism permeates all parts of my life. Because of its divisive power, if I do not challenge racism, it determines my chosen friends and networks. . . . (p. 1)

I think it is hard for liberal feminists to own their own racism and the role they play in the oppression of women of color. I, therefore, commend Carter Heyward, Peggy McIntosh, and Ann Russo, as well as my colleague, Jan Surrey, for their work and bravery; for this work must be done if we are to accomplish the task at hand.

POLITICS

All of the above is political, is it not? It's about economics; the haves and the have-nots, the deserving and the undeserving. Miller (1986) uses the terms dominant and subordinate. She explains, "Once a group is defined as inferior, the superiors tend to label it as defective or substandard in various ways. These labels accrete rapidly. Thus, Blacks are described as less intelligent than whites, women are supposed to be ruled by emotion, and so on" (p. 6). When this book was written, the subordinate was seen as female or Black, and no distinction was made between the different experiences of women. I, therefore, want to emphasize that status and the power are relative. Although white women are subordinate, in most instances, to white men, white women are typically dominant with respect to women of color. Likewise, given my educational background, I have some privileges that other Black women do not have. We are not unidimensional. Issues of race, class, and gender interact, and we must acknowledge these multiple and complex realities of women's lives.

INABILITY TO MANAGE CONFLICT

In addressing these issues, which stir up anger in Black women, and anger, resentment, and guilt feelings in white women, conflict arises.

What do we do with this conflict, especially since women are socialized to avoid, ignore, and deny conflict? First, I think the persons involved need to be highly motivated to work through the conflict. Each person has to believe that she will get something personally out of the time, energy, and risk taking that is necessary in order to look at the truth, and own one's own "stuff," in order to work toward resolution. In so doing, one has to tolerate feeling vulnerable.

Jordan (1990) suggests an interpersonal and psychological definition of vulnerability as that experience of self in which we are open to the influence of others, at the same time that we are open to our need for others; what we reveal of ourselves is relatively undistorted by defense. We also need a safe space/place in order to do the work. There needs to be a mechanism in place that gives some structure, and safety to do the work and take the necessary risks.

FEARS OF THE LOSS OF SELF

Black women fear losing themselves as they assimilate. They fear becoming alienated from their histories, their Blackness, their mothers, fathers, and grandmothers. They wonder whether their view is being diluted, whitewashed, and whether they are being brainwashed. They wonder whether they are selling out. In our history of racial slavery and oppression in this country, the mulatto or light-complected person was allowed to stay in the master's house. I now know that that was because the master felt guilty about his mixed-racial child being a field hand, while his other children lived in luxury and privilege. These slaves eventually became a privileged group, just by the nature of the white blood that ran through their veins and their white-like skin. They became known as "house-niggers," "the creme of the crop," while their mothers (who usually had been raped by the masters), remained field-hands, "field niggers." African Americans carry this history with them, so, the question of who you are, and whether you remember where you came from, remains a critical one.

This fear of the loss of self is also shared by white women and other women of color who connect across racial-ethnic lines. just as African Americans are accused of being an Oreo (Black on the outside and white on the inside) if they are perceived as becoming too assimilated, I have heard Asian women say that they have been accused of being a banana, yellow on the outside and white on the inside. Likewise, white persons who take risks to help Blacks are referred to as "nigger lovers." These experiences are real, these fears are real, they get in the way, they hold us back.

INABILITY TO ACCEPT DIFFERENCE

Nobody wants to be different. We all want to be like the other because we experience being like the other as being accepted by them. We all want to be valued. Unfortunately, our experience has typically been that different means less than, or not good enough. Being alike has come to mean being normal and different as being abnormal. Our culture tends to polarize and dichotomize; to be seen as different triggers unconscious attitudes and fears that are deeply engrained in our culture and in ourselves.

So, I ask, must we be identical in order to understand the other, in order to trust or be trusted? Given our different histories there will be disagreements and differences of opinion. Can we as human beings tolerate disagreement? In sum, *I believe that, if we are truly going to develop mutual relations across cultures, we must own our differences and the incredible impact of racism and classism, and, in so doing, address the inevitable conflict.*

JAN SURREY

I speak here tonight as a white, heterosexual woman with a strong cultural identity as Jewish. My four grandparents all came to the United States in the early 1900s from Russia, and both my parents were born in New York City. The Judaism I was introduced to was politically socialist and antireligious. The shadow of the Holocaust and the dangers of anti-Semitism encircled my birth, and I was encouraged towards assimilation in a very white, middle class, semi-suburban city in upstate New York, where my Judaism and my white privilege were fairly invisible to me. I did attend Jewish Sunday School where I was exposed to what felt to me embarrassing but exhilarating notions of Jewish specialness and chosenness. Extreme emphasis on learning, education, intellectual pursuit, and philosophical inquiry as well as liberal politics, political activism, and a commitment to social justice were my Jewish heritage.

When I was sixteen, I had an argument with the rabbi of our temple who claimed that the central fact of the lives of all Jews was the presence of anti-Semitism. I told him that the discrimination and prejudice most salient to me in my daily life was related to my being female. (Historically this was the dawning of the women's movement, although for various reasons I had already declared myself a feminist by age 5!) The rabbi refused to listen or take my experience seriously, and I subsequently left the temple. As a white, Jewish woman coming of age in the "60s," my own immediate experience of confusion and injustice centered around the issue of gender, and this issue was not validated within a liberal, deeply patriarchal religious system.

These facts have shaped my life and my work and my own feminist journey. For me, this journey is not only about struggling for justice in the world, but is also deeply related to the psycho-spiritual journey of coming to appreciate and embrace women's ways of being and being together. The Stone Center work has been a powerful force in my life for supporting the development of a positive gender identification and reversing the power of internalized sexism through the revaluing and refraining of women's strengths in relationships. This development has been evolving for me over the past 15 years through my life-giving and empowering connections with women here.

Yet, I recognize how my own early experience may have left me enthusiastically seeking solidarity and alliance with women, especially women of color, without as deep an appreciation for the need to work through the complexities of race, class, culture, religion, and ethnicity as they shape our relationships and our politics. I have, over the years, been educated to this by other women, and I have increasingly appreciated my own ethnic roots and cultural dilemmas as a post-Holocaust Jewish woman.

In the past year, as the adoptive mother of a Chinese baby girl, my own experience and consciousness of white racism, Anglo-centrism, and issues of difference have been raised exponentially! The primacy and centrality of race in every situation and every interaction is something I could never have experienced before. From the frequency of racist comments we hear about our daughter, often so-called "positive" racist comments ("She's such a china doll!"), or learning, as I take her at 16 months to her first gym class, to scan the environment within the first moment to see if there are any other Asian or nonwhite children or adults there and to watch people taking in the biracial adoptive relationship between us. All this in one glance, as I begin to see the white world through the eyes of the mother of an Asian daughter. I know that we are only beginning to learn about living as a biracial family, as I commit myself to the ultimate connection through diversity—within the mother–daughter relationship.

The theory groups at the Stone Center have started to explore questions of how our own ethnic particularities and social location as white, privileged, middle-strata, professional, North American women have impacted our models of development: our language, concepts, and visions of mutuality and connection. I can no longer say that our model represents women's development without naming our particularities and potential blind spots, seeking opportunities to educate myself about these blind spots and to engage with women of different experience in an open dialogue.

Over the past seven years, my work with my partner Stephen Bergman, in running intensive workshops focused on creating mutuality in male–female relationships, has moved me to appreciate the dynamics of the struggle for mutuality within the context of inequalities of power and privilege. I have seen over and over again the resistance of the more powerful group to truly hearing, taking in, and being moved and changed by opening to the real experience of the subordinate group. Through watching men relate to women, I have become greatly sensitized to my own limitations in relating to other groups of women. I have experienced a growing sense of the meanings of my whiteness and white privilege and am learning about myself as a member of a dominant group which, like men in relation to women, relies on the subordinate group to keep the issues in the foreground and which has a vested interest, though not necessarily an intentional motivation, in maintaining the status quo. Men's lack of interest and inattention to gender is itself a sign of privilege and is inherently oppressive. Seeing how men behave has helped me to accept the inevitability of my own white power and privilege and what Pheterson (1990) has labeled our "internalized domination" and, therefore, our participation in systemic white racism, often through "not seeing" or "not noticing." As a result I have been moved to work with other white women to educate ourselves about our privilege, to examine how it impacts our lives, our theories, and our clinical as well as our political work. Such internalized domination also takes the form of unrecognized class privilege, heterosexual privilege, married privilege, able-bodied privilege, and others, all of which need to become part of our awareness of ourselves and of how our relationships are affected.

CLINICAL APPLICATIONS

Every relationship, including the therapy relationship, is fraught with the impact of these interlocking differences and blindspots. For example, when I work with an African American client, I must be able to hold her profound anger at white racism, be aware of and open to her concern about my potential for color blindness, and be available and capable of talking about all this in the therapy without imposing my need to do so. (I do not believe this can be done without some prior personal work on confronting racism.) The attention to difference is essential, for example, in working with another Jewish woman, where it may be extremely important to explore our religious, class, or family's country of origin differences, and where there is potential for internalized anti-Semitism to impact the movement of connection and disconnection in our work together through transference and countertransference. And, it is also true in working with a white, Anglo-Saxon Protestant client, where my Jewishness may be very present, as well as the possibility that, as white women, we may miss the significance of our shared privilege and its impact on the client's life story, her relationships, and the quality of our connection.

For example, in my work with a very affluent, white, anorexic woman, we were able to make a profound connection around a picture of a starving Somalian mother and child which she brought with her into a therapy session. She began to talk about the meanings of her own "starvation" in the context of her family, as well as her guilt and confusion about the affluence and privilege she had grown up with. This provided a framework for our exploration of her eating "disorder." She was strongly identified with the starving child and the powerless mother, and she was also experiencing a real sense of guilt about her contribution to creating starvation in the world. I took all sides of her experience seriously and did not interpret or reduce her guilt to family "pathologies." We explored her privilege as a real and significant issue for her, especially as a backdrop for her experience of emotional and spiritual deprivation.

I am learning the necessity, as well as the tremendous resistance, to keeping these cultural perspectives in mind, in every hour, with every client, as I have been learning to do with my gender awareness.

RELATIONAL MUTUALITY

As we talk of building connections through difference, we are using the Stone Center relational model of mutuality as a theoretical framework. My own vision of building healthy, growth-fostering connections involves a process of direct engagement and authentic interchange between groups or individuals, where each participant can speak from their experience and can attend and respond creatively to the other. This is a direct perception, connection, and joining with the subjective experience of the other—what Belenky et al. (1986), describe as connected knowing—the building of knowledge based on empathic connection. As Stone Center theorists (Jordan et al., 1991) have described, such mutually empathic connection is the basis of relational growth and healing. Intensity of feeling and powerful conflict are frequently part of this process. When the struggle for mutuality (we think struggle is a good word to describe this process) involves individuals or groups with unequal power in the world, especially the power to "name" reality, we see what Bergman and Surrey (1991) have described as the "double standard" on the road to mutuality between the genders. Members of the dominant group have particular work to do in recognizing their own internalized domination and resistance to change, and how they assume their own experience is normative.

In the relational model, the struggle for mutuality is a transformative process as power dynamics change, and both groups can feel enlivened and empowered in new ways through the connection. When working through cultural differences, the particularities of each experience become more clear, yet the appreciation of the common experiences of oppression and internalized oppression can ultimately lead to a greater understanding of the interlocking systems of race, gender, class, and ethnicity. This vision of growth though connection has important implications and applications for theory building, for developing cultural competence in clinical work, as well as for building political alliances.

RELATIONAL IMPASSES

In the struggle for mutuality in relationships, papers by Stiver (1991) and Bergman and Surrey (1991) have described impasses that create disconnection, that is, that stop the movement of relationship towards mutuality. I will suggest a few key impasses in the struggle for mutuality among women, especially focusing on what I have experienced as difficulties mainstream white women may contribute.

1.   White middle-class women have to do the work of coming to terms with our own internalized domination and our personal and collective history of exposure to, and participation in, "power-over" relationships. When our power to oppress remains invisible or unexplored, we can feel blamed and then get personally defensive when it is pointed out. With this, we take ourselves out of relationships as we become unreceptive and unwilling to hear, be moved, or have our consciousness raised by the experience of women of color.

The whole American emphasis on individualism and psychology's over-emphasis on personal motivation promotes a failure to develop a mature sense of self in the context of the larger forces of systemic power. In our colloquium last year, Heyward, Jordan, and 1

(1992) described this consciousness as central to the ethical task of therapy—generating knowledge of our lives in the context of knowledge of the world.

Further, we have learned to see the white experience as normative and all others as other. We must learn to see our own particularities as simply part of the spectrum of cultural diversity and not the measure by which others are judged. For example, as we sit in our offices seeing white clients, how much is our consciousness of our ethnicity and our class privilege impacting our understanding of our work at the moment and of our clients' concerns in general?

2. For many white feminists, the consciousness of white male dominance and the power of sexism in our lives and relationships is historically relatively newly acquired and may feel tenuous. This feeling contributes to the difficulty we have dealing with the complexity of our double identity as both victim and oppressor which is necessary for engaging in this dialogue. It is especially hard for many of us as women to confront the ways we may be participating in destructive or harmful actions partly because of the strength of our identification with the victim and the difficulties we have in -thinking of ourselves as hurtful, especially as we try so hard not to hurt others. Among women, there is also a kind of hierarchy of pain, where women feel they must give up their own feelings when someone else's pain seems more intense or deserving of attention. We need to learn to hold our own and others' feelings simultaneously.

3. As we come to explore the particularities and commonalities of our experience as women, white, heterosexual women have to directly confront our complicated and often obfuscated relationships to white men—fathers, husbands, sons, teachers, brothers, bosses—with consideration of both the social and economic subordination we experience and the significance of the access to power and privilege we gain through these relationships.

4. Another major impasse to staying engaged in the struggle for mutuality is the emotional response of shame and guilt in many white women in dialogue with women of color. As Jordan (1991) has written, shame is characterized by movement into isolation, and an experience of feeling wrong and unworthy of being in connection. Shame gets in the way of relational movement, and leaves the person feeling helpless or dependent on the other for release from this painful state, and can lead to withdrawal or avoidance. Women of color have rightfully been angered and frustrated by this experience with white women and need to be able to trust that we are doing our own working through of these feelings, so that we can remain open and connected while discussing racism. It is essential for white women to do this work togeth-

er, to some extent, prior to undertaking real engagement in intergroup confrontation and dialogue.

5. Finally, the power of opening up to the pain and anger in the relationship sometimes leaves white women feeling afraid of real engagement. Avoidance of real connection results in superficiality and caution about saying anything because it might be misunderstood or interpreted as insensitive or racist. This keeps relationships from the creative power of shared authenticity and growth through connection. The fear of not being safe and our difficulties receiving and holding anger keep the real, mutually empowering connections from happening. We must have safe enough and structured enough opportunities to do this important work, but we must also give up our expectations of absolute safety and protection, as risk and vulnerability must be a part of all creative and transformative struggle.

WORKING THROUGH IMPASSES

What do we need to build such connections? Commitment, persistence (what Dorothy Soelle calls "revolutionary patience"), and structure. We need to appreciate the inherent value and richness of cultural diversity and to see the enormous significance and urgency of working through difference and the possibilities of psychological and political empowerment emerging from this work. We need to educate ourselves and also to create opportunities to work together to build cross-cultural connections. Such work requires that we create enough structure and support for relational processes so that difficult subjects and feelings do not lead to disconnections or angry impasses, but rather can be supported, sustained, and worked through to some new and shared understandings. A prior commitment to staying through the process is essential. I hope to see the Stone Center take a very active part in helping to create such opportunities through ongoing groups, workshops, and continued colloquium presentations.

My experience has been that working at a group level is more possible and powerful than between individuals. Nearly all the diversity work I've participated in suggests the value of alternating intragroup with intergroup dialogue. Working with differences within groups and developing a sense of group support is essential to complement the process of working with intergroup differences. The potential impasses, disconnections, and violations that we have all inherited and bring with us into the struggle for mutuality are very powerful, but I believe that we can learn to rechannel the power of the forces that divide us into energy for connection and change.

DISCUSSION SUMMARY

After each colloquium presentation a discussion was held. Selected portions are summarized here. At this session, Dr. Beverly Tatum joined Drs. García Coll, Cook-Nobles, and Surrey in leading the discussion.

Question: Hi. I'm a student here at Wellesley. I've noticed that when these discussions come up in class or in social settings that a lot of my white women friends who are not Jewish make the comment that they feel they have no culture, no ethnicity. I was wondering if you could address how that could be an obstacle to overcome in making these connections.

Surrey: There is nobody who does not have ethnicity, but the sense of being empty implies that there is a norm versus ethnicity. That's the whole shift we're talking about, the shift has to be "we are all ethnic." Most people need to explore a couple of generations back into their families and really tap into the richness that's there. We all need to begin to appreciate the roots and to really explore, to become sensitive to our own ethnicity, to the family traditions, even to the class issues.

Cook-Nobles: In a workshop about these issues that I participated in recently, what came out was that for some white people, to celebrate pride in being white conjures up images that they're not comfortable with, such as the KKK. That was the first time that I was in touch with some of the shame and guilt involved in white pride.

Tatum: This is a very common response that white students in my classes will talk about—the fact that they feel embarrassed about being white once they become aware of the racism in this society. European Americans really had to give up their European identity when they came to this country in exchange for whiteness, and so part of the healing process is really to go back to reclaim that connection to being European-American.

The book *Ethnicity and Family Therapy* has chapters from almost every ethnic background you can imagine. It's written about what it means to be from a particular cultural background in terms of your own heritage, and it helps students to realize a lot of things that took place in their families really were rooted in particular cultural heritages. Only then can they have other ways to think about being white. In addition, there is a history of resistance, for example, to racism, the abolitionist tradition or white allies, but most people don't know what that history is, and that's a history that needs to be reclaimed.

Surrey: In teaching ethnicity in therapy we always have trainees break up into their different cultural backgrounds, and we usually have a WASP group. They talk about the expectations for therapy and how white Anglo-Saxon Protestantism might be interfering with coming to therapy and with the ability to express emotions. Also, they acknowledge this is a culture and that it has implications for who they are as therapists.

Cook-Nobles: One of the most powerful exercises that I ever did in coming to consciousness about racism and culture and ethnicity was as part of multicultural issues training for staff in which we did an exercise where each of us brought an object which represented part of our cultural background and presented that object to the group. Each of us had to claim a culture as part of us, and what came up was that each of us felt different and a sense of isolation. Whether that was because of ethnicity or race or class or sexual orientation or immigrant status or educational level or family quirks, whatever, it brought a generic sense that everybody has a culture and everybody has some sort of cultural identity.

Comment: I wanted to thank you for introducing the issue of power into the discussion of difference, and the whole realization that we are, at the same time, oppressor and oppressed in different contexts. I want to recommend James Baldwin's essay, "Being White and Other Lies," which was given to me by an African American student in my clinical doctoral program as we struggled with whether or not she would hate me for having nothing to teach her but white people's psychology. Baldwin's point is that this is a nation of immigrants and of people who were oppressed somewhere. The deal that we cut with the dominant culture when we got here is that we will trade our legacy of oppression in our countries of origin for the opportunity to be white at the expense of Black folks. This essay states that we have to give up the position of power and privilege and exchange it for a more honest kind of vulnerability, if we are to make genuine crosscultural connections.

Question: I'm Mexican, I was born in Mexico and I came over to this country when I was six. One of the things that's always seemed very strange to me in this country is the polarization between Black and white. In my country, there are all shades and there is racism. People there do look down on people who are darker, but it's not as polarized as it is here. It's not like here where if you have one molecule of Blackness in you, you're a Black. I wonder if some of you could comment on that?

Cook-Nobles: Well, I think it has to do with the history of slavery in American history in that that molecule of Blackness made you able to do labor. Did anyone see the movie "Queen"? It didn't matter that she looked white, once it was found that she was Black then the anger and the abuse and the rejection were there. She kept saying, "I'm white, I'm Black, I'm both." It wasn't until she accepted her Blackness, because it was the Black community that accepted her, that she came to some kind of resolution; so I do think it's rooted in that history.

Question: I have noticed that when we talk about solidarity of women of color, white people see people of color as a term that's an insult. They think it's a revolution in disguise because people of color are out there and they're united by being people of color and then there are white people who are out here on the other side. Was this addressed in your work at any time?

García Coll: We are struggling with how to name ourselves. The Stone Center's work has always talked about the use of language and how precise we have to be; yet we can't come up with a term we feel comfortable with. We feel, as women of color, uncomfortable with the term "women of color." There are two problems with it: one is the implication of minority or colored as something pejorative; the other is the implication that we are homogeneous. The dilemma is: do we try to come up with a term or do we just resist coming up with a term because there's really nothing to be termed? The critical notion is (1) that diversity reflects something that actually comes very much from the biological sciences in which there's an incredible variability in genotypes, phenotypes, and species, and (2) that the beauty of human beings is the variability in shades and rainbows and permutations and combinations, and (3) that the notion of trying to put us into strict categories is wrong, because strict categories come from a political struggle of trying to put people in categories that they won't be able to move away from. So, as you see, we have been struggling with it.

REFERENCES

Belenky, M., et al. (1986). *Women's ways of knowing.* New York: Basic Books.

Bergman, S., & Surrey, J. (1991). *The woman-man relationship: Impasses and possibilities.* (Work in Progress No. 55.) Wellesley, MA: Stone Center Working Paper Series.

Cannon, K. G., & Heyward, C. (1992). *Alienation and anger: A Black and a white woman's struggle for mutuality in an unjust world.* (Work in Progress No. 54.) Wellesley, MA: Stone Center Working Paper Series. (Reprinted as Chapter 13, this volume)

García Coll, C. (1992). *Cultural diversity: Implications for theory and practice.* (Work in Progress No. 59.) Wellesley, MA: Stone Center Working Paper Series.

Heyward, C., Jordan, J., & Surrey, J. (1992). Ethics, power and psychology. Stone Center Colloquium Series. Tape No. A8.

Jordan, J. (1 990). *Courage in connection: Conflict, compassion, creativity.* (Work in Progress No. 45.) Wellesley, MA: Stone Center Working Paper Series.

Jordan, J. (1991). The meaning of mutuality. In *Women's growth in connection.* New York: Guilford, pp. 81–96.

Jordan, J., Kaplan, A., Miller, J. B., Stiver, I., & Surrey, J. (1991). *Women's growth in connection: Writings from the Stone Center.* New York: Guilford.

Jordan, J. V., Surrey, J. L., Kaplan, A. G. (1991). Women and empathy: Implications for psychological development and psychotherapy. In *Women's growth in connection.* New York: Guilford, pp. 27–50.

McIntosh, P. (1988). *White privilege and male privilege: A personal account of coming to see correspondences through work in women's studies.* Working Paper No. 189. Wellesley, MA: Center for Research on Women.

Miller, J. B. (1986). *Toward a new psychology of women* (2nd edition). Boston: Beacon Press.

Pheterson, G. (1990). Alliances between women: Overcoming internalized oppression and internalized domination. In L. Albrecht & R. Brewer (Eds.), *Bridges of power: Women's multi-cultural alliances.* Philadelphia: New Society Publishers, pp. 22–39.

Russo, A. (Winter 1992). White women and racism. *Boston Area Rape Crisis Newsletter.*

Soelle, D. (1978). Revolutionary patience. Maryknoll, New York: Orbit Press.

Stiver, 1. (1991). *A relational approach to therapeutic impasses.* (Work in Progress No. 58.) Wellesley, MA: Stone Center Working Paper Series.

Tatum, B. (1992). Talking about race, learning about racism: The application of racial identity development theory in the classroom. *Harvard Educational Review, 62,* 1–24.

Tatum, B. D. (1993). *Racial identity development and relational theory: The case of Black women in White communities.* (Work in Progress No. 63.) Wellesley, MA: Stone Center Working Paper Series. (Reprinted as Chapter 5, this volume)

This chapter was presented at a Stone Center Colloquium on March 3, 1993. © 1993 Cynthia García Coll, Robin Cook-Nobles, and Janet L. Surrey.

10

Rethinking Women's Anger: The Personal and the Global

JEAN BAKER MILLER
JANET L. SURREY

WHAT IS ANGER?

We would like to explore the possibility that anger can take on a different quality in the hands of women—or when women take on full participation in the conduct of all the world's affairs and when women's experience enters fully into the construction of our culture's framework of thinking and feeling. In the literature, great confusion has existed about anger, especially in psychoanalytic and psychodynamic writing, but also in psychological material. Anger is often linked with aggression, and aggression has been defined in a variety of ways. We prefer to separate anger from aggression. We would say that anger is an emotion. Aggression refers to action with the intent to be destructive to others or to control others through force, which may or may not follow from anger (Miller, 1983). For example, someone may cooly produce, buy, sell, or use guns or even nuclear weapons on the order of someone else who may or may not be angry. Today, several leading psychological researchers on anger make this distinction, for example, James Averill (1982) at the University of Massachusetts and Charles Spielberger in Florida (1983).

The confusion between aggression and anger has arisen because the latter has been strongly associated with aggression in our culture.

Instead, if we thought of anger first off as a part of relationships, we would have a very different view of it. The reason we have not understood anger as part of relationships probably lies in the fact that relationships have been relegated more to the domain of women than of men. Despite all of the development of the psychological fields, we have not recognized the full value of relationships—even though they are, of course, the source of all human development. We would like to propose some ideas about how we may create a new vision of anger if we were to see it within the context of relationships, that is, within a context in which connections between people are given their full and primary value.

First, we would perceive anger as a necessary part of the movement of relationships. I want to stress the movement because when we talk about relationships that is what we really are talking about. The essential feature of good, that is, growth-fostering, relationships is that they are in motion. There has to be a flow. If relationships are static, they are usually bad for the people in them, not fostering growth.

Another way to put this is to say that emotional development for children and adults occurs basically in the context of relationships where there is a possibility for us to be moved by another person or persons, and for us to affect them. The relationship changes along the way. It moves with us. We are moved by many emotions, and certainly anger is one of them.

Anger occurs when anyone feels unable to express her/his experience or feels not heard, at least to some degree, or feels unable to hear the other person(s). She/he then begins to feel that something is wrong. Something hurts. That is what I believe anger is—an emotion which arises when something is wrong or something hurts and needs changing. Of course, if one person obviously mistreats or violates another, this too means that something hurts or is wrong and leads to anger. If, as a result of the expression of anger, the flow of action in the relationship alters in a way that allows each person to include her/his important experience, the anger often can dissipate quite readily. Here, as Teresa Bernardez (1988) has suggested, anger seems to be an emotion we possess which inevitably prompts us to act against wrong treatment or violation of us, against injustice.

We can think of many examples of anger occurring in this direct and straightforward way. Suppose, for example, a ten-month-old child begins to feel tired or hungry and tries to convey this to her parents. They are preoccupied with something else and don't respond immediately. The child then becomes angry because something is wrong and demonstrates this with crying or thrashing about. She has now more forcefully notified her parents that something hurts, and they now try to attend to it. In doing so, they respond to both the initial physical need and to the psychological situation, the child's need to feel she has an impact, that she can reach the people in her relationships and that they can hear and respond to her. This, of course, represents a relatively uncomplicated example.

Because anger arises when something is wrong or hurts, it usually occurs along with other emotions, with a mixture of feelings. These are usually painful feelings such as hurt, disappointment, humiliation, and others. Most of the time we experience a combination of feelings with mixtures of meanings, not one simple feeling devoid of content. Some writers, for example, Paula Caplan (1989) have written about anger as a secondary emotion, meaning that it follows after we are first made to feel one or more other painful feelings.

COMPLICATIONS

Next we have to consider what happens when a relationship cannot allow the appropriate expression of anger, that is, when a child or adult cannot express anger, or the others in the relationship cannot respond in a way that will bring about a change in what is happening. Here, people begin to move into all of the complications which occur when the relationship does not provide well for the expression and reception of anger. These patterns can vary with different cultures, classes, and ethnic groups. In general, however, for men in this culture and certainly in several others, a prominent substitute for anger is aggressive behavior, either physical or verbal or both. I believe that this kind of behavior is an attempt to circumvent the experience of anger as part of the flow of relationships. Anger is a vulnerable feeling. An angry person usually also feels hurt and in pain and opens this up for and to others. By contrast, aggressive behavior is an attempt to prevail by force and to end the flow of the interaction. It is very different from real engagement with difficult feelings.

Of course, there are other forms that men's anger can take, for example, withdrawal, but overall, I believe boys and men have been encouraged, indeed overstimulated, from early childhood to engage in aggressive action as a way of avoiding the real, interpersonal experience of anger, and of many other emotions, too (Miller, 1983).

Some people have developed a strategy of appearing to express anger in a way which is intimidating to other people. However, this aggressive display usually does not represent an expression of anger about what really matters or what really hurts, but often reflects a learned behavior, a set of accusations and attacks. This behavior is frequently a strategy for control or power over others, often used by those in dominant positions. While this pattern can occur in women, it is more common in men.

Women, for our part, tend to develop many of the various forms of indirect expressions of anger. These can include a range of psychological and physical symptoms or complaints, as described recently by Teresa Bernardez (1988) and Irene Stiver (1988), complaints which are not about the really important sources of pain.

For some or many men in this society, overt displays of aggressive behavior can feel as if they gain the aggressor a much more powerful and invulnerable position than would allowing others, or themselves, to know the disappointment, hurt, or sadness which has occurred. For women this can be the case too. However, to be openly angry has been so taboo that women are more likely to resort to the indirect forms. Thus, in both cases, for men and for women, anger and its meaning can be lost. I believe the reason we find anger so difficult is that it concerns our feelings of not being able to represent our experience, to be heard, engaged with, and responded to—and all of this means to be *valued* in the important relationships in our lives. That pain can feel almost unbearable. It can seem easier and as if we are less vulnerable if we keep up the nonrelational forms of anger in either repetitive, aggressive forms or more disguised forms.

ANGER AS A RESOURCE

If we could create a climate in which we could bring forward and value growth-fostering relationships, rather than aggression, as the primary, necessary, and most valuable ability of human beings, I believe we could begin to transform the nature of anger. I think we could see it as a resource in relationship rather than a danger. For anger to be a resource, we need a context of relationships in which we are safe to express anger and, most importantly, the real reasons for it. We need relationships in which we are safe to hear the other person's anger without experiencing it as an attempt to attack or diminish us. Anger, seen in this way, notifies the people in the relationship that something is wrong and needs attention, and moves people to find a way to make something different come about. Anger, then, can become the energizing initiator for transforming the relationship to something better.

If people believed that anger could function in the service of moving a relationship towards a better connection, it would make a huge difference. This is especially true for women, who tend to be afraid that anger will create a disconnection or end a relationship. In order for women to believe in another possibility, we would need to construct a cultural context which defines anger as a resource to improve connection. This would necessitate major change, but we can make a start by talking to each other about this possibility in some of our personal relationships and even in some organizations and institutions. We cannot begin to express anger in this way except in relationships based in mutuality or, more accurately, based in the search for mutuality. In relationships in which one person has more power or is aiming for more power or for nonmutuality, it usually is not safe for the less powerful person to express anger.

Next in changing our cultural context, we would all have to practice a great deal to learn how to express anger just as anger, without all the distortions we've developed about it. All of us, I believe, are very backward on this score. Probably even more difficult, we would have to develop ways to hear and receive anger directed to us, to understand that it is a message that something is wrong or hurts and that a change is needed. We all need to learn to respond better to anger. Experience can teach us that the process of expressing and responding well to anger enhances connection, adding focus, clarity, and energy for empowerment of our relationships. As we proceed, it is important to have a perspective of patience, recognizing that most of us are just beginning to take faltering steps along this path.

We must emphasize that the expression of anger in this way is very different from just "sounding off" or "ventilating." Carol Travis' book provides a valuable critique of expressing anger for its own sake (1982). The essential difference is that we are talking about anger in the context of relationships and anger as one of many feelings which can move the relationship to something better. The goal of the expression of anger should be that the people in the relationship become better connected rather than less connected. The aim is not the expression of anger per se, but the recognition of the value of anger as a step in working together in relationship to clarify the source of the pain and to do something about it—to right what is wrong.

I don't mean by any of this to water down the power of this emotion. I suspect, too, that this all may sound idealistic or unreal, but I believe that impression may be an indication of our cultural conditioning or brainwashing. People believe anger is linked with aggression and destruction because that is the tradition fostered in this culture by those in positions of power. They have influenced all of our thinking. This is so in any society; those in power determine our experience to a large extent and, thus, exert a major influence on the creation of our very feelings. They, then, provide the labels for these feelings.

I want to stress here two points: (1) Once any group in society establishes itself as dominant, it would have to utilize aggression as a disproportionate part of its way of acting in order to maintain its dominance. (2) Simultaneously, it cannot develop fully the cultural forms which threaten its dominance. Relationships among people are the key forms which potentially threaten dominance. They are absolutely essential for human life and development, and relationships formed in mutuality and based in empathy and responsiveness are inevitably incompatible with a system of dominance. In such a system, anger, a powerful emotion with the potential to right wrongs and to play a valuable role in changing hurtful relationships, would likely be suppressed and distorted. Our culture has yet to appreciate the value of relationships, and as a result they cannot yet flourish fully and well for all of us. Our society has often treated the need for relationship almost like a necessary evil, one which women have been encouraged to fill.

To summarize thus far, despite the fact that the psychological fields have long said that everyone develops only within relationships, we are suggesting that professional thinking has yet to grant full weight to the primary value of growth-fostering relationships and to the processes which create these relationships. This situation probably reflects the fact that our culture, in general, cannot fully recognize their value, and it has put the work of making and building relationships into women's domain. The usual way of thinking in this culture has not fully encompassed anger in the context of relationships, but linked it with aggression. Changing the usual thinking, we can begin to "re-envision" anger as a valuable part of relationships. Doing so is particularly important because it can be a powerful force for movement within relationships and for movement to better relationships. Seen in this way, and separated from the connotations of aggression, anger would be encompassed by many women with much greater ease. This ability would go a long way, not only towards enhancing women's mental health, but towards building our full place in society, towards diminishing aggression and violence, and towards making the world a better, safer place. Janet will now elaborate some of these points.

ANGER IN A RELATIONAL CONTEXT

During the time I was preparing this presentation, the story of the Carol Stuart murder was unfolding.[1] Therapy hours with clients were

---

[1] Carol Stuart was murdered in Boston in 1989. She was seven months pregnant at the time. Although the police and press all focused on a young black man, her husband now is suspected to be the murderer.

filled with responses, conscious and unconscious, to this murder. It evoked deep anger, fear, and compassion, and stimulated personal memories and associations related to these feelings. One client began to talk about an incident that confused her. While she and her boyfriend were watching TV, she began to feel unsafe and angry. Suddenly she stood up and said, "We have to end this relationship." Although she did not end the relationship, she was puzzled about what this reaction represented. I asked her if this had anything to do with the Stuart case, and she remembered that they had been watching a TV news story on that case. This vignette is not described here to begin a discussion of the client's loose boundaries or her borderline psychopathology or the externalization of her fear and anger. I took her response very seriously, and in the therapy hour we worked on how it did and did not resonate with her feelings in this particular relationship as well as in relationships with other men in her life currently or historically. We talked further about what the communications and consequences of this murder and others like it were for all women, what these meant to my client, and the cumulative impact this violence had had on her life decisions. To discuss the connection between the personal and the collective level of experience, it is necessary to work from an enlarged clinical paradigm, beyond the isolated individualistic self.

I would like to consider tonight how our shared anger and vulnerability (around which we are profoundly, empathically connected) can be a resource for positive action, instead of becoming suppressed, stuck, distorted, unfocused, or exaggerated—and, ultimately, isolating and disempowering.

Further, I hope to initiate discussion about the *importance* of enlarging our clinical frameworks and paradigms to encompass an appreciation of the larger relational dynamics which shape all our experience. Jean has presented a reconstruction of women's anger as a resource for change. She has described the potential value of anger in creating forward movement in relationships under certain conditions—when these relationships are rooted in the search for mutuality, that is, relationships moving in the direction of mutual empathy and empowerment. Alternatively, anger generated in the dominant person in hierarchical, "power-over" relationships can stop the interplay and flow of feelings. It can rupture the connection and may be used as a coercive threat or lead to violent or destructive action. As Miller (1983), Stiver (1988), and others have described elsewhere, anger in the subordinate member in such emotionally disconnected, hierarchical relationships becomes suppressed, disguised; or it may turn into somatic complaints, general emotional instability or irritability, or free-floating, unfocused rage directed outward or against the self. Under mutual relational conditions, anger can function to indicate that "something is wrong" *in the relationship.* Frequently, this is a sign of nonmutuality and arises out of the desire for healthy connections. Anger can lead to a shared focus of attention on what is wrong; a "looking together" which validates and legitimates the experience, often diffuses the immediate emotional reaction, moves the experience into greater clarity, sharpens perception, and deepens understanding. ·

This suggestion assumes that both or all persons can be expressive of and receptive to anger as it arises in the relationship. It is this interplay and exchange between people that moves anger into a framework of shared understanding. (This may not happen immediately, but may occur over a period of time.) By maintaining connection or dialogue—often around very difficult emotions—the anger can keep moving in a constructive direction. Real responsiveness in relationship does not always mean agreement, but may well lead to conflict or a stated unwillingness to accept a hurtful, destructive outburst. Under relational conditions where connection and movement are maintained, anger can generate a sustained energy available for action and change. The movement of relationship can help people move through immediate angry feelings to come to handle a difficult situation effectively

An alternative model, based in a "separate self" paradigm, was described by a male colleague in a discussion of anger as a "positive emotion." He described anger as arising when "something gets in the way of what you want." He said that the positive value of anger is that it provides energy to mount an "attack" or "strategy" to get what *you* want. The problem in this analysis is evident when the "something" that gets in your way happens to be another person. From a relational perspective, anger can be seen as a resource for action and change in relationships, rather than for self-interest alone. Such a relational model has direct application to empowerment models of therapy.

For example, a client of mine had been raped by a patient in her work as a psychiatric nurse. She has moved through a long period of terror, shame, and isolation into a shared, connected experience of fear, vulnerability, and anger. In addition to her psychotherapy, this evolution has involved her work in a group with other rape victims. She has joined with other women to speak out publicly about her experience in lectures and testimonies before legislative committees. She also has undertaken efforts to have a discussion of this subject included in the nursing education curriculum.

Her experience has become a resource for relational empowerment for herself and others. She has come to appreciate that her experience was not an isolated event, but rather one shared directly and indirectly with other women. She believes that her original shame and silence about the horror of the rape and how it had been handled by other professionals kept her feeling alone, depressed, and stuck in her angry feelings. In Stone Center language, she has moved from a position of "condemned isolation" to authenticity and empowerment in connection. Judy Jordan, in her work on shame, has beautifully described the movement out of shame as a powerful, liberating energy (1989).

Such an empowerment model highlights the value of anger moving in relationship to constructive and creative action. Lyman (1979) has described anger as an essential political emotion. Teresa Bernardez (1988) and Carter Heyward (1984) have described anger as a sign of or a response to injustice, which implies a vision of and desire for a better, just, or mutual relationship. Action towards creating or holding such a vision or desire supplies the important energy for justice-making and peace-making activities. As Beverly Harrison (1985) writes, "Such is the power of anger in the work of love." This is true on the personal and global levels in the work towards creation of a safe, just, life-affirming, and relationship-affirming world.

The organization called MADD, Mothers Against Drunk Driving, offers a vivid example. Energized by the tragedy of their personal pain, these women have joined together in action. Linked in an understanding of the roots of the loss and violence in their lives, they have extended beyond their immediate anger at the individuals responsible for the death of their children and have moved into educational, political, and legislative action.

The acronym, MADD, sounds especially relevant here. It represents the mothers' shared anger—but also hints at the possibility of anger leading to feelings of insanity under conditions where anger isolates and separates and when constructive arenas for action are not possible. When people can share anger and build connections that allow ongoing movement and interplay around feelings of great intensity, the power of such experience can lead to deeply passionate and constructive, long-term action.

It is essential to remember that our discussion of anger is based on a particular definition of anger as an emotion arising inevitably in development, which can, under conditions of mutuality, move the relationship towards greater connection. In women, much anger as we know it today can become seriously distorted by relational disconnections and unresolved internal and external conflict. In contrast to the Eskimos' many words for snow, we subsume too many different experiences, emotions, and behaviors in the word "anger." We should work on a good phenomenological typology. As Jean has said, aggression, hostility, hatred and destructive, violent behaviors are not necessary outcomes of anger, but rather result from an avoidance of vulnerable emotions, intrapsychically and relationally.

As noted earlier, we usually experience anger as part of a complex mixture of feelings, and we should not study it as an inherently differentiated emotion. Anger is often connected with feelings of fear, vulnerability, loss, and great caring. Frequently women cry when angry because of this mixture of emotions. Women's anger has often been misunderstood, trivialized, invalidated, exaggerated, or pathologized as "strident," "bitchy," or "narcissistic." Such judgments become internalized and complicate the healthy movement of anger. Bernardez (1988), Lerner (1985, 1986), Greenspan (1983), and Miller (1983) have described the "feminine" ideal in our culture which excludes anger as a legitimate feminine emotion.

MATERNAL ANGER

The "maternal ideal," the "good mother" construction of this culture excludes the possibility of healthy anger from mothers. We believe this reflects a deep cultural belief that anger and nurturance cannot coexist (Miller, 1983). Dinnerstein (1976) and Miller have discussed the origins of this terror of maternal anger. Dinnerstein suggests this fear is fundamental to the child's narcissism and sense of powerlessness in light of the caretaker's apparent omnipotence. Miller suggests it is a culturally-based gender arrangement. Since women are the assigned carriers of the responsibility for care, empathy, and maintaining connection, they represent the only refuge from a dangerous, hostile world. I agree with Jean that this deep cultural split is not fundamental to development, and both men and women need to work to integrate nurturance and healthy anger. For women, this must involve new and more realistic constructions of mother as empathic *and* angry. Angela McBride (1973) and Adrienne Rich (1976) have both written as mothers about the deeply paradoxical experiences of love and tenderness coexisting with anger, and of the rage of unprocessed, disconnected frustration, exhaustion, and felt insufficiency.

The current uncovering of sexual abuse in families often becomes focused on the mothers' lack of protection and healthy anger. Beyond the dangerous problem of "mother-blaming" in psychological formulations, I think there exists a deep collective call by daughters to mothers for protection—reflecting the need to recreate and envision their mothers as capable of responding with appropriate anger, clear-sighted, and courageous, responsive action—all as part of maternal love. We must consider further *under what relational and political conditions* this is possible for mothers.

Such a reconstruction of "mother love" has a long history in women's peace, antiwar, and antinuclear activism. In her work on feminism and nonviolence, Pam McAllister (1982) considers the significance of integrating love and anger:

> Together these seemingly contradictory impulses (to rage against yet to refuse to destroy) combine to create a strength worthy of revolution. To focus on rage alone will exhaust our strength, force us to concede allegiance to the path of violence and destruction. On the other hand, compassion without rage stifles our good energy. Without rage we settle for slow change, ask for something mediocre like "equality." It is with our rage that we find the courage to risk resistance and it is with our intimate connection to the life force which pulses through our own veins that we insist there is another way to be. By combining our rage with compassion, we live the revolution everyday. (1982, p. iv)

Mothers' anger has mobilized women to political activity, when the women have been able to create a relational context which validates this anger and provides an arena for action. I think of a poem written by a Cambodian mother to her daughter entitled, "Revolutionary Lullaby" (we don't usually hear these two words together) or a letter by a Nicaraguan mother explaining to her daughter her commitment to the revolution as part of her commitment to her daughter:

> My greatest wish is that one day you become a true woman with pure feelings and a great love for humanity. And that you know how to defend justice whenever it is being violated and that you defend it against whomever and whatever. (Anonymous)

I think about Argentina's Madres de Plaza de Mayos—the mothers of the disappeared—for whom the emotional response to the disappearance of their children was translated into organized, extremely courageous political protest, a refusal to be silent or silenced about the atrocity of their government's activity. Such transformation of deeply personal emotions means moving out of isolation into profound connection. The movement of emotion in such a context becomes the source of validation, depth of understanding, and action. Personal experience generates the ongoing resource for action and cannot be split off from "political activity." In this way, the personal and political are inextricably connected.

ANGER AS A RESOURCE FOR PERSONAL
AND GLOBAL CHANGE

We need to create empowering relational contexts in therapy and beyond to validate and "recontextualize" women's experience by linking
the personal and the global (Conn, 1990). I use the word global to emphasize the degree of our existential and empathic connection as
"earth creatures" and our mutual economic, political, and ecological
planetary security. The emergence of a global psychology challenges
old paradigms of separate, bounded, self-seeking power, control, and
dominance and builds on new visions of a relational, interdependent,
and ecological self. Psychotherapy practiced from this global perspective seeks to uncover the connections between personal pain and global crises—to empower individuals to act with awareness of the larger
world, to "act locally and think globally"[2]

We need to consider the limitations of old paradigms which focus
singularly on the intrapsychic world of the individual or, at best, the
individual family system to understand psychopathology. For example, if a woman's anger is viewed only from the perspective of her
own family history and the interactions within her own marriage, she
may well seem "too angry" or "over-reacting." She does need to understand how her anger and fear as a woman are being continually
evoked and then unrepresented in many of her life activities and experiences because of women's position in society. Frequently, this anger
becomes focused on one individual—often it is her husband, and
sometimes her mother or her children. A client of mine recently told
me that she did not want to come to hear this talk since she tries not to
focus on her anger as a woman because it seems to lead only to anger
and conflict within her marriage.

This decade has witnessed an event of extraordinary significance:
the uncovering, remembering, and naming of the reality of childhood
sexual abuse, violence, and incest—and their psychological impact on
women's lives. Such an event, according to Judith Herman (1989), has
evolved in large part from the women's movement and the sharing
and validating of experience between women, frequently between
women therapists and women clients. That this is a global phenomenon became clear to me when a psychiatrist in Amsterdam said to me
last year, "We're about five or six years behind you in the States in un-

---

[2] I'd like to acknowledge here the contributions of my global psychotherapy
group, Sarah Conn, Miriam Greenspan, Mary Watkins, Ann Yeomans, who
have begun meeting and working together to develop these themes.

covering and dealing with the prevalence of incest and early sexual abuse."

I believe we are in the midst of a deeply personal and collective process in which women are uncovering women's memories of abuse, along with the accompanying pain, terror, and anger through the building of connection among women. This is why survivors' groups have been so significant in helping individuals move out of shame and isolation. This collective *re-membering* calls for personal and political levels of understanding and arenas for action. Women clients are on the front lines of this revolution; they are doing work that is changing the consciousness of us all—both men and women. That their experience represents a severe point on the continuum of "normal" experience needs to be represented in our thinking and clinical work. We must work deeply and in a respectful way with the anger being unleashed so that it both validates individual experience and seeks the underlying collective and historical experience of women in patriarchal systems. Such systemic and historical understanding moves beyond blaming individual men (or women)—although, clearly, individuals are responsible for their behavior—and makes the larger connections that can point to new arenas for action on legal, legislative, political, as well as on personal levels. These connections must reflect our understanding of the structural and systemic violence that impacts all of us in different ways, i.e., sexism, racism, classism, heterosexism, nationalism, and the violation and abuse of the planet. This must become an integral part of our understanding of the larger context of child sexual abuse.

The naming of sexual abuse and violation committed by psychotherapists is part of this revolution. In Boston we have witnessed the formation of TELL, Therapist Exploitation Link Line, a support network for women who have been abused by psychotherapists. TELL provides a context for personal sharing and recovery. According to this model which views action as an essential part of recovery, the meetings include presentations of educational information about legal action and discussions of possibilities for legislative advocacy work.

We can all begin to relate to the larger context of such abuse by mental health professionals and to look carefully at the modal power and gender relations at the root of all patriarchal systems or power-over, hierarchical relationships. We need to explore the implications of such a power analysis for the therapy relationship. As we do so, we may be called "too political," or "not clinical," "underpathologizing," or "overidentified with the victims"—all comments that we have heard. It seems to me that a deep emotional response is appropriate and necessary for clinicians working with women survivors. A young psychiatric resident recently reported that she was told she should not work with a particular client because she was "too emotionally affected" by the horror of this woman's experience.

As clinicians, we are part of this revolution in consciousness. How can we deal effectively with our own experience and emotional responses as we work with clients who have been physically and sexually abused? One day last week I reviewed my day's experience. Several hours of therapy, supervision, and a case conference all focused primarily on the experience and impact of childhood physical and sexual abuse. I suspect many of us are experiencing a tremendous amount of anger and sadness as we take part in this work. There is potential for depression, unfocused anger, or for placing the weight of the anger on particular individual perpetrators. One woman psychologist recently told a colleague that she was becoming too angry, upset, and burnt out by her work. She stated that she knew she didn't want to see the depth and prevalence of the problem and what this really meant about our world. She pointed to the birth of her daughter as a possible reason she felt this so much more intensely.

I think we clinicians need to create relational conditions *for ourselves*, contexts that can help our anger become a resource for personal and political change—that can lead to our empowerment and not to isolation, burnout, clinical detachment, ineffective, angry outbursts, hostility, and emotional numbing or leaving our work. Jean and I suggest that such a context would include opportunities for in-depth personal sharing, relational interchange towards focusing and sustaining attention, clarity and understanding, and liberation of energy for action. We further need to create larger arenas for action towards social change.

As therapists, we have been empowered by our clients' courage to see, speak out, and break the silence, and we too can struggle together to become deeply responsive, empathic, and empowered clinicians. In doing so, we can move towards a mutual empowerment model which is fundamental to therapeutic and healing relationships (Surrey, 1987).

I hope we can continue to address these questions tonight and in subsequent colloquia. I look forward to hearing about your experiences working with and thinking about these issues.

DISCUSSION SUMMARY

A discussion was held after each colloquium presentation. Selected portions of the discussion are summarized here. At this session Judith Jordan, Alexandra

*Kaplan, and Irene Stiver joined Jean Baker Miller and Janet Surrey in leading
the discussion.*

Question: How can anger be expressed relationally in a relationship in which there is an imbalance of power, e.g., in a man–woman
relationship in which the woman is economically dependent on her
husband?

Jordan: It's very hard. As Jean said, if one person is dominant,
you can easily have coercion. You can have the subordinate person trying to express a grievance and the other person using power to silence
that expression.

Surrey: If both people in a man–woman relationship are really
trying to work towards mutuality, it may be possible. For example, in
couples work we sometimes see that men and women are on a different developmental path. If the man uses anger in a coercive way, he
may have to change the way he uses it or even cut it out for a while,
and the woman may have to learn to bring it in. So there may be a
double standard on the road to mutuality.

Kaplan: Perhaps to say something similar in slightly different
terms, for men a basic factor may be their assumed privilege which
becomes confounded with anger. What we may think of as anger as
an emotion can be for men, in some contexts, the expression of a
sense of entitlement—or their reaction if this entitlement is not granted. I think there can't be the relational use of anger in a situation of
power imbalance—at least, it takes enormous work to overcome that
factor.

Stiver: Some women in such marriages come to therapy with depression. They often find it easier to work on their sadness first. Of
course, the sadness is tied to not feeling free to express anger, or to put
it more fully, to acknowledge the degree of disappointment or hurt in
the relationship. Once they can touch the sadness, they often find
more clarity and more ability to begin to move the relationship to
something better.

I want to say, too, that anger—and all emotions—are not considered to be legitimate communication. You're supposed to just communicate some kind of objective content. The emotion is seen as getting in
the way of communication, rather than as expressing a meaning about
the communication. Anger is not just something that says something
hurts or is wrong; it says this is so important to me. Any emotion says
that.

We all see this in the work arena too, where we're supposed to
leave feelings out of communication as if the feelings were not a communication.

Question: How is this view of the separation between anger and aggression informing your own therapy?

Miller: I believe it makes a very big difference in the basic way I view anger. The traditional view of seeing anger linked with an instinct called aggression has acted to keep us with an underlying sense of anger as dangerous, always questioning and worrying about anger in our clients and in ourselves. It makes a very big difference to see it as a reaction, often very justified, to something that is wrong, rather than the expression of an aggressive instinct, that is, linked with a need to destroy.

Surrey: I would emphasize the importance of the interchange around anger. So often no one has engaged with a person about the anger. People have been left feeling all alone with the anger.

This approach has really helped me to keep my courage up and stay engaged with clients in their anger—including sometimes to express my anger back when something is hurting me. It's helped me to stay in the relationship, to really confront and stay engaged with the feelings.

Question: How can we raise our sons and daughters so they can be more comfortable with anger and we can be too?

Surrey: I think that what we were just saying about therapy is also true with children—staying engaged, actively responding and inquiring about what's wrong and about all of the feelings involved. Even if we can't always do this so well, we can look towards trying to really stay open, stay in the process, in the dialogue over time about these issues.

Question: It seems that you are using aggression to be almost synonymous with violence. What about the use of aggression in the sense of assertion? Also, what do you think of the idea of someone being passive-aggressive?

Miller: Some people still agree with the traditional Freudian idea that all constructive action comes out of an aggressive instinct by way of psychological mechanisms such as neutralization, transformation, and the like. Others believe that there exists something very different which can be called something like assertion. Gerald Stechler, for example, believes that babies exhibit these two different forms of behavior from early in life. Assertion is something like taking action in the world, a kind of forward movement. The other, which I believe he calls aggression, is a result of frustration, of being impeded. This kind of discussion has been going on in the field for a long time, and it continues. In most cases, however, I think anger is still linked with aggression.

In response to the second part of your question, I think that being passive-aggressive is one of the many ways that people can develop to deal with anger when they have not had the possibilities of dealing with anger directly and well in the relationships they've had.

Surrey: Just to add a word about assertion—the concept of self-assertion arises from a "separate self" paradigm and does not place the action in a relational context in which the intersubjective meanings and consequences are considered. I think it is more descriptive to call this action in a relational context or action in relationship.

Question: Why do adult women often have so much trouble expressing anger to their mothers? Do you think they feel that it will be seen as betraying their mothers' love?

Miller: Yes, that can be one major factor. I think many of us come to feel that where there is anger, there is a loss of love. This belief can exist for women both as recipients and expressers of anger. We need to learn to place anger as part of relationships, as part of love and, ultimately, of building better connection. I think we all have a long way to go in learning this.

REFERENCES

Averill, J. R. (1982). *Anger and aggression: An essay on emotion.* New York: Springer-Verlag.

Bernardez, T. (1988). *Women and anger: Cultural prohibitions and the feminine ideal.* (Work in Progress No. 31.) Wellesley, MA: Stone Center Working Paper Series.

Caplan P. (1989). *Don't blame mother: Mending the mothe—daughter relationship.* New York: Harper and Row.

Carlson, K. (1989). *In her image. The unhealed daughter's search for her mother.* Boston: Shambhala.

Conn, S. (1990). Protest and thrive: The relationship between global responsibility and personal empowerment. *New England Journal of Public Policy, 6*(1).

Dinnerstein, D. (1976). *The mermaid and the minotaur.* New York: Harper and Row.

Greenspan, M. (1983). *A new approach to women and therapy.* New York: McGraw Hill.

Harrison, B. (1985). *Making the connections.* Boston: Beacon Press.

Herman, J. (1989, June). Unpublished lecture. Stone Center/Cambridge Hospital Conference on Women, Boston, MA.

Heyward, C. (1984). *Our passion for justice.* New York: Pilgrim Press.

Jordan, J. (1989). *Relational development: Therapeutic implications of empathy and shame.* (Work in Progress No. 39). Wellesley, MA: Stone Center Working Paper Series. (Reprinted as Chapter 7, this volume)

Lerner, G. (1986). *The creation of patriarchy.* New York: Oxford University Press.

Lerner, H. (1985). *The dance of anger.* New York: Harper and Row.

Lyman, P. (1979, August 25). On rage and political memories. Paper presented at the Society for the Study of Social Problems, Boston, MA.

McAllister, P. (1982). *Reweaving the web of life: Feminism and nonviolence.* Philadelphia: New Society Publishers.

McBride, A. (1973). *The growth and development of mothers.* New York: Harper and Row.

Miller, J. B. (1983). *The construction of anger in women and men.* (Work in Progress No. 4.) Wellesley, MA: Stone Center Working Paper Series.

Miller, J. B. (1988). *Connections, disconnections and violations.* (Work in Progress No. 33). Wellesley, MA: Stone Center Working Paper Series.

Rich, A. (1976). *Of woman born: Motherhood as experience and institution.* New York: Norton.

Spielberger, C. D., Jacobs, S. A. & Crane, R. S. (1983). Assessment of anger: The state-trait anger scale. In J. N. Butcher & C. D. Spielberger (Eds.), *Advances in personality assessment,* vol. 2. Hillsdale, NJ: Erlbaum.

Stiver, I. & Miller, J. B. (1988). *From depression to sadness in women's psychotherapy.* (Work in Progress No. 36.) Wellesley, MA: Stone Center Working Paper Series.

Surrey, J. (1987). *Relationship and empowerment.* (Work in Progress No. 30.) Wellesley, MA: Stone Center Working Paper Series.

Travis, C. (1982). *Anger: The misunderstood emotion.* New York: Simon and Schuster.

This chapter was presented at a Stone Center Colloquium on March 7, 1990. © 1990 Jean Baker Miller and Janet L. Surrey.

11

From Depression to Sadness in Women's Psychotherapy

IRENE P. STIVER
JEAN BAKER MILLER

Current literature tells us that twice as many women as men experience depressive periods, and one out of ten women can expect to have a serious depression in her life[1] (Weissman & Klerman, 1977). Married women in particular are more prone to develop depressions than both married men and single women who are heads of households (Radloff, 1986). Some workers stress difficulty in the marital relationship as a precipitant of depression in women rather than the marital status per se (Weissman & Klerman, 1987).

Traditional theoretical and psychodynamic approaches to depression do not adequately take into account this greater incidence of depression in women, nor do they help us understand these striking findings. Newman (1984) has raised questions about the accuracy of the diagnostic methods which lead to the findings of higher rates of depression in women. While this point awaits further clarification, we know that depression is certainly very common in women. In papers which emphasize a relational conception of women's development, Kaplan (1984) and Jack (1987) have offered new views on depression.

---

[1] The exception is manic depression which occurs at an equal rate in women and in men. This finding is consistent with other data which suggest a greater biological component to this condition (Weissman & Klerman, 1987).

Kaplan notes that some of the key elements of depression, such as inhibition of activity, inhibition of anger and low self-esteem are in fact encouraged in women's development. They are very similar to the characteristics used to describe women in our culture, e.g., the need to please others, to accommodate to the expectations of others, not to listen to one's own wishes and to blame oneself for one's unhappiness. Jack describes women's relational self coming into conflict with societal and familial social norms of the "good woman" and "good wife." These views lead the women "to lose themselves in the process of trying to establish an intimacy they never attained" (p. 179) because others were not there for them, nor allowing and encouraging them to engage authentically.

We would like to continue the exploration of why women become depressed. We will do this through a focus on sadness, and consider some therapeutic implications of this emphasis.

SADNESS AND DEPRESSION

Depression has been classified and divided in a variety of categories including depression as a personality type, neurotic and psychotic depressions, and endogenous and reactive depressions. Although we will be discussing clinical depressions which are reactive to a range of life events, we will also be talking about those women who have a history of an underlying depression and are vulnerable to become more acutely depressed when existing coping methods are disrupted by stress in their current lives. We believe that many women have been depressed over long periods of time, largely as a consequence of disconnections in their day-to-day experiences with the people important to them. As Kaplan noted (1984), the losses in women's lives are not of "oral" and "narcissistic supplies" as the traditional literature indicates, but rather of the *opportunity to participate* more fully in relationships, with both authenticity and a sense of empowerment.

The kind of chronic depression which many women experience occurs along a continuum of dysphoric reactions from mild to more severe expressions of underlying hopelessness, low self-esteem, a sense of helplessness or powerlessness in effecting any change in their lives and with a more or less constricted self-concept. These characteristics become more intense and more symptomatic when an acute depressive episode develops; in addition, depressive symptoms would then include a profoundly dysphoric mood, retardation of functioning, suicidal ideation and the potential for suicidal behavior.

We would like to delineate depression as a clinical syndrome from the emotion of sadness. This distinction will help to clarify the psychological meanings of each. In addition, the distinction between sadness and depression has important implications for the psychotherapy of depressed women.

Considerable confusion exists in the literature in the variety of terms used to talk about dysphoric experiences, such as sadness, sorrow, melancholia and mild and severe depression. Some writers use sadness, sorrow and depression interchangeably, while others carefully distinguish sadness as "a normal emotion" from depression as a pathological state. With the exception of those more biologically oriented who view depression as a distinct illness with particular biochemical and genetic characteristics, most writers tend to see sadness on a continuum leading to depression.

Freud, in his classic paper, "Mourning and Melancholia" (1917/1961), said that mourning was characterized by "normal grief" in response to a major loss, while melancholia was a more pathological reaction. Unlike normal grief, it was accompanied by a significant lowering of self-regard and an intensification of guilt feelings. Gutheil (1959) believes that pessimism adds the element that changes sadness to depression. Arieti and Bemporad (1978), in talking about "mild depression," say that it "is difficult to differentiate it from the feeling of depression as a normal emotion, generally called sadness, which is part of the gamut of feelings of the average individual" (p. 63).

We would like to suggest that, phenomenologically, significant and qualitative differences exist between sadness and depression. It is a difference between a "feeling state" and a state in which feelings are hidden; what is left is a "nonfeeling state" but with clear dysphoric components. Although we do not see sadness and depression on the same continuum, we do believe that when there is not an adequate relational context in which sadness can be experienced, expressed and validated, depressive reactions develop.

The relative lack of attention to sadness and its role in depression may occur because sadness is a powerful emotion. Intense affect is often seen as more characteristic of women's experience than men's. It is both devalued in our culture and threatening to those who are more defended. Not only does no entry exist for sadness in the indexes of many major books on depression, but our own professions give little attention to helping trainees (and more experienced clinicians) recognize, identify and experience their patients' sad feelings with them. The tendency in our culture to admire and value more stoical responses and to devalue intense open expressions of sadness and grief occurs in family settings and to a large extent in the practice of traditional psychotherapy as well.

In particular, the resistances in families to help others, especially children, stay with their feelings of sadness and disappointment probably follow from the readiness with which parents experience their children's feelings of pain as accusations which lead mothers and fathers to feel they are bad parents. Also, parents sometimes find it intolerable to endure what they imagine their children experience when they do feel sad. In any event, when children find that the very people to whom they look for support when they encounter disappointments in life are not truly available to them and do not legitimize or even tolerate their feelings, they often conclude that they should not have such feelings, that they are somehow to blame for whatever led to those feelings, and they soon learn to hide and defend against the feelings.

We believe that the major task in therapy is to help our women patients who are depressed move from that nonfeeling and defensive state to an affective experience in which their sadness can be recognized and validated. We often ask patients who are diagnosed as depressed whether they are feeling sad or depressed. At first, they often look confused and indicate that they don't know the difference or that they feel both. Then we elaborate, "When I ask if you feel sad, I mean something like do you feel close to tears, are the tears connected with sad images, losses of important people, do you feel a lump in your throat, does your heart feel like it's breaking sometimes, does it sometimes feel like unbearable grief? These feelings," we add, "may be different from feeling 'depressed'; that may be more like feeling in a black pit or a deep tunnel, bleak and heavy, with no sense of any hope or light at the other end, without many images other than doing away with oneself, seeing no way out of the muddle, and feeling that one is a bad person and that nothing can change that." Patients sometimes have further elaborated this description of depression with such phrases as, "feeling dead inside" and "feeling like I am always under a black cloud."

When we have asked these questions, many people can differentiate immediately between sadness and depression. Some are able to say they know both states and can remember instances in which they felt one or the other. For example, one of us interviewed recently a 30-year-old married mother of two young children who was acutely suicidal. While she believes she has been depressed for many years, the suicidal ideation has escalated over recent months. Most significant, for many years, beginning at age four, she was sexually abused by her brother-in-law. Although she told her mother and sister about the abuse, they left her feeling unprotected and did not acknowledge her deep fears. When asked whether she was feeling sad or depressed, with the elaborations outlined above, she stated very clearly, "Depressed." She went on to say she saw no purpose in continuing to live; she was "a torture to her husband," and if she died, she would save her children from her "terrible influence."

She said she felt completely trapped in her marriage since she could not bear to have her husband touch her. However, she could not see herself existing without him. Similarly, she could not bear her worries about her children's well-being and felt that she deserved to be punished by God who would take away her children. As she said all this, she maintained a completely flat and matter-of-fact mood as though she had thought it all out logically, and that's how it was. When asked if she remembered feeling sad sometimes, she responded immediately, saying, "Yes, only two weeks ago when I visited my father-in-law in the hospital after he had a heart attack." She really cared for her husband's family; and as she sat with her father-in-law, she held his hand to reassure him, wanted to cry and felt very sad. We might speculate that the threat of losing her father-in-law put her momentarily in touch with her yearnings for a father who would have been more protective of her and as caring as her father-in-law, but those yearnings were too painful for her to tolerate.

Another woman's father had been in a coma for months. She had been anticipating his death for some time but rarely felt in touch with her sadness about losing him. Typically, she did not acknowledge the importance of this imminent loss and reported, instead, that she had no energy, felt tired all the time, and was oversleeping. She missed appointments and "didn't give a shit" about anything. Alternatively, she became enraged at the ways she felt her life had been wasted because her father did not recognize that she had such a need for his help when she was younger. At those times she couldn't hold any caring feelings for her father.

These reactions can be described as depressive or as some ineffectual attempts to flee from both her depression and the underlying sadness. The therapeutic work at times does lead her to an awareness of her terror of losing her father, her shock and sorrow at seeing him change from a person of enormous stature into a "wizened little man, paralyzed and unable to speak, like a nonperson." She then talks of missing him and of those times when they were connected and he talked to her and tried to help her plan her life. At these times she becomes tearful, and on rare occasions she sobs as she acknowledges how much she loves him and how unbearable it was for her when he was not responsive to her.

Although both women seemed to ward off sadness more than depression, they reported feeling less empty, more substantial and less alone when they experienced the sadness more directly. Indeed, we believe that if therapy moves productively, a shift occurs from depression to sadness which, in turn, leads to a shift away from hopelessness. A major increase in the woman's sense of worth occurs when she feels she has feelings, a change from the kind of person who has no feelings. Although all people feel great relief when they can feel again, women are often particularly self-condemning when they believe that they have no feelings. The optimal therapeutic situation would allow for a legitimizing of the woman's painful feelings, being truly with her as she "stays with the feelings" and seeing these feelings in the context of her relational needs and the pain she experienced when these needs were not met.

Perhaps the major difference between sadness and depression is that the depressive experience is very isolating and nonrelational. It is exquisitely self-centered in that the person has withdrawn from others and has focused on her personal defects, often around concerns about appearance and performance; essentially, this focus represents displacements from the more important concerns associated with feelings about those significant relationships which have been deeply disappointing or have been lost. Thus, the person may often feel stupid, ugly, evil, not likeable, etc. A deep sense of hopelessness, helplessness and self-blame accompanies these self-perceptions since she believes that nothing can change them.

On the other hand, genuine feelings of sadness enhance the experience of connection with others and increase self-esteem. Sadness, unlike depression, allows for more direct awareness of the meaning and importance of lost relationships or disappointments in existing relationships. This, we believe, follows from the woman's increased sense of connection with her self through the direct experience of feeling something "real." This feeling leads to an increased sense of authenticity as well as increased empowerment which, in turn, begins the process of moving away from the depressive and isolated position.

Without a safe relational context which is responsive to the depth of a depressed person's underlying sadness, the depressive position is in some sense preferred, since one often has the illusion of being less vulnerable in isolation than one feels when in danger of abandonment. This state of alienation, however, maintains the person in the depressive position; it becomes more and more threatening to expose one's vulnerability to a world which is perceived as either unresponsive or hostile and critical. Simultaneously, the person feels more and more undeserving of help from others.

AN ILLUSTRATION

Our basic notion is that many women who suffer depression have not been able to experience their sadness and, most important, have not been able to experience it within a context of empathic and validating relationships. There is one major reason why this occurs: The people in the surrounding context of relationships (and often society in general) do not recognize that a disappointment or loss has occurred. Alternatively, they may recognize that some kind of loss has occurred, but they do not recognize its significance or magnitude *for* the woman. Not only do they not help the woman acknowledge the loss, they often actively prevent her from doing so and, therefore, contribute to severe confusion and self-doubt. Sometimes the woman initially may have some sense of her feelings, but people around her are conveying the strong message that she shouldn't have them. There's no reason to have them; so if anything is wrong, it must be that something is wrong with her.

One of us worked on a project on stillbirths some years ago which illustrates this point. This study was begun by Bourne (1968) and Lewis (1976) in London in the 1960s. They had observed that women who suffered stillbirths often became depressed and/or experienced a great deal of trouble with the next baby. They also noticed that almost everyone connected with the stillbirth acted as if it hadn't happened and fled from the whole experience as quickly as they could. It was what they called a "nonevent." Almost no one in the woman's life would allow her her sadness nor be with her in it. This included the husband or male partner, the woman's mother, father, sisters and other family members as well as friends, the nurses and certainly the doctors. Almost everyone said platitudinous kinds of things like, "Cheer up. You're young. You'll get pregnant again and have a baby soon." However, the woman couldn't forget about it and couldn't cheer up.

Hospital procedures reinforced the definition of the situation as a "nonevent." The dead child usually was not given a name; there was no funeral or any ritual; the child was not brought to the parents and thus was never seen by them.

Bourne and Lewis believed that the mothers' depression and the troubles with the next child could be prevented if the mothers could experience their sadness. Lewis tried to work with hospital staff members to convince them to bring the baby to the mother and father, to encourage the parents to give the child a name and to have a proper funeral and burial. He was not making much headway with hospital staffs. In many instances, staff members became very angry and often characterized the proposals as cruel. (We believe that staff members reacted this way because they had not been trained in dealing with the sadness and were afraid to have to deal with it openly in their work.)

Almost by chance a woman newspaper columnist heard of this work. She herself had had a stillbirth and had gone through the same depression and terrible feelings of isolation. She wrote one column on the topic, and hundreds of letters from women poured in to the newspaper, all confirming her experience.

After this public expression, real change occurred. The recommended alterations in hospital routines came about, and now there are self-help groups for women who've experienced stillbirths, as well as other reproductive losses. In general, because some societal institutions now recognize this event, the people around the women (their partners, families and friends) are beginning to acknowledge that something has happened and to be with the women in their experiences of loss. That is, society now has defined what is happening in a fashion which includes more of the truth of the women's experience. This new societal definition of events renders other people more able to recognize their sadness too. The whole picture has improved.

Before these changes occurred we saw some of the women in treatment, sometimes along with the whole family. The woman's depression was very striking. Usually her sense of isolation and of being alone with these feelings was very powerful. Sometimes the husband's sadness appeared very obvious, but he rarely could stay with it and not veer off. Thus, the woman was usually "carrying" the sadness that the husband (and sometimes other family members too) did not let themselves experience together with the woman.

We thought that this story would help to illustrate our central point because this issue now appears so clear, although it was not at all clear initially. Further, it offers an example of how preventive work, and even some change in societal definitions of reality, can come about. However, it is not a good example in other ways. For one, it may be clearer because it concerns a discrete and dramatic event. It is not like the many disappointments and disconnections which occur over long lengths of time throughout many women's lives. These are causes for sadness which are much harder for others to understand, and even the woman herself to recognize. Second, the frequent causes for sadness in a woman's life usually are not physical like a stillbirth; rather, they are the actions of the people closest to the woman, often members of her immediate family or her partner. We will describe a woman whose experience illustrates these much less obvious points.

CLINICAL EXAMPLES

Mrs. A. is a 48-year-old woman, married to a very successful lawyer. She has two daughters, ages 19 and 24. She entered therapy with symptoms of a clinical depression, including tearfulness, insomnia, loss of appetite and irritability. She was described by her husband as "difficult" at home. She talked about what a bad mother and bad wife she felt she was, although she had many complaints about her husband. The husband had contacted a psychiatrist he knew personally who made the referral, describing these depressive symptoms and suggesting that issues about aging were probably the underlying precipitant.

At the first session Mrs. A. said she was "an alcoholic," that she had been trying to tell her husband this for some time, but he did not take her seriously. She had told one other person, her physician, who told her he took it very seriously and would call her husband and discuss it with him. He never called, and she never returned to see him.

Although she attributed much of her bad feeling about herself to her alcoholism, she stated clearly that she was not prepared to stop drinking. She believed she would never have the courage to do so. She often became quite tearful but without any sad content to her thoughts; instead, the tears usually accompanied her feeling powerless to change her life and her deep feelings of frustration about her husband and her problems at work. She was always having angry outbursts and creating scenes at home which she saw as "childish" attempts to get her husband's attention or to get him to take her seriously. After each of these scenes, her depression intensified.

Early in our work together I had remarked several times that she looked very sad to me. She told me much later that she hadn't any idea what I was talking about, and she did not then know what being sad meant. She did know, however, that she felt awful and desperate. She stated that she wanted to stop drinking, which she did secretly and alone, but she could not imagine existing without the numbing effects of alcohol. Although she did not understand what I meant by "sadness," she felt that I did take her seriously and in particular knew that I appreciated how much she both wanted to continue to drink and to stop drinking.

I continued in a very low-key fashion to suggest that she attend some Alcoholics Anonymous meetings and gave her a meeting book. I told her she did not have to stop drinking until she was ready, but she could go to AA meetings and would get help there learning how to stop, how to move from the stuck position she was in currently. Six months after she entered therapy, she began to attend some selected AA meetings, and three months after that she did, in fact, stop drinking. She became quite actively involved in AA and also joined a women's substance abuse group.

One day she was telling me that the previous evening she had felt an urgent need to phone each of her two daughters who were living in different cities at some distance from her. The daughters had spent the previous weekend visiting each other. The main reason for this urgent need to call them was that she felt very sad about the effects her alcoholism may have had on them, and she wanted to persuade them to attend Adult Children of Alcoholics meetings.

In the phone conversation her older daughter told her that she wished she had taken time off from school some years ago as had her younger sister. My patient remembered then that there had been some discussion about this several years ago, and both she and her husband had been dead set against it. Remembering it all, she felt even sadder and began to weep. She said to her daughter, "I wish I had been able to be there for you then, to listen to your wish to do that then, but I could not hear you—all I cared about was how I was going to get my next drink. I feel so sad that I failed you then."

This encounter seemed to both my patient and me a clear indication that she had just taken an enormous step. Precisely *through* her ability to be sad, she was more empowered than ever before to establish a more mutual relationship with her children, who certainly felt closer to her as a consequence of these changes in her.

As Mrs. A. moved out of the depressive position and as she no longer numbed her feelings with alcohol, she was able with genuine sad affect to speak about those disappointments in her life that really mattered. For example, she felt her husband was very much the center of her life, yet saw in a variety of ways how little she was the center of his life. She viewed him as a good and decent man, but felt he could not listen to her. Instead, he expected that she be available to meet his needs. His needs included her hostessing social events important to his career, even when she felt it put her in jeopardy to participate in situations which involved serving alcohol.

As we talked about this issue, she brought in a letter from her mother which she felt was typical although she had never truly noticed it before. Her mother had suffered from recurrent depressions for many years and had always deferred to her father. The striking thing about the letter was that it was replete with phrases such as, "your father thought," "your father said," "your father would like." She began to see some similar patterns in her own marriage. Another moment of genuine sadness occurred when she was talking about a special occasion in the past when she had wished her father had given her a fur coat. At first she berated herself for being so petty and then began to weep, which astonished her. She was surprised that she felt so deeply about what seemed to her to be such a trivial matter. She was able to stay with the sadness when I suggested that what she wanted from her father, who was a very reserved and withdrawn man, was an expression of his caring for her, a sign that he valued her and wanted to respond to her needs.

A year later when her father died and she went to see her mother, her mother's first words to her were, "I am free!" Although my patient was amazed to hear this from her mother, she had done enough work around her own depression and sadness and the struggles in her marriage, to hear what her mother said in the context of her mother's depression and the nature of her life with her father. It proved very liberating and it allowed her to feel more empowered in her relationships with her mother, husband and children.

Two other brief illustrations highlight the ways in which current life events precipitate more acute depressive reactions in women. The meanings of these life events in the context of the woman's experience are often misunderstood. For example, a woman in her 50s, married to a very powerful businessman for 30 years, became acutely depressed after a family argument. The marriage had been difficult from the start, but she had learned to accommodate to her husband's many demands, including performing as hostess of large parties and accompanying him on many business trips. She felt considerable underlying resentment towards him and often felt used and exploited by him. But she played her part, and she in turn was given many material things in the form of jewelry, fur coats and the like. She had a very close relationship with a younger sister who lived nearby and who was frequently at her house.

As a result of a major family argument between her husband and her sister's husband, her husband banished the sister from the house and insisted that her name never be mentioned again. The patient's more chronic depressive state developed into an acute clinical depression at that point. We would speculate that the major impetus to the depression was less the friction with her husband, her anger at him and her "identification" with her sister (which were certainly all there), but more the loss of her relationship with her sister. This relationship had allowed her to tolerate her sadness and profound disappointment in the marriage, and she could, therefore, stay on the nonsymptomatic side of her depression. The loss of her sister confronted her more dramatically with the disappointments she had with her husband, and she felt completely alone to cope with her vulnerability about all the feelings stirred up in this situation.

Another woman who was also in a disappointing marriage became depressed after her mother died. A more traditional understanding of this case would suggest that her depression represented a pathological grief reaction to the loss of her mother with whom she had an ambivalent relationship. Closer scrutiny suggests another story. This woman came from a very protected, conservative background. At age 18 she fell in love with her husband who was very handsome and charming; she looked forward to a romantic and sexual relationship with him and to having many children. She learned very early, however, that her husband was not very interested in sex or children. After 10 years they finally did have one child.

She felt sustained by her relationship with this daughter, with whom she was very close, but also by frequent telephone contact with her mother, whom she saw as her closest friend. They spoke to each other often, and she felt her mother was the one person who helped her, as she said, "keep my head on straight." When her mother died, she lost the one person who helped her tolerate her deep disappointment in her husband and offered her an empathic relationship to counter the isolation she felt in her marriage. Again, this case could easily be misunderstood, and she would be identified as too dependent on her mother.

THEORETICAL ISSUES

We will examine briefly the current theoretical understandings of the dynamics of depression. They are based largely on early psychoanalytic formulations with modifications introduced by ego psychologists and object relations theorists. None of these dynamic formulations addresses why depression is so prevalent in women nor explores the role of sadness in the therapeutic work with seriously depressed women.

Although our interest here is in the psychological rather than biochemical and genetic aspects of depression, it is important to note that hormonal, biological and genetic hypotheses offered to account for these gender differences have not to date yielded consistent findings (Weissman & Klerman, 1977; Weissman & Klerman, 1987).

While there are a number of important differences among the various theorists, there are some common themes which reflect the prevailing assumptions about the etiology of depression. The early psychoanalytic writers recognized the significance of loss as a major precipitant of depression. However, they believed that those most vulnerable to depression were fixated at the oral stage where they had experienced the first major loss through deprivation and rejection. Abraham (1927), Freud (1917/1961) and others thought that the depressed person's earliest relationship with the mother was characterized by a profound ambivalence in which loving feelings were blocked by hateful feelings. The hateful or angry feelings were, however, repressed because of fear of further loss and were expressed through self-recriminations, guilty feelings and the like.

The recurrent themes are that those people vulnerable to depression were fixated at the oral stage and were, therefore, unusually dependent and needy; these individuals regressed to this dependent, needy state when confronted with losses later in life. Since their relationships with their mothers were characterized as "ambivalent and narcissistic," they were unable to sustain loving feelings; and their intense, hostile and angry feelings were too dangerous to express; anger was then repressed and turned inward, and thus contributed to the depressive symptomatology of low self-esteem and guilt.

Bibring (1953) offered a somewhat different model of depression. He saw it as a state of helplessness of the ego which arose when there was too great a discrepancy between the appraisal of one's own abilities on the one hand and one's level of aspiration on the other. Although he postulated a range of life circumstances which could create such a state of helplessness—from aspirations to hold on to the lost person even in the face of death, to entertaining grandiose expectations for recognition and success—he believed there needed to be an earlier vulnerability based on fixations at any one of the psychosexual levels of development. Even later writers of the interpersonal school, such as Arieti and Bemporad (1978), also came down to a model which goes back to the early years when the vulnerability for depression was firmly established.

Most important, through focusing so consistently on early loss and fixation, these theories do not acknowledge the *power* of those life experiences which precipitate or trigger appropriate sad reactions. In this chapter we are suggesting that the very lack of recognition of the legitimacy of the sad responses to life events results in the sadness going underground and the ultimate development of depressive symptomatology This sequence was illustrated in the examples of women whose sorrow and sadness about their stillbirths went unacknowledged, and who became depressed; and in the vignettes of women who were profoundly disappointed in their relationships with their husbands but did not feel entitled to their sadness and thus became depressed.

Epidemiological studies of depression suggest that life events and social connections correlate significantly with depression (Belle, 1982; Paykel, 1982; Turner et al., 1974). The classic Brown and Harris study (1978) found four vulnerability (background) factors for depression in their samples of depressed women: having three or more children under 14 living at home, lacking employment away from home, loss of a mother before the age of 11 and lack of an intimate, confiding relationship with a husband or boyfriend. While there are no comparable findings with samples of depressed men, these vulnerability factors do speak to some of the significant life circumstances confronting many women; it is also likely that there is little recognition in the day-to-day lives of these women of the power of these events to evoke sorrowful and sad reactions. The stage is then set for the women to develop more severe depressive reactions when faced with a loss or traumatic event in their lives.

Other empirical studies have raised questions about the roles that dependency and anger play in depression. As noted earlier, most psychodynamic explanations of depression have stressed early deprivation of "oral supplies," rejection, abandonment, etc., which resulted in a lack of resolution of dependency needs. Such individuals, usually women since women are most vulnerable to be labeled dependent in this pejorative way, are considered at risk to become depressed in response to later life events which recapitulate these earlier deprivations. However, Weissman and Paykel (1974) report that although dependency was a characteristic of the depressed state, it was not an enduring feature of the depressed women. When the depressed women recovered they were not found to be more dependent than the nondepressed women. It is also likely that a misunderstanding of behaviors labeled as "dependent" in depressed women contributes to maintaining the woman in the depressed state.

We would like to suggest that when a woman is depressed this "nonfeeling state" keeps her out of touch with her true emotions. As a consequence, she becomes more and more fearful of making a move to effect any kind of change and might certainly appear "passive," "dependent," and "stuck." In reviewing the literature on depression, it is impressive to see how highly pejorative and judgmental is the language used to describe the so-called "dependency" of the depressed person, e.g., clinging, demanding, greedy, voracious, devouring, and the like.

Empirical observations also do not support the assumption that depression is a consequence of repressed anger. Weissman and Paykel report that the depressed women they studied were in fact more hostile and angrier than the women in the control group. Interestingly they found that indications of the hostility of depressed women were rarely apparent to the psychiatrists interviewing them or seeing them in treatment but were reported to be observed readily by family members. In particular, children were often the targets of the depressed women's anger.

We believe that the anger does erupt more forcefully for some women as they become less defended and more depressed in response to significant life events, but that the anger feels dystonic, threatening and guilt-provoking. When women experience disappointments in the important relationships in their lives, feelings of deep frustration and anger develop but are shut out of awareness for several reasons. We know that women have a history of difficulty feeling entitled to their anger and coping with it (Bernardez-Bonesatti, 1978; Miller, 1983), and that they are very afraid that expressions of anger will jeopardize what relational possibilities they believe they do have. Also, women are threatened by the possibility of hurting those they care about.

What is perhaps even more central is that the depressed woman has not dared to be fully aware of the nature of her disappointments. A lifetime of not listening to her own thoughts and feelings and a lack of belief that she is entitled to feel bad keep her disappointments out of awareness. We believe that many women find after marriage that they do not have the kind of relationship they have expected all their lives, in which their husbands want to know their experiences and value the whole relational process. Because the depressed woman then is not clear why she is angry, she often finds reasons in the form of complaints, tantrums and irritable outbursts over apparently trivial matters (Bernardez, 1988). All of these behaviors confirm her sense of herself as unreasonable, bad and unworthy and contribute to self-sabotaging behaviors in her relationships.

As a result, expressions of anger are not liberating, but rather maintain the depressive spiral of isolation, guilt and self-hate. The therapeutic techniques many of us learned to use with depressed people, to help them get their anger "out" instead of turned inward, often has disastrous consequences. We have seen instances of depressed women becoming more suicidal after they have been encouraged to be more expressive of their anger in therapy sessions.

Instead, therapeutic work should help women patients to appreciate why they are angry and to understand why it is so hard to be angry. Through this approach women often can see more clearly how angry they have been for a very long time, why they did not understand it and consequently felt helpless and powerless to move with it.

The therapeutic encounter can then offer a safe place to risk the expression of authentic feelings, such as sadness and anger. When this relational context is characterized by empathic understanding, women begin to clarify what they are feeling and appreciate the meaning and legitimacy of what they are sad about. Through this process they can begin to feel empowered to move out of the position of isolation and self-hate.

As stated earlier, we believe that many women become depressed when there is no place for them to experience the anguish associated with significant disappointments and losses in the important relationships in their lives. We suggested too that culture at large, and family settings as well, do not readily tolerate and legitimize women's painful feelings in response to life events.

Married women in particular often feel that they have no right to "complain" if their husbands are decent men, offer financial security and if their children are healthy and "OK"; yet we know many such women do get depressed—and they typically blame themselves and are blamed by others as wanting too much, being too dependent or having many "complaints." Rubin (1976) reports that working-class women, asked what they value most in their husbands will say, "He's a steady worker, he doesn't drink, he doesn't hit me" (p. 93). However, we also know that among the significant variables countering depression in these women is having a husband or boyfriend who can be a confidant.

In fact, many women feel deep disappointment in the important relationships in their lives, but they often feel unable to act to change the situation because the important people and the whole surrounding culture do not provide the framework of thoughts and words with which they can even begin to formulate—let alone express—what they are feeling and seeking. They cannot become empowered. It is the very experience of being disempowered that contributes to lack of self-worth, a deep sense of failure and self-blame and an inability to identify and feel entitled to those things which really matter—i.e., connections in the way women are seeking them. This is, of course, the set of conditions which will inevitably lead to further immobilization and depression.

The most growth-enhancing therapeutic encounters are those that provide for the mutual experience of connection through the therapist's readiness to be with the patient in her pain. All of us have our sorrows, and all of us need the relational opportunities to feel them. It is the process of being truly moved by whatever our patients are experiencing that contributes to the mutuality of the relationship and the empathic experience. And it is this process which empowers both therapist and patient to move out of the depressive position.

All of us who have worked with depressed patients know how readily the therapist begins to feel hopeless, disempowered and depressed in the face of the patient's isolation and disconnection. The patient is unable to identify what she is truly feeling and does not feel entitled to her sadness; instead, she feels unworthy as well as deeply resentful and consistently defies any offer of help. This maintains the depressive spiral.

This constellation can be interrupted through the therapist's efforts to help identify the underlying sadness and by "bearing" together with the patient what appear as unbearably intense emotions. For it is the very expression of authentic feelings which strengthens the connection between patient and therapist and allows them both to move in a mutually empowering way. The patient then is no longer feeling alone and bereft. As she feels more understood and as her own feelings develop more clarity and expression, she can experience more positive self-worth and can begin to hope for and move towards more gratifying connections in the future.

DISCUSSION SUMMARY

After each colloquium presentation a discussion was held. Selected portions of the discussion are summarized here. At this session Drs. Judith Jordan, Alexandra Kaplan, and Janet Surrey joined Dr. Stiver in leading the discussion.

Question: I wonder if you could say something about sadness and anger in the therapy with women who are recovering from sexual abuse and also from battering relationships.

Stiver: That is a very relevant question since women who have been sexually abused or battered often have had to split off many feelings, particularly their sadness and anger.

The sadness will be difficult to touch for some time. Instead, there are the more depressive symptoms—despair, self-hate and isolation.

Still, I believe the sadness needs to be addressed before the anger. The anger probably would be the more dangerous feeling to experience, at least early in the treatment since it would be experienced as threatening the relationship with the abuser or the batterer, despite how horrendous that relationship may be. Often that person is the only person the woman feels any connection with—and she cannot tolerate the possibility of jeopardizing it.

Jordan: One of the reasons that groups for incest victims and battered women are so powerful is that as women begin to listen to stories told by other women who have experienced similar horrible situations, they begin to get in touch with their own feelings—they begin to develop some empathy for their own experiences as well. This becomes a very meaningful way to bring the feelings back into connection.

Kaplan: For abused or battered women the sadness is particularly profound because it is related to a loss of self, of feeling so bad and so tainted and without any self-worth. I think the anger comes only later, after there is some distance from the relationship with the abuser and more of a sense of self.

Question: In the stillborn situation you said that the father was also sad but not expressing the sadness. Why didn't he get depressed? Also, why does the mother take on the father's sadness along with her own?

Stiver: That's a very big and complicated question; it relates to the still unsettled question of why depression, in general, is more common in women than in men. I think there are major differences in the developmental paths for men and women which lead women to be more in touch with feelings in many ways and to have a greater awareness of how important relationships are to them, while men are raised to be less in touch with their feelings and less aware of how important relationships are to them.

Some people think that men defend against depression in other ways, for example, in alcohol abuse or acting out in more antisocial behavior because they take flight from feelings into action. However, I think that's a bit oversimplified. I think that men have found other avenues in which they can direct their energies such as the work arena. They become involved in performance and in doing things which can serve as ways of avoiding feelings and not dealing with what's going on in relationships. At the same time, men are usually better taken care of. Although they don't have to acknowledge relationships as important to them, they often are surrounded by those who provide relationships for them.

Comment: In my experience working with many babies who were born deformed, I think there was a lot of denial by the fathers—more by the fathers than the mothers. I think the men tended to wall off the grief. To experience the grief would be to admit that "something in my seed could have caused the deformity." There was a need to deny that responsibility. The women were much more open to experiencing it. In addition, the mother carried the child for nine months and had a relationship with it.

Stiver: I'm reminded of Zetzel's notion. She didn't distinguish between sadness and depression, but she talked about gender differences in depression. She described women as much more able to tolerate and stay with the experience of painful feelings but then not able to move out of them; while men avoid the subjective experience of painful feelings but move into instrumental action prematurely. With the stillbirths, the men's tendency more often may have been to rush to some action, some "solution," instead of knowing how they felt. Women are often caught in a more disempowered position of feeling bad and not knowing how to move out of it.

Surrey: I also think the painful feelings would be much more dystonic for men because of the way men are raised. Often there wouldn't be that much relief for a man to cry with somebody because it would cause so much conflict for him.

Kaplan: I think you're suggesting, too, that the actual experience may be a different one for the woman and the man. The woman had a relationship with the baby she carried for nine months. For the man it was more of a question of whether he "failed" if he thought that something was wrong with his sperm.

Comment: We have to look at the ways in which society at large makes it difficult for men to express their feelings and to be in a relational mode, to show their vulnerability.

Stiver: I think that's absolutely true; and, further, there's a cycle that follows from that. When men have been raised for so many years in that way, they need to ward off those expressions of feelings in others too. A kind of spiraling effect follows. The men have much more trouble tolerating these feelings in women; then the women feel more and more frustrated and unheard and in turn find it very hard both to honor their own feelings and to understand the hidden feelings in men. This spiral leads to depression.

Question: It sounds like you are implying that traditional marriage is a very sad business. If that is so, what would you suggest we do about it?

Stiver: The literature is not totally clear, but some studies suggest that marriage is more of a protective experience for men and more risky for women. Other studies suggest that marital difficulties correlate very highly with depression in women. Women go into marriage hoping to have "a mutually empathic relationship" with all that implies. Often the women meet with frustration and disappointment.

In order to appreciate this familiar experience, it's important to see how men and women usually enter marriage from very different pathways with different experiences and expectations. Although we can assume that men also hope to find in marriage a partner responsive to their relational needs, I don't think this is consciously experienced in quite the same way. And paradoxically men more often do have their relational needs responded to without having to acknowledge them. Also, men have found other avenues of trying to find gratification in their lives, which is what they have been taught—that is through work, performance, etc. It is difficult then for them to be responsive to their wives' relational needs.

As to what to do about it, that's the big question. I can respond to the individual situation rather than to the larger societal question. Certainly we all know that in our work with some couples the men do begin to feel more comfortable with their feelings and as a consequence more able to honor their own and their wives' relational needs. In other couples there sometimes is little change, and the men are not motivated to continue the work. Perhaps more innovative changes need to be developed.

Surrey: There are some recent data which show that the state of women's friendships, whatever their marital situation, is predictive of overall mental health—and also depression.

Kaplan: We know that women often say that if they really want to talk, they'll talk to their women friends. Women often seek out a relational context and friends outside of their marriage, and there are certainly women who choose women as partners and don't try to work out a relationship with men. The finding that Gilligan and her colleagues report is relevant. Women tend to be more anxious in the face of isolation and more comfortable with intimacy, but with men it's the reverse.

Jordan: I think a lot of the work has to be done with the men, helping to increase their tolerance for affect, particularly for the kinds of affect we're talking about today—sadness and other vulnerable feelings. The men in our culture are so socialized against feeling these feelings. If we could help men to open up to these feelings in themselves, they could then be open to them with their partners. The other need is to help open up an increased relational awareness in all people. We're not talking about you versus me—self-sacrifice versus self-glorification—but about developing a consciousness of the relationship of "we."

Surrey: I would say that women also have difficulty managing close relationships, all kinds of relationships, sexual and nonsexual. As a culture we have a lot of work to do in all relationships, not just male–female relationships. Mother–daughter relationships are especially significant. So I don't think we should totally focus on the male–female relationship.

REFERENCES

Abraham, K. (1927). Notes on the psychoanalytic investigation and treatment of manic-depressive insanity and allied conditions. In *Selected papers* (pp. 137–156). London: Hogarth Press.

Arieti, S. & Bemporad, J. (1978). *Severe and mild depression: The psychotherapeutic approach.* New York: Basic Books. Belle, D. (Ed.). (1982). Lives in stress: Women and depression. Beverly Hills, CA: Sage Publications.

Bernardez, T. (1988). *Women and anger—Cultural prohibitions and the feminine ideal.* (Work in Progress No. 31.) Wellesley, MA: Stone Center Working Papers Series.

Bernardez-Bonesatti, T. (1978). Women and anger: Conflicts with aggression in contemporary women. *Journal of the American Medical Women's Association.* 33(5), 215–219.

Bibring, E. (1953). The mechanisms of depression. In P. Greenacre (Ed.), *Affective disorders: Psychoanalytic contributions to their study* (pp. 13–48). New York: International Universities Press.

Bourne, S. (1968). The psychological effects of stillbirths on women and their doctors. *J. Royal College of General Practitioners, 16,* 103–112.

Brown, G. W. & Harris, T. (1978). *The social origins of depression: A study of psychiatric disorders in women.* London: Tavistock.

Freud, S. (1961). Mourning and melancholia. In J. Strachey (Ed. and Trans.), *The standard edition of the complete psychological works of Sigmund Freud* (Vol. 14, pp. 243–258). London: Hogarth Press. (Original work published 1917).

Gutheil, E. A. (1959). Reactive depressions. In S. Arieti (Ed.), *American handbook of psychiatry* (1st ed., Vol. I., pp. 345–352). New York: Basic Books.

Jack, D. (1987). Silencing the self: The power of social imperatives in female depression. In R. Formanek & A. Gurian (Eds.), *Women and depression: A lifetime perspective* (pp. 161–181). New York: Springer.

Kaplan, A. (1984). *The "self-in-relation": Implications for depression in women.* (Work in Progress No. 14.) Wellesley College, MA: Stone Center Working Paper Series.

Lewis, E. (1976). The management of stillbirth: Coping with an unreality. *The Lancet 2* (pp. 619–620).

Miller, J. B. (1983). *The construction of anger in women and men.* (Work in Progress No. 4.) Wellesley, MA: Stone Center Working Paper Series.

Newman, J. P. (1984). Sex differences in symptoms of depression: Clinical disorder or normal distress? *J. Health & Social Behavior, 25,* 136–159.

Paykel, E. S. (1982). Life events and early environment. In E. S. Paykel (Ed.), *Handbook of affective disorders* (pp. 148–161). New York: Guilford.

Radloff, L. S. (1986). Risk factors for depression: What do we learn from them? In J. C. Coyne (Ed.), *Essential papers on depression,* (pp. 405–430).

Rubin, L. B. (1976). *Worlds of pain.* New York: Basic Books.

Turner, R. J., Noh, S. & Levin, D. M. (1985). Depression across the life course. In A. Dean (Ed.), *Depression in multidisciplinary perspective,* (pp. 32–59). New York: Brunner/Mazel.

Weissman, M. M. & Klerman, G. L. (1977). Sex differences and the epidemiology of depression. *Archives of General Psychiatry, 34,* 98–111.

Weissman, M. M. & Klerman, G. L. (1987). Gender and depression. In R. Formanek & A. Gurian (Eds.), *Women and depression: A lifetime perspective* (pp. 3–15). New York: Springer.

Weissman, M. M. & Paykel, E. S. (1974). *The depressed woman.* Chicago: University of Chicago Press.

This chapter was presented at a Stone Center Colloquium on April 6, 1988. © 1988 Irene P. Stiver and Jean Baker Miller.

12

On the Integration of Sexuality: Lesbians and Their Mothers

WENDY B. ROSEN

In both my personal experience as a lesbian and my professional experience as a therapist working with lesbians, I have been privy to countless coming out stories and have been struck by the centrality of concern regarding the impact of the disclosure on the mother–daughter relationship. "What did your mother say?" is a commonly asked question that can easily spark a string of responses among a group of lesbians, ranging from hilarity to tears. Neutrality is virtually absent in the repertoire of possible reactions to this issue. While there are certainly lesbians who deem their experiences in disclosing their sexual identity to their mothers as positive and productive, more often this is the exception, rather than the rule, especially in the initial stages of the disclosure.

What is there about the particular nature of the negotiation between the lesbian and her mother, and why is this issue so profoundly charged and the impact potentially so damaging to their relationship? In an effort to answer these questions, I have chosen to retrospectively explore the lesbian's relationship with her mother and her evolving experience of herself over the course of several years prior to, during, and following her disclosure of her lesbian sexuality to her mother. This is not to suggest that all lesbians do come out to their mothers, but rather that with or without disclosure, it is a preoccupying theme in the lives of most lesbians.

The ideas in this chapter are based on some of the findings from a

recent exploratory study I conducted as part of my doctoral dissertation, in which I focused on the normal developmental experiences of
lesbians. It is a well-known fact that the bulk of the clinical literature
on homosexuality is couched in heterosexist and homophobic assumptions, and thus, inevitably casts lesbianism in a pathological
light. Secondly, most of the literature, whether biased or gay-affirmative, is focused on gay men. That lesbians are underrepresented in the
literature has obvious parallels to the literature on women's developmental experience, in general. Just as women's psychology simply
cannot be extrapolated from male-based theoretical constructions, so
the developmental experiences of lesbians cannot be understood by
studying gay men. Both cases are as clearly off base as is the assumption of a uniform similarity of developmental process between hetero-
sexuals and homosexuals. Heterosexist assumptions in the realm of
sexuality present ramifications as dangerous and damaging as sexist
assumptions with regard to gender. Such biases, nevertheless, are
rampant and ubiquitous in this culture. It should be noted that all the
women who volunteered as subjects, and who are represented in this
study, are white.

AN ILLUSTRATION

As a way of illustrating the lesbian's experience of disclosure to her
mother, I will sketch a not-so-brief, but highly elaborate vignette. Barbara is a thirty-two year old, white lesbian, who is currently enrolled
in a doctoral program. She has been in a relationship with the same
woman for seven years, and they have been sharing a home together
for five of those years. Barbara is the second of four children and grew
up in an Italian Catholic, middle-class family. Her father is an engi-
neer, and her mother, who completed secretarial school, devoted her
earlier married years to raising a family. When the youngest child was
in high school, her mother began to work part-time. All of Barbara's
siblings, consisting of an older, married brother and a younger brother
and sister, are heterosexual. Her sister, one and one-half years
younger, is currently engaged to be married.

Barbara described her childhood as relatively uneventful, except
that she never felt very close to her mother. She had no concrete explanation for this, only that she always perceived herself as somewhat
"different' within the family context. Barbara characterized herself as
"a strong-willed, active and independent child, bright and athletic."
One thing she recalled that really set her apart from her Italian
Catholic family was that she, unlike her siblings, never entertained a

fantasy of or desire to get married. This was a serious family departure, since talk often focused on family, marriage, and weddings. She recalled:

> I never thought about marriage ever! I remember, in my family, you learned as a girl to make tomato sauce, so as a woman, when you get married, you would have that important skill. But I learned it, because I was growing up, and I thought it was just part of that. It was different . . . for *me*, it felt different. I felt like a different person.

The perceived estrangement from her mother was quite painful for Barbara, and she often suffered confusing bouts of sadness and loneliness. She recalled making extra efforts at being a "good girl" by working excessively at her schoolwork, excelling at sports, and trying to entertain her mother, getting her to smile or laugh. On the whole, however, she felt quite alienated and sensed that she somehow must be a fundamentally bad or defective kid.

During adolescence, Barbara had several close girlfriends and periodically dated boys, which involved some heterosexual sexual experimentation. Her strained relationship with her mother continued during this period, and Barbara remembers that her mother was particularly interested in the quality of her daughter's social life, especially regarding boyfriends. This was disturbing to Barbara, since it never felt central to her, especially in contrast to her friendships, academic work, and athletics. Once again, then, she felt out of sync with her mother. Often, she would get drunk in order to endure going out on dates and "getting with the program." It's not that she disliked boys, but rather that she often felt as if she was "going through the motions" of dating them without ever feeling any appreciable intensity of emotion or sexual desire for them. As Barbara put it:

> I really just wanted to chum around with them. I thought there must have been something wrong with me. I remember saying to someone that I just didn't get it, the whole world of dating and attraction. Some people are born blind. Some are born not being able to hear, and I was born without this . . . whatever the "this" is.

The relationship with her mother was particularly strained, since Barbara felt compelled to date boys, like other girls, in order to please her. But she could not find a way to tell her mother about her conflict, and she began to hate herself for not being like other girls. Her mother was in the dark about Barbara's pain and saw her daughter as willful and withholding. The tension between them continued. Barbara recalls that her sister and mother grew quite close during this time, and that they would often have conversations about marriage, children, and so on. She described her sister as "kind of boy crazy." Barbara, on the other hand, had very intense attachments with her girlfriends, and, overall, preferred their company to that of boys. Since this was not a popular position to acknowledge openly, she would often manage it by spending long lazy, loving afternoons with a girlfriend discussing boys.

Barbara began to be aware of her feelings of sexual attractions to other young women when, at about eighteen, she went off to college. At first she was enormously conflicted. I'll let her words convey the essence of her very powerful feelings:

> I panicked. This was a conflict, a major conflict. I didn't tell a soul for a year and a half. I was denying that I was a lesbian. I was ashamed and afraid of what my family would say and think. I grew up thinking I must be some kind of terrible person . . . suddenly horribly immoral. I was horrified. It seemed unnatural. I had the most violent self-hate. I couldn't even look at myself in the mirror. My drinking became heavy during this time. I cried. I was angry. I thought, "Oh my God. I'm a lesbian. I'm not going to get married. I'm not going to have kids. What am I going to tell my grandparents?"

Barbara described her fear and self-loathing, as her feelings towards women went against absolutely everything she was raised to believe was valuable and acceptable including the tenets of her Catholicism and the strongly heterosexual system of values and prescribed modes of relating for a young woman. Barbara felt wracked with guilt, especially with regard to her mother, whom she felt she was hurting, disappointing, and in jeopardy of losing altogether. She saw her mother as having devoted her whole life to raising her family and preparing her children to marry and raise their families and felt that, as a lesbian, she represented a glaring and shameful failure in her mother's life task. Barbara was terrified of the rift that easily might ensue.

Furthermore, Barbara felt adrift in the world of social interaction. Despite the fact that she never fully embraced the world of heterosexual dating and romance, she at least knew what a heterosexual girl was supposed to do. As a lesbian, she knew about her love for women, but had always understood it to be the man's job to initiate a more intimate, sexual relationship.

During this time, Barbara's contacts with her mother diminished markedly. Calls and visits were infrequent. Barbara felt she had less and less to say to her mother, less and less that she comfortably could tell about her life. When her mother would ask questions about Barbara's social life, Barbara could speak only of the women in her life, focusing on various activities with "friends." She would dodge the issue of dating, saying that she did not have time for it, that there was no one particularly interesting, and so on. Barbara's mother began to register consternation and worry, wondering openly if Barbara ever would get married and raising questions about whether Barbara was afraid of men or of intimacy. She began to question whether her daughter was destined for the religious life; perhaps she had a calling. She also was confused about Barbara's increasing aloofness and withdrawal, feeling hurt and angry about it. At the same time, she remained unaware of her daughter's tension and mounting despair at the two lives she was feeling forced to live simultaneously, one public and one private. Over time, increasing periods of silence replaced the awkwardness of these painful interactions between mother and daughter.

Barbara turned more and more to the new and expanding network of women friends that she met through the lesbian and gay organization at her college, and also, within the local women's community. She found enormous solace and relief in discovering that a community of lesbians existed, that she was not an isolated freak of nature, and that an alternative to heterosexuality was viable. Barbara also sought counseling at this time. It was only when she began to establish and maintain these connections that her depression gradually began to dissipate. In particular, her first relationship with a woman lover served an essential function with regard to her evolving sexuality. Barbara described it this way:

> I really needed someone who could take me by the hand and lead me out, and I knew that. I met someone who was that . . . someone who was comfortable with her sexuality. It was like coming back to a place in myself that I hadn't been in a really long time. It felt really welcome. It felt innocent in that it was free from pretense, and it seemed to be me remembering me, rather than someone I was trying to be. With boys and men I always felt I was playing a particular role. . . . The light finally went on. I knew I wasn't crazy.

As Barbara further established herself in a community of relationships, she became increasingly comfortable and open about herself as a lesbian. She came out more publicly at college and even ventured to tell one of her siblings, her sister. Her sister was not at all surprised, had suspected it for some time, but did not feel invited by Barbara to ask about it. Barbara, at the same time, felt increasingly pained and dissatisfied with the distance in her relationship with her mother. She felt she was living at best, a half-truth with her mother and that this was terribly compromising for each of them and for the relationship.

On the other hand, she was terrified of telling her mother that she was a lesbian. Barbara feared her mother's possible horror and fury and ultimate wholesale rejection. Furthermore, Barbara never really had presented herself to her mother in the context of her sexuality. It was not the kind of relationship they shared, and suddenly, this information was to be the central topic of a potential disclosure. This left her feeling strangely both saddened and embarrassed.

How can we understand Barbara's experience? What has made the relationship between lesbian daughters and their mothers so painfully strained? Why is the anticipation of Barbara's disclosure of her lesbian sexuality to her mother such a charged and dreaded one?

RELATIONAL DEVELOPMENT IN WOMEN

To answer these questions, I will begin by turning to the Stone Center's work, which, over the past decade, has afforded us an evolving conceptualization of women's development that posits the importance of relational movement as the lifeblood of self-growth. In particular, the mother–daughter relationship represents the earliest model of, and serves as the paradigm for, all future empathic connections. Before I begin an exploration of the relational rupture experienced by Barbara and her mother, I will review briefly a few of the central dynamic features of the mother–daughter relationship that capture relational development. From there, I will move on to describe the particular nature of the lesbian's developmental path as it, of necessity, diverges from the general developmental course for heterosexual women in this culture.

Three key relational concepts emerging from the work of the Stone Center form the main threads of the following discussion. The first of these is "mutual empathy," which Jordan (1984, 1985, 1987, 1989), Kaplan (1988), Mencher (1990), Miller (1982, 1984, 1986, 1988), Stiver (1986, 1990), and Surrey (1985, 1987) have variously described as central to the definition of relationship. Mutual empathy implies a relational flow that is grounded in the capacity of each person to be "attuned to and responsive to the subjective inner experience of the other, both at a cognitive and affective level" (Jordan, 1984). Surrey (1985) captures the mutually empathic experience as one in which "'being with' means 'being seen' and 'feeling seen' by the other and 'seeing the other' and sensing the other 'feeling seen.'" Miller et al. (1991) has described it in her words as "the attempt to be with the truth of the other person's experience in all of its aspects." I would phrase this as the capacity to know and be where the other truly lives.

This capacity for mutual empathic processes ideally originates within the matrix of the mother–daughter connection and is founded on the early experience of mutual attunement (Chodorow, 1978). This is not to suggest that the mother–daughter relationship is the only source of mutual empathic processes, but rather that it is typically the earliest model and most likely the clearest example of such a relationship. Empathic development can and does occur in the context of other important relationships throughout one's life.

A second important concept, and one that follows from mutual empathy, is that of "relationship authenticity," defined by Surrey (1985) as the "ongoing challenge to feel emotionally real, connected, vital, clear and purposeful in a relationship." It describes the ongoing and mutual need in a relationship to be seen and recognized for who one really is. Relationship authenticity, like mutual empathy, refers to a process, rather than a static state, particularly as a relationship, of necessity, must change to meet the growth of each person within it. Miller (1986) speaks of the ability to continuously "represent one's experience" within the relationship as such experience arises.

The third concept, one proposed by Surrey (1985) to describe relational development and put forth as an alternative to the object relations theory concept of separation-individuation is that of "relationship differentiation." She describes differentiation as "referring to a process which encompasses increasing levels of complexity, choice, fluidity, and articulation within the context of human development." The challenge is to maintain connection while fostering, and changing with, the growth of one another. With regard to the mother–daughter relationship, failure of this capacity to both continue in, and change within, the relationship leaves both feeling shamed and devalued. Jordan (1985) extends the notion of differentiation and suggests that movement towards personal integration occurs within a relational context. I would further emphasize that a derailment of relationship differentiation, an incapacity to maintain connection while adapting to one another's growth and changes, leads to complications in the realm of personal integration. I think one often sees evidence of such complications during adolescence, when a range of functional capacities is rapidly emerging and simultaneously bumping up against a system of values and beliefs that affect the fluidity of relational resilience towards change.

In summary, three central features of relational development for women that typically find their source in the mother–daughter relationship are those of mutual empathy, relationship authenticity and relationship differentiation. Referring back to the vignette, in her relationship with her mother, Barbara was, in fact, derailed in all three of these relational processes. What can account for such ruptures of connection? What are the obstacles for Barbara and her mother?

THE CULTURAL CONTEXT: SEXISM AND HETEROSEXISM

In further setting the stage for this exploration, it is important to consider a few central issues related to psychological development in general and to the societal context in which it occurs. If one thinks of human beings as having the potential to evolve in increasingly articulated ways, and further, if one thinks of the environment, that is, the culture and the context of relationships, as joining with this potential so as to produce a range of possible outcomes, then one can begin to outline a framework for understanding certain detours in the process. Among the myriad potentialities in the human template is that of sexuality. If you postulate that the self in all of its many aspects flourishes in the context of relationships, you include the realm of sexuality. In the mother–daughter relationship, as the earliest example of such a meeting between growth potential and the environment, it is the mother who ideally nurtures with openness and receptivity the full range of emergent possibilities for her daughter. I say "ideally," because clearly, this is often not what happens in reality.

It goes without saying, at this point, that the larger cultural context contributes a great deal to processes of personal development, and that families typically serve as the primary conduits for the transmission of cultural definitions and messages. Western culture, as many have noted (Kaplan, 1988; Miller, 1986; Singer, 1977), predicates its system of values and beliefs on a hierarchical arrangement of dichotomous constructions—differences are set up as "either-or" and "better-worse." Examples include, to name a few, those of masculine-feminine, independent-dependent, white-black, Christian-Jewish, heterosexual-homosexual—the list is endless. Of particular importance to this discussion and the obstacles faced by Barbara and her mother, are the insidious, powerful, and pervasive cultural conditions of sexism and heterosexism. These value systems assume that men and maleness are better than women and femaleness. Further, they suggest that heterosexuality within this sexist culture is better than and preferable to homosexuality, which, by definition, challenges the balance of power that defines sexism. Homosexuality is seen as a threat to a sexist system in at least two ways: two women together suggests that a man might not be necessary for a woman to be fully competent and functional; two men together threatens the stereotypic and sexist assignment of gender roles in that it posits that one man in such a relationship is serving the devalued function of a woman. In general, and most importantly, both sexism and heterosexism, as the combined basis for a system of pervasive power imbalance and abuse, are each sources of severe relational damage in our culture.

Now, back to Barbara. Barbara's representation of her preadolescent and, especially, her adolescent years is not an unusual one for many lesbians. Previous studies (Rosen, 1990; Troiden, 1979) have described a similar constellation of retrospectively recalled feelings and perceptions of unterpersonal relationships, marked by confusion, isolation, fluctuating self-esteem, and an overall sense of being somehow different in inexplicable ways. As the eldest daughter in a rather traditional Italian Catholic family, Barbara's early environment contained certain expectations and messages regarding who she was to become. These included, among other things, heterosexual, married, and sexually somewhat naive and unassertive. At the same time, certain possibilities, among others, were absent from the repertoire presented by her mother, such as lesbian, unmarried, and sexually both curious and active. Barbara's experience vis-à-vis her mother is an extraordinarily familiar one and clearly contains the early seeds of a painful developmental set-up with multiple ramifications.

First, as a heterosexual woman, a wife and mother, Barbara's mother comes to her tasks with a packaged set of predetermined criteria for her success in these roles. Such criteria are dictated by the tenets of both sexism and heterosexism, which demand that mothers in this culture pass the baton of the traditional woman's role to their daughters, and thus assure the continuation of the existing balance of power in a patriarchal structure. Her own self-esteem and the stability of her "place" rest upon her capacity to fulfill her task of raising her daughter to carry on this role. In this way, the culture demands the active disavowal of a whole range of possibilities that Barbara's mother could include as developmental "fits" for her daughter—in particular, those possibilities that challenge the existing cultural arrangement. It follows from this that Barbara's mother will engage in an inevitable empathic failure for her daughter whose sexuality is gradually evolving in a wholly different direction. That her daughter could become a lesbian is simply not a culturally permissible image to which a mother can be openly receptive without threatening both the larger system and her own personal sense of order. The meaning of this is powerful—Barbara's mother will unavoidably miss the cues regarding her daughter's sexuality, in general, and her lesbianism, in particular, throughout Barbara's development. She will be, of necessity, selectively inattentive, and thus remain minimally attuned to the emotional manifestations of Barbara's evolving sexuality. She will be unable to serve as an empathic resource for her daughter in this aspect of her growth.

It is essential to note that the reverse is also true; that is, Barbara unavoidably will fail her mother empathically. As a lesbian, and thus as a woman who, of developmental necessity, claims active rights to and ownership of her own sexuality, Barbara is a living representation of her mother's culturally determined failure in her role and the task assigned to that role. By not moving in the direction of heterosexuality and marriage to a man, and further, by evolving sexually in the absence of a man as the active catalyst of her flourishing sexuality, Barbara is defying the cultural prescription for a woman. She is not providing a comfortable 'fit" with her mother's requirements towards the cultural dictates for homeostasis. This creates friction and forestalls empathic resonance with the mother's evolving needs as a heterosexual woman and mother in a sexist and heterosexist culture.

What, then, are the implications for Barbara and her mother of such cultural demands on women? The developmental setup goes as follows. For her mother to be truly empathic towards Barbara as she develops and matures requires that she fail in one of her major culturally defined tasks as a heterosexual woman and mother. For Barbara to be truly empathic towards her mother requires that she disavow certain internal realities and remain inauthentic in the relationship. In other words, this culture, by virtue of its sexist and heterosexist underpinnings, violates the relationship between the lesbian and her mother, and, in most cases, ensures the lack of mutual empathy between them. Painful evidence of this deficiency abounds in Barbara's story. For years, Barbara felt marginalized and disconnected. During her adolescence, especially, she found herself struggling to feel and behave in ways that were fundamentally dystonic, such as trying to date boys and to act as if her feelings of friendship with girlfriends included no sexual desires whatsoever. In order to sustain this heterosexual persona, Barbara resorted to dangerous means, such as heavy drinking. Eventually, she succumbed to feeling quite depressed, and it was only when she consciously realized that she was a lesbian that she could begin to make sense of her experience, one that forcefully had been couched in inauthenticity. Living had become increasingly a question of endurance. Barbara's culturally induced maladaptive efforts were designed, in part, to find some kind of mutually empathic resonance with her mother, who also was a victim of a damaging and inherently divisive cultural prescription. During these same years, Barbara's mother, while living with the illusion of success in her task as a heterosexual woman and mother, was also suffering with confusion at her daughter's pain, depression, drinking, and "failures" at sustaining heterosexual intimacy beyond her infrequent dating. She was unable to be empathic with her daughter's internal struggles; thus, her seeming "success" at passing the baton of heterosexual womanhood to her daughter was tantamount to relational failure as a mother. It is painful for mothers to fail their daughters empathically, just as it is painful for daughters to challenge and oppose their mothers' feelings. For a lesbian and her mother, this culture determines that such relational pain is almost a certainty.

SEXUALITY AND SHAME

What feelings can be expected to accompany the disconnection associated with such ruptures of mutual empathy? The primary concommittitant feeling is typically one of shame, given the central importance for women of relationship and the movement towards connection to others. Jordan captures succinctly the experience of shame as follows:

> ... shame is most importantly a felt sense of unworthiness to be in connection, a deep sense of unlovability, with the ongoing awareness of how very much one wants to connect with others. While shame involves extreme self-consciousness, it also signals powerful relational longings and awareness of the other's response. There is a loss of the sense of "empathic possibility"; others are not experienced as empathic, and the capacity for self-empathy is lost. One feels unworthy of love, not because of some discrete action which would be the cause for guilt, but because one is defective or flawed in some essential way. (1989, p. 6)

The principle point here is the deep feeling of isolation, the sense that one's very essence is damaged and is the source of relational disconnection.

Women in this culture are highly susceptible to feelings of shame (Jordan, 1989; Lewis, 1987). This is the case for many marginalized groups, and particularly true for lesbians, both as homosexuals and as women. Barbara's depression, her heavy drinking, her efforts at heterosexual pretense, were all manifestations of shame. Lesbians often experience shame at some point in their development with regard to their burgeoning sexuality. Often it is an amorphous feeling without a clear source, one that occurs prior to the conscious awareness of one's lesbianism. The conclusion that "something is wrong with me . . . I'm just not like other girls" is a typical deduction. In the context of the lesbian's relationship with her mother, as the case of Barbara so poignantly highlights, there are many relational ruptures that result in feelings of shame. In the realm of sexuality, the particular developmental path for a lesbian provides a ready setup for a shame-ridden interchange with her mother. Among other places, it is here where the lesbian's experience departs from that of a heterosexual woman's. The assumption that men are the bearers of active sexual desire and women the objects and the passive recipients of that desire (Jordan, 1987) suggests that men are the essential catalysts for and definers of women's sexuality, or to put it another way, women are coaxed into their sexuality by virtue of men's sexuality—reflected in the stereotypical image of the virginal bride in white being "deflowered" on her wedding night.

The lesbian's developmental path, on the other hand, clearly defies this patriarchal construction. Lesbians, by necessity, are forced to confront and actively own the existence of their sexuality in a way that heterosexual women are not. The assumption of heterosexuality together with the silencing of women's own active sexual "voice" provides a developmental obstacle for lesbians which can be negotiated only through conscious redefinition and some form of public rectification. Lesbians are forced to voice their reality in order to represent authentically their own truth (Miller, 1988). Such an open declaration of one's sexuality is not a necessity for heterosexual women because heterosexuality is assumed, and thus, their sexuality is not subject to the same kind of scrutinized, and often shamemaking, exposure as is true for lesbians. It is an all-too-common experience for the lesbian to be in the position of coming out, only to be met with the private or not-so-private musings about just what it is she does in bed.

How does all of this translate for Barbara and her mother? In what ways does shame come into play for each of them? What meaning does this hold for their relationship and the capacity for growth and change within it? Barbara and her mother never really had discussed sexuality in any way. There had been talk of marriage, husband, and future children, and thus, some aspect of sexuality was at least implied, albeit couched in heterosexist assumptions. Barbara was not at all encouraged to notice, be curious about, or rejoice in her own sexual capacities, except as they were designed to fulfill her prescribed role as a heterosexual woman and future wife and mother. In order to correct the erroneous assumptions that her mother held about her daughter, and also to rectify the painful breach of silence between them, Barbara was faced with the need to acknowledge openly the truth of her lesbianism. Suddenly, and for the first time in her life, Barbara's sexuality was to become a focus of discussion between her and her mother. Any discussion of sex was thoroughly at odds with the nature of their relationship and with the heterosexual Catholic upbringing of which they were both a part. Barbara anticipated feeling exposed, embarrassed, and vulnerable. Barbara's mother conceivably would feel forced to face both her failure in her role, and her likely awkwardness about sexuality, particularly her own. Most importantly, there would be exposed that feeling of disconnection between them, a very frightening moment of relational truth. The anticipation of such a disclosure typically precipitates two possible choices for lesbians. One, because of unbearable shame, is to hide and remain secretive about the truth. The other is to risk disclosure in the potential service of some kind of relational reparation with the mother. Successful negotiation in the latter case presents an enormous challenge, though far from an impossible one, to the lesbian daughter and her mother in a sexist and heterosexist culture.

Jordan states that "in the extreme, shame contributes to dissociation and inner fragmentation as the person struggles to be free of the experience of personal defectiveness" (1989, p. 6). It is precisely in this respect that both relationship differentiation and personal integration suffer, at least in the realm of sexuality, for the lesbian and her mother. The inevitable presence of culturally induced shame associated with one's lesbianism, and by extension, one's acknowledgment and articulation of sexuality as a woman, serves as an obstacle in the path of relationship differentiation for mother and daughter insofar as the culture impinges in its demands for disavowal. Cultural requirements make it almost impossible for mother and daughter to adapt and grow and maintain connection in the face of these particular changes in the developmental realm of sexuality. Taken a step further, such circumstances contribute to a forestalling of integration with regard to the lesbian's sexuality. To me, successful integration, that is, the antithesis of dissociation and fragmentation and the antidote to shame, relies upon the capacity for successful relationship differentiation, beginning with the mother–daughter relationship. Where, then, does this leave the growing lesbian and her mother? Do Barbara and her mother have, as they say, a "snowball's chance"?

That processes of empathic development, in fact, can and do evolve in the context of other important relationships is an extraordinarily important factor for lesbians, and one that manifests itself with some regularity in most, if not all, their lives. This was certainly the case for Barbara. At the same time that she went to college and began to be consciously aware of her lesbianism, Barbara was approaching rapidly the height of disconnection with her mother and the depth of her own despair. It was at this point that she began to make relationships with other lesbians and eventually became involved in a fully intimate relationship with a woman lover. As a result of these connections and the reparative experience of mutual empathy that they offered with regard to her evolving lesbian sexuality, Barbara gradually could begin to feel whole, to become an integrated, competently functioning and feeling, active presence in the world. Her sense of shame began to dissipate, especially as her isolation decreased and was replaced by relationships that offered the opportunity for mutually empathic processes to develop further. Such opportunity was clearly essential to Barbara's continuing growth and integration in a context of sustained connections that could remain resilient to change. The developmental experience of most lesbians in this regard strongly endorses mutuality in relationships as a fundamental necessity in the movement towards personal integration.

So, why would Barbara choose to disclose her lesbianism to her mother at this point? She was able, after all, to compensate for the limitations in her relationship with her mother through the establishment of other important, empathic connections with women. She was able to move towards increasing levels of integration with regard to her sexuality, as these relationships allowed for growth in her capacity to be adaptive and resilient. She was able to establish an intimate relationship with another woman that felt stable and promising. Why wreak havoc in her currently distant, but otherwise, nontumultuous relationship with her mother?

The answer is a simple one. The disconnection between Barbara and her mother felt bad. Disclosure, for Barbara, was very much in the service of connection. The relationship felt compromised by virtue of a sustained period of secrecy which left Barbara feeling inauthentic vis-à-vis her mother and left her mother feeling confused, hurt, angry, and unempathic towards her daughter. While Barbara did not really know with certainty all the reasons for their uneven relationship all along, she did know now that the hidden fact of her lesbianism was, at the very least, a contributing factor to the current distance between them. Disclosure to her mother, as she perceived it, offered the possibility for some clarification for each of them as to who they really were to one another, as well as for shedding light on just what the relationship could expand to include. Barbara felt that the issue was important unfinished business for each of them and that such an essential truth was fundamental to the authenticity and integrity of the relationship. Any possibility for reparation and further relational movement depended upon the disclosure. Although Barbara knew that coming out to her mother held absolutely no guarantee of growth in the relationship, it was important to her, nonetheless. She no longer could tolerate living a lie.

Did Barbara's disclosure make an appreciable difference? Did it enhance their relational growth? The answer is yes and no. Barbara's mother was extremely dismayed and disappointed to learn that her daughter was a lesbian. She felt embarrassed and did not want her to share this news with the extended family. She was angry with Barbara for what she saw as her daughter's forsaking the Church and all of their cherished, traditional family values. Although not stunned by her mother's response, Barbara nevertheless was pained. She never really expected her mother simply to accept and welcome her lesbianism, given her understanding of all the cultural values and beliefs to which her mother adhered and with which Barbara was raised. She recognized that acceptance would entail a substantial and highly conflict-laden leap for her mother; but on the other hand, this was her *mother* . . . and Barbara was her eldest daughter. That very fundamental connection should count for something and bear up against any assaults to it. Over time and with help, Barbara was able to feel that the important point was that the disclosure provided greater clarity about each of them, about some of the strengths and limitations of their relationship and about more realistic expectations that each of them could hold. Barbara had other essential relationships to fill in some of the gaps, and her mother found a way to appreciate Barbara, albeit in a somewhat circumscribed way, making it clear that her daughter could place emphasis on her sexuality elsewhere in her life. Each was left sadder and wiser.

Barbara and her mother's disclosure experience is not at all unusual for lesbians. A more or less mutually agreed upon level of relational compromise occurs between mother and daughter that, in some respects, resembles their predisclosure relationship. It typically does not predict monumental changes, but rather provides an opportunity for possible change, reparation and growth. As Heyward suggests, "the coming out process is a paradigm . . . for healing" (1989, p. 9). Such growth as does occur is not necessarily manifested as a deepening of the connection between mother and daughter nor as an increase in relational resilience and adaptation. Rather, it makes possible another kind of integrity in the relationship—one that allows for the relational bearing of differences, but often not without significant mutual loss and grief. There is a wound to the relationship and a degree of scarring in its aftermath. In the context of the strong sexist and the heterosexist cultural demands that exert their influence through so many institutionalized channels, such as the church and the traditional family structure, among others, it would seem almost impossible for any other mother–daughter relational outcome. A permanent sense of loss and grief associated with the relational rupture is seemingly the only logical extension.

The fact is, however, that alternative outcomes do occur. Sometimes permanent rupture and total loss are the result of disclosure. On the other hand, there are those mother–daughter relationships that do emerge with greater relational strength and flexibility, an enhancement of mutual empathy, as well as substantial movement towards increasing relationship differentiation, authenticity, and integrity. These relationships demonstrate a capacity to integrate a missing piece, in this case, that of lesbian sexuality, so that the relationship becomes clearer and less rigid, stereotypical, and static. Given the insidious and pervasive sexist and heterosexist culture within which mother–daughter relationships occur, it is remarkable that certain mothers, in fact, are able to transcend these obstacles. As much as it takes a stunning degree of courage and belief in the power of relationships for the lesbian not only to come into her truth, but then to live it authentically, I believe there should be equal admiration for those mothers who, for whatever reasons, are able to find some power in themselves within their relational contexts to embrace a rather complicated truth, only to discover deeper truths hidden beneath it.

CONCLUSION

In conclusion, I am suggesting that the relational experience of lesbian daughters and their mothers is an extraordinarily complicated one to navigate in a culture that rests firmly on the foundation of sexism and heterosexism. In particular, I am asserting that lesbians and their mothers and the relationship between them suffer markedly as a result of these pervasive cultural influences. Shame, like a virus, invades the relationship and threatens to leave the lesbian and her mother locked into a dynamic of blame, self-recrimination, and overall, mutual empathic rupture. In the meantime, the real culprit, the patriarchal system of oppression, continues the spread of cultural disease.

I believe it is at this point that important questions arise. Is there a way in which the experiences of lesbian daughters and their mothers provide a window through which to view the experiences of women, in general, in this culture? Do we see the cultural damage imposed by a patriarchal system of sexism and heterosexism as a form of psychic trauma to all women, insofar as such trauma severs one's capacity to feel and to be in connection? Are mothers and daughters, by their very natures, inevitably doomed to be in conflict as a result of so-called oedipal disillusionment, preoedipal fears of engulfment, and other facile constructions derived from sexist and heterosexist assumptions? Or rather, have mothers and daughters, both lesbian and heterosexual, long been pitted against one another as collective victims of disempowerment as women? Mothers and daughters, women in relationship to one another, can form a remarkably powerful bond.

I will close with a brief disclosure story told to me some years ago by a lesbian friend in response to my query: "So, what did your mother say?" My friend described the following:

> My mother said, "How could this have happened to you?!" I thought for a minute, smiled and answered, "Just lucky I guess!"

DISCUSSION SUMMARY

After each colloquium presentation a discussion was held. Selected portions are summarized here. At this session, Mses Mencher and Slater and Drs. Stiver and Heyward joined Dr. Rosen in leading the discussion.

Question: What did you do in your work with Barbara and her mother? Did they get anywhere? What have you done with other mothers and daughters to help them effect a reconciliation?

Rosen: Barbara was a woman in my study, not a client. However, I have worked with other mothers and lesbian daughters and it is often very complicated and painful. It is a process that can take quite a long time. My aim largely is to help them listen to one another, to find their capacity to be empathic with regard to a mutual experience of pain and to lift the experience out of the blaming mode. The important point is for the two of them to realize the force of larger cultural issues impinging on their relationship and the resultant rigidified, stereotyped images that have been formed of one another.

Mencher: When I have worked with mothers and their lesbian daughters, the most powerful experience for the mother is when I validate that she has a right to her pain and shame and all her many feelings of yearning and longing and rage and envy. I think in many cases that a mother feels her daughter's lesbian path to be a rejection of her and her path as a heterosexual. The mother feels that she has made many compromises in her life in pursuit of her particular path, and her daughter's suggestion that there may be an alternative way to go is a real challenge to the mother's confidence in her own compromises. I try to help the mother see this as an opportunity towards greater authenticity for both herself and her daughter in their relationship to one another.

Rosen: I would emphasize here that it is the sense of failure that becomes contained in the mother–daughter relationship that is in need of reframing, such that the empathic failures of the culture are not erroneously felt as either individual or relational failures.

Slater: What Wendy is outlining here is, for most mothers, that inarticulated sense of loss. It is very rare that a mother can identify that her real pain is about something deeper than "I am in pain because you are a lesbian." That very non-mutual framing of the problem leaves mother and daughter feeling very stuck. To do some of the naming that has been described here tonight would be very useful in terms of generating greater fluidity and movement between the two of them.

Rosen: I had the experience of supervising a family treatment in which a young adult lesbian came out to her parents, and her mother's reaction was extremely severe and regressive, falling to the floor into a fetal position. It emerged through therapy that, in fact, there were serious, longstanding marital difficulties between the parents that were being masked by the overdetermined focus on the daughter's lesbianism.

Stiver: You've implied this issue, but I do think that mothers in bad marriages are really terrified that they will be left absolutely alone without a mate and without a daughter. The terror is one of disconnection, which feels devastating and which comes out in many forms.

Comment: This is part question and part comment. What do you hear empirically in your therapy work and your research about the majority of lesbians' experiences in coming out? Is it always negative with shame, shock, and the like? Are there positive receptions by mothers? I had the experience of being told by a group of friends to come out to my mother, that it was "no big deal" and to just "get over it already." Well, of course it was a big deal to my mother, but she eventually did get over it. This is my comment: I agree that it is an enormous energy drain, and I really encourage women to get on with it and do it, because otherwise it is a much bigger deal than it needs to be.

Rosen: There were women in my study who had remarkably positive coming out experiences with their mothers, but they were extremely afraid going into it. That's where I think you see some of what I've been talking about. Even if the coming out experience turns out to be okay, there is an initial anticipation that is filled with fear and a lot of wasted time and misunderstanding between mothers and daughters. There were a number of mothers who were not merely receptive, but experienced a real sense of mutual growth along with their daughters. These mothers managed to use the information as a catalyst for taking personal inventories regarding those ways in which they felt inauthentic in their own lives and began attending to repairs. I felt those to be some of the most heartwarming responses.

Mencher: I think that one of the things that Wendy is implying is that at the very moment of the exposure of disconnection that occurs in coming out to a mother, there exists the only possibility for true, authentic future connection.

Slater: I might add that even in the occasional situation where someone is immediately responded to positively by her mother, that didn't change at all what it took to get to that point of bringing the relationship to a place of potential rupture in order to offer that authenticity and eventual healing. Even if it does go very well, I think that, regardless of the outcome, many of the components of lesbians' experiences prior to the disclosure are largely the same.

Question: I'm working with a woman in her sixties who has a daughter in her thirties, and as we have talked together, it seems apparent to both of us that the daughter is a lesbian. She, however, has not been able to raise the issue with her mother, who I think is quite ready to hear this information and realizes that the conspiracy of silence really creates a disconnection between the two of them. She very much feels that this discussion needs to be initiated by the daughter. I'm wondering how you feel about it and whether she can bring this to her daughter.

Rosen: Why does she feel it has to be initiated by her daughter? It's a very interesting story. One of the ways we can think about this is that this woman is very worried that she openly will fail her daughter empathically, that she will have missed something by asking her the wrong question. In fact, it would be no worse, really, than failing her by ignoring something altogether.

Heyward: This question helps me realize how much I think this whole issue really transcends the roles. Mother and daughter can become a lens into a larger relational quandary and possibility. Wendy has asked if it can become a window into all women's lives. I think the answer is yes, I think that is partly true, because so much has to do with the inauthenticity of both persons, and that's what I hear you saying, Wendy. Which one initiates does not seem to me finally to be the point, so much as the breakthrough into the realm of possibility. Sometimes mothers come out to their daughters, and a lot of the same issues are there when that happens. It seems to me that somewhere right in the middle of it all is largely unmet yearning that is bred into all of us in the heterosexist patriarchy for the intimacy and authenticity with women, with our mothers, with our friends, with our lovers, with ourselves. This is a quandary we all share, and I think it is unavoidable for all of us in a heterosexist patriarchy. So, I think that for a mother who is sitting on something that is authentically with her, to imagine initiating an empathic conversation with a daughter is a very beautiful possibility.

REFERENCES

Chodorow, N. (1978). *The reproduction of mothering. Psychoanalysis and the sociology of gender.* Berkeley: University of California Press.

Heyward, C. (1989). *Coming out and relational empowerment: A lesbian feminist theological perspective.* (Work in Progress No. 38.) Wellesley, MA: Stone Center Working Paper Series.

Jordan, J. (1984). *Empathy and self-boundaries.* (Work in Progress No. 16). Wellesley, MA: Stone Center Working Paper Series.

Jordan, J. (1985). *The meaning of mutuality.* (Work in Progress No. 23.) Wellesley, MA: Stone Center Working Paper Series. (Reprinted as Chapter 3, this volume)

Jordan, J. (1987). *Clarity in connection: Empathic knowing, desire, and sexuality.* (Work in Progress No. 29.) Wellesley, MA: Stone Center Working Paper Series.

Jordan, J. (1989). *Relational Development: Therapeutic implications of empathy and shame.* (Work in Progress No. 39). Wellesley, MA: Stone Center Working Paper Series. (Reprinted as Chapter 7, this volume)

Kaplan, A. (1988). *Dichotomous thought and relational processes in therapy.* (Work in Progress No. 35.) Wellesley, MA: Stone Center Working Paper Series.

Lewis, H. (1987). *The role of shame in symptom formation.* Hillsdale, NJ: Erlbaum.

Mencher, J. (1990). *Intimacy in lesbian relationships: A critical examination of fusion.* (Work in Progress No. 42.) Wellesley, MA: Stone Center Working Paper Series.

Miller, J. B. (1982). *Women and power.* (Work in Progress No. 1.) Wellesley, MA: Stone Center Working Paper Series.

Miller, J. B. (1984). *The development of women's sense of self.* (Work in Progress No. 12.) Wellesley, MA: Stone Center Working Paper Series.

Miller, J. B. (1986). *What do we mean by relationships?* (Work in Progress No. 22.) Wellesley, MA: Stone Center Working Paper Series.

Miller, J. B. (1988). *Connections, disconnections, and violations.* (Work in Progress No. 33.) Wellesley, MA: Stone Center Working Paper Series.

Miller, J. B., Jordan, J., Kaplan, A., Stiver, I., Surrey, J. (1991). *Some misconceptions and preconceptions of a relational approach.* (Work in Progress No. 49.) Wellesley, MA: Stone Center Working Paper Series. (Reprinted as Chapter 2, this volume)

Rosen, W. (1990). *Self-in-relation development in lesbians and the mother–daughter relationship.* Unpublished doctoral dissertation, Smith College School for Social Work, Northampton, MA.

Singer, J. (1977) *Androgeny: Toward a new theory of sexuality.* Garden City: Anchor.

Stiver, I. (1986) *Beyond the Oedipus complex: Mothers and daughters.* (Work in Progress No. 26.) Wellesley, MA: Stone Center Working Paper Series.

Stiver, 1. (1990). *Dysfunctional families and wounded relationships—Part 1.* (Work in Progress No. 41.) Wellesley, MA: Stone Center Working Paper Series.

Surrey, J. (1985). *Self-in-relation: A theory of women's development.* (Work in Progress No. 13.) Wellesley, MA: Stone Center Working Paper Series.

Surrey, J. (1987). *Relationship and empowerment.* (Work in Progress No. 30.) Wellesley, MA: Stone Center Working Paper Series.

Troiden, R. (1979). Becoming homosexual: A model of gay identity acquisition. *Psychiatry, 42,* 362–373.

This chapter was presented at a Stone Center Colloquium on December 4, 1991. © 1991 Wendy Rosen.

13

The Woman–Man Relationship: Impasses and Possibilities

STEPHEN J. BERGMAN
JANET L. SURREY

As the work of the Stone Center (Jordan, Kaplan, Miller, Stiver, & Surrey; 1991), Gilligan (1982,1989), and others has evolved over the past decade, we have begun to appreciate the different gender-related pathways of psychological development. The stage is set for a crucial dialogue to begin—for men and women to come together to describe and explore the impact of these differences and to struggle not only for equality but for mutuality in relationship. By mutual relationship we refer to what Miller (1986) and Surrey (1985) have described as growth-fostering relationships characterized by mutual engagement, mutual empathy, and mutual empowerment.

As old systems of relationship break down, new visions are called for. The historical roots of the male–female relationship are thousands of years old and are embedded in a patriarchal system which has shaped our institutions, our thinking, and the patterning of our relationships. As we work towards change, we must recognize the weight and depth of this history. Clinically as well as culturally, we see many couples struggling with very similar relational impasses. It is essential for both women and men to move out of a sense of personal deficiency, pathology, or blame—as we are *all* called on to participate in this cultural transformation of the dynamics of relationship. So far there have not been adequate opportunities to work *together* on these challenges.

In an effort to meet this need, we led our first gender workshop in 1988, "New Visions of the Male–Female Relationship: Creating Mutuality." Since then, we have conducted this workshop more than two hundred times, and its evolution has involved 15,000 people, including men and women clinicians, college and medical students, and couples, in Holland and Istanbul, Turkey, and four-year-olds in an American preschool. Usually the men and women do *not* come in couples, except in workshops designed explicitly for couples. The workshops are designed for specific periods of time, from three hours to three days. Almost without exception, it is the first time in their lives that participants have come together with members of the other gender for the purpose of exploring gender differences and relationships.

In this chapter we'd like to describe what happens in these workshops and what we are learning about how women and men struggle for mutuality. We believe that the workshops are a microcosm of the larger culture, suggesting contexts for facilitating positive growth and change in relationships. We will also discuss implications and applications for clinical work with individuals and couples.

The workshops were originally designed on the model of relational mutuality—namely, that healthy, growth-enhancing relationships are built on experiences of mutual engagement, mutual empathy, mutual authenticity, and mutual empowerment. In designing the workshops, we were also influenced by political workshops created at the Center for Psychological Study in the Nuclear Age in Cambridge, MA to foster Soviet–American relationships. In those workshops *intergroup dialogue* was a central facilitating structure. Constructive conflict and *struggling with difference* are inevitable in relationships. They stimulate growth when the creative tension of *staying with the differences* is supported by the relational context. What Miller has called "waging good conflict" (1976) can lead to growth and enlargement of relationships. The gender workshops are designed to bring out prototypical conflicts and impasses between men and women, and then to offer structures and strategies for breaking through the impasses and for building connection.

Our work up to his point has been primarily with white, middle-class, highly educated men and women, although in most workshops there are members of various ages, sexual preference, race, class, and ethnicity, who have spoken up to represent their different perspectives. We are hoping to find ways to explore more explicitly the impact of diversity on the dynamics of woman-man relationships. The men who have come to these workshops represent a highly select sample—those who will risk doing such work.

Riane Eisler, in her book *The Chalice and the Blade* (1987), calls for the creation of a new form of relationship—moving beyond the pow-er-over, "dominator" model to what she calls the new "partnership" model, which finds its roots in the pre-Bronze Age, prepatriarchal cul-tures she has studied. Eisler views this evolution as part of a whole paradigm shift, corresponding to new models of science, physics, and biology, as well as shifts towards global awareness.

In our workshops, we emphasize the qualifies of creativity which contribute to mutuality. Moving beyond old models of self-develop-ment as the basis for healthy relationship, such as consolidating iden-tity, healthy narcissism, assertiveness, or firm ego boundaries—we emphasize the relational and creative qualities which foster growth-enhancing connection. To name a few: curiosity, flexibility, spontane-ity, freedom of movement, patience, persistence, humility, playfulness, humor, and also intuition, risk taking, trying out new perspectives and configurations, paradoxical thinking, holding opposites simultaneous-ly, knowing when to hold and when to let go, and openness to change.

The importance of creativity has not yet been fully recognized in the study of human relationships. Like most psychological characteris-tics, it has been studied primarily in traditionally male realms—the arts and sciences—and not yet in its fundamental forms in daily life and relationships, where women's creativity has often gone unrecog-nized.

THE WORKSHOP

The workshop begins with a discussion of the larger cultural context, and how important we feel it is for peacemaking and global survival. We discuss the range and limits of our own particular experience, and how issues of class, race, age, and heterosexual orientation make sig-nificant differences. We also take up the issue of stereotyping, empha-sizing that we are working with *group differences* between men and women, cognizant that these will not describe any particular man or woman. Recognizing our own particularities, we begin to articulate a relational perspective on women's and men's psychological develop-ment, assuming a basic underlying motive and desire for human con-nection in both groups. Janet describes the Stone Center relational model of development and the paradigm shift that we will be using in the workshop. This involves a complex model, encompassing a sense of self but also a sense of the other and a sense of the relationship, stressing what Stern calls "self-with-other" experiences (1985).

Healthy connection implies an awareness of and care for self, other, and the relationship, and none of these can be sacrificed in the search for mutuality. Janet also describes the connections, disconnections, and violations that shape women's experience in this culture, including women's carrying the one-sided responsibility for the care and maintenance of relationships.

Steve then speaks about reframing men's psychological development from this same relational perspective (Bergman, 1991) and describes "male relational dread," a man's sense, in a close relationship, that he is not enough and therefore must withdraw or attack. As one man described it: "When my wife says 'I love you,' my back starts to sweat." It is essential to provide a common language—conflict, connection, mutuality, empathy, power and dread are named and defined and can then be used as the basis for communication throughout the workshop.

In the second phase of the workshop, men and women are asked to go into separate rooms to answer a prepared questionnaire. Then, breaking each larger gender group into smaller groups of three or four, participants are asked to respond to three questions, with one person recording each small group's answers. The three questions are:

1. Name three strengths the other gender group brings to relationship.
2. What do you most want to understand about the other gender group?
3. What do you most want the other gender group to understand about you?

The rationale for this is to give each gender group the opportunity to give voice to its particular experience and to stimulate respect, curiosity, interest, and empathy for the other group. The answers to these questions later become the basis for the intergroup dialogue.

When the genders separate for the first time to answer the questions, there is a palpable sense of relief—how much easier it is for members of both genders to be with their own!

The women easily form small groups and seek a group process to answer the questions. They readily engage with each other, and Janet observes the clear relational energies and responsive movements, verbal and nonverbal—there is much hand waving and head nodding—all around the room.

The men, while relieved to be with each other away from the women, begin more slowly, starting with jokes and sarcastic banter, of-

ten about having to be there. Many have begun the workshop by holding themselves apart, assuming a critical, contemptuous, or bored
stance. Actually, many of the men have been brought under some
duress by women—as one said, "dragged kicking and screaming."
However when they get with the other men, they become enlivened
and energetic. Filling out the questionnaire in the small group, frequently each man will first write down his *own* list of answers in silence and then join in compiling his list with other individual lists.

Next, all the women come together into one large group with
Janet, and the men with Steve, to share their responses with each other
and with each of us. Typically, a strong sense of connection between
the women evolves quickly. Often the women talk about how much
easier it is to be with other women than in a *mixed* group, how much
safer and more confident they feel. They speak of how much anxiety
and attention go towards monitoring the men's responses.

The men, when they get together in one large group, are often
surprised at how similar their individual responses to the questions
are. Hearing that other men share the same thoughts and feelings in
their relationships with women is a tremendously important step and
helps the men to feel accepted and validated by other men for doing
this work—what one man jokingly referred to as "the wimp-work of
relationship." This men's group eventually becomes energized and cohesive.

We have found that this same-gender group experience is a vitally
necessary precursor to the next phase. Janet and the other women are
always amazed at the difference in the men when they come back into
the mixed gender group, after being together in the men's group: they
are no longer stiff or holding back, but energized and curious, and, as
Janet once said, "looking so much more *dimensional*."

MEN'S ANSWERS TO QUESTION 1

"Name three strengths the other gender group brings to relationship."
This question is always the *easiest* for the men to answer. Some of
the men's answers about women are: nurturance, capacity for feeling,
sensitivity, speaking emotional truth, realness, self-revealing, interest
in working on relationships, courage to raise issues, ability to deal
with more than one thing at a time, capacity to ask for support, seeing
both sides of a situation, warmth, tenderness, skill at noncompetitive
interaction, women are the "waker-uppers" in relationship, women
have more patience with children.

WOMEN'S ANSWERS TO QUESTION 1

"Name three strengths the other gender group brings to relationship."

This, the easiest question for the men, is inevitably the most *difficult* question for the women. (Some groups have said, "None.") It is difficult because the women soon realize that some quality of men— say, "objectivity"—may be a strength or not, depending on whether or not it is in the service of the relationship, that is, it depends on "the relational context." Here are some of the women's answers about men's strengths: caretakers; deep loyalties; relationship through action and projects; lifting heavy objects; rational thinking; focusing on one thing at a time; honesty; directness; can let things go and move on; breadwinners; protectors; know how to deal with fear; alliance builders; not so overwhelmed by feelings; strategic; product makers; purposeful; stabilizers of the relationship; killing spiders; their sex-drive; they make us feel frisky about sex; they have internal heaters at night.

MEN'S ANSWERS TO QUESTION 2

"What do you most want to understand about the other gender group?"

This question is invariably the hardest for the men. The reasons for this are multiple. Women are usually more forthcoming about their experiences, so men have less to ask about. Also, men have been trained away from a curious, open, empathic stance about others and often are concerned that if they ask questions, they won't know how to deal with the emotions stirred up and unleashed. For many men, opening up a connection by asking questions about a woman's experience feels dangerous. As one man said, "I may get caught in an emotional bog;" another, "an emotional swamp." (This "wetland" imagery is quite common.) Men's questions tend to be about women's anger and what women's relational processes are like:

"What are you so angry about? What do you want from me? Why do you expand your processes *ad infinitum*? When you're with your friends, how do you know when to end a conversation?—do you ever actually get anywhere? What is it like to be oppressed? How do you come to personalize relational failure to such a degree? What supports you? What is it like to have your cyclical bodily functions? Why is the sharing of feelings so important? How can your emotions be so fluid? How can you do three things at once? Why do you fake orgasm? How to understand your sensitivity to subtle cues, verbal and nonverbal?

How do you stay with your feelings so well? How do you care so much without losing your self? What's this intense need in a relationship? Why do women tend to tolerate men's behavior? What's it like to have babies?"

WOMEN'S ANSWERS TO QUESTION 2

"What do you most want to understand about the other gender group?"

This, the hardest question for men to answer, is invariably the *easiest* for the women, who have many, many questions. One woman answered, "Everything! I've been waiting my whole life to hear this!" The questions women ask of men center on men's fears and vulnerabilities and the effort to understand men's emotional and relational life:

"What are men's real fears? Why is it so hard to talk about relationships? How can you disconnect actions from emotions, how can you have sex without being emotionally involved? Why the urgency for sex? What is the burden of needing to be successful? What moves you deeply? Do men feel? If so, how and what? What do sports really mean? What do jokes really mean? What helps men overcome their experience of dread? Why won't men go to doctors? Why won't men stop and ask directions? What are you so afraid of in relationships? Why do you have trouble listening? What is the most effective way to teach the harms of patriarchy? How can we engage men in dialogue? What goes on between men that you don't want women to know about? What is it between sons and their mothers? What happens between receiving a message and sending back your response? How can you put yourself first so much of the time? What would it take to get men to become relational without major bloodletting? What's it like to live in a man's body?"

As the women and men return from their separate groups, we ask them to sit on opposite sides of the room. At this point, there is a lot of anxiety and often anger from the men, who begin to complain about the separation—"in a workshop on relationship you shouldn't separate us!"—and often to question our competence as leaders.

We asked one man, who seemed terribly anxious, what was wrong. He said, "I'm afraid that *something might happen!*"

The women are often leaning forward in their chairs, curious, expectant, and one woman replied, "I'm *hoping* that something might happen!

The men experience the face-to-face setup as an invitation to confrontation, possibly leading to disconnection and maybe even physical withdrawal or violence. Compared to being in the men's group, this is a kind of living hell. As one highly motivated, caring man said, with a mournful sigh, "It was so much easier the old way. You didn't have to work so hard."

This intergroup encounter is the most powerful and poignant time in the workshop. Whether we work for two hours or eight hours (depending on the time available), certain predictable impasses and breakthroughs occur.

Almost invariably, the women will ask the men to go first and to read their responses to Question 1, three strengths women bring to relationship. One small group of men will answer hesitatingly, the women will respond enthusiastically, and then ask more questions, wanting to go deeper. At this, the men will experience the women's questions as (to use the language of three different groups) "bullets," "arrows," or "darts" and will start to feel judged as inadequate, under attack, and criticized. Dread is generated, and the men withdraw and fall silent. This stimulates the *Dread/Anger Impasse*: the men retreat, the women begin to get angry and feel abandoned and misunderstood, and then the men either withdraw further or attack the women for being angry. Things stop, dead. After a while the women will read their responses to Question 1, often beginning by saying, "We found it really *difficult* to answer this question." Since this is the easiest question for the men, the men feel more criticized, often saying, "You couldn't even come up with *three* strengths?" The women reply, "It depends on how they're used." The men: "You can't even name three without *qualifying them?*" In this hostile atmosphere the men find it hard to grasp that a strength may also be a weakness, *depending on how it's used in relationship, the relational context*. This is a consistent gender difference, often invisible to men. Stuck in the impasse, there follow attempts to avoid further conflict. One man suggested to a woman that she go and listen to herself alone with a tape recorder until she modified her anger to a level to which he could respond. (An example of how women are supposed to go off, get therapy, or read self-help books to change themselves to fix the relationship.) This comment made the impasse worse.

WHAT IS A RELATIONAL IMPASSE?

An *impasse* occurs when a relationship is stuck, static, unmoving, with a sense that it may never move again. Things go dead, each participant retreats into his or her self. Everyone feels the relational space close down, and the closing down closes down more space, and a negative spiral is created; increased dread leads to increased anger leads to increased dread. Things become more polarized, and often fall into more gender-stereotypical behavior, resulting in disconnection and the loss of the possibility not only of contact but also of *working with the conflict*. An impasse is *relational* in the sense that it cannot reside only in one person or the other, but *in the process* between them—it's not a matter of him or her, but how they are interacting. While there may be a transferential component, the impasse is not mainly transferential, but rather the result of one relational style meeting another, quite different one—the result of everyone's learnings over many years, about what happens in relationship. Yet in the workshops, when individuals and couples start to see that these group impasses are clearly recognizable in their own lives, there is a sense of relief. In our workshops for couples, people often are astonished to hear other couples using their exact same words or phrases.

Another striking gender difference, also mostly invisible to men, is the way that there is a continuous flow towards the group focusing on the *men's* experience. Partly this is because the women keep asking more questions, partly it is because the men do not. Over and over, like the ballast of a ship, the attention tips to what's going on with the men. If you remember, Question 2—"*What do you most want to understand about the other gender?*"—was quite difficult for the men to respond to. Again and again we see how, in the end, the problem of mutuality is not only the men's inability to talk about their experience in relationship, but also their disinclination to explore and their difficulty in searching out the women's experience, in asking questions that would open up the relationship, what Jordan, Kaplan, Miller, Stiver, and Surrey (1991) have called "approaches to empathy" or "relational intersubjectivity" or simply "curiosity about the experience of the other, the other's interiority." The process of "trying on the feelings" of the other as a way of knowing and connecting, so essentially familiar to women in relationship, is often foreign to men. In one group, after Steve over and over urged the men to ask the women a direct question about their experience, one man asked, "What do you want from us?" Group observation of whose experience receives the most attention can lead to a constructive discussion of how power imbalances are played out—without any conscious intent.

In addition to the *Dread/Anger Impasse*, two others are invariably present in our workshops, and often in couples, that we can only mention here: the *Product/Process Impasse*, where the women want to keep opening up the process while the men are trying to complete the task. One couple related a conversation they had when they were moving to a new house, carrying a box to the car:

WOMAN: It's sad to say goodbye to this house.

MAN: Yeah, but think about where we're going (*the woman slows down and starts to cry*).

MAN: Uh-oh.

WOMAN: Please—can we talk?

MAN: Not now. We've got to finish this.

WOMAN: I really need to talk. I need to know where you are.

MAN: (*exasperated*): I'm right here. Moving. How can we talk when we're trying to move?

WOMAN: How can you just go about moving without any feeling?

The third impasse we call the *Power-over/Power-with Impasse*, where the men experience conflict as a threat or an attempt to control, while the women want everyone's voice to be heard and attended to and retreat from what seem like definitive stands. An example, based on one medical student's dilemma brought up in a workshop, is around something as simple as going to dinner:

WOMAN: Where shall we go to dinner?

MAN: Let's go to Miguel's.

WOMAN: How about Pintemento?

MAN: Okay, let's go to Pintemento.

WOMAN: But it sounded like you wanted to go to Miguel's.

MAN: No, no, it's okay—let's go where *you* want to go.

WOMAN: But I want to go where you want to go, too. (*pause*) Why don't you want to go to Pintemento?

MAN: I just want to decide.

WOMAN: We *are* deciding.

MAN: We're not getting anywhere. (*tensely*) Let's just make a decision.

WOMAN: (*screaming*) Why are you yelling at me?

MAN: (*screaming*) I'm not yelling.

All three impasses may occur in any particular aspect of a relationship. Think, for example, of how any or all of these impasses might get played out around sex.

THE SHIFT TO MUTUALITY

What happens to break through these impasses? What we consistently try to introduce into the process is the value of *staying with conflict* and

staying in connection, holding to and moving with a sense of "the relationship," the "We," which includes but also transcends the "You" and
the "Me." Acknowledging the importance of mutual responsibility for
the relationship can be a very new and fresh level of thinking for many
people. Sometimes the concept is not easy. We suggested to one man
that when he felt like retreating, he think about taking care of the relationship. He replied, "How can I think about the 'We' when I'm thinking about the 'Me'?" We felt he was speaking for all of us.

And yet it is just at the point when the participants are deadened
and flattened by the anger and dread and pain of an impasse that to
talk not of a particular person but of "the relationship" is of the most
use. Those of you who work with couples know that, in the pain and
rage of the initial visit, to focus on one—or each—person's failings or
pathology is to invite disaster. But when both members of a couple focus on "the relationship," the idea that "the relationship is not working and we are going to address that, together," often brings a sense of
relief, movement out of the impasse, away from blame or shame and
towards a new sense of possibility.

In an impasse, the polarization and rage can be extreme. One
man, enraged, said to a woman, "I've had enough of women's anger,
and if I hear the word 'patriarchy' one more time, I'll kill! It's not *me!*"
In this kind of impasse, other men and women try to offer empathic
responses to those who have become polarized, and the group begins
to find ways of holding the conflict, and the different perspectives, to
move towards some enlarged understanding that encompasses the
differences. The work stays in the here and now, and, when it moves,
stays away from a "self-centered" perspective. We encourage group
members to make "I-statements"—speaking from each one's personal
experience, beginning a statement with "I feel" or "I think," but we
have learned that it is not enough to just "get your feelings out." Participants have to be aware of the effect of their statements on the tenuous web of connection that is being created by the group. "I-statements" made *with awareness of the relational context and an intention to
build connection* move the group towards greater clarity and authenticity, "I-statements" made without this awareness and intention solidify
the impasse.

The group moves back and forth through power struggles, polarization, emotional reactivity, defensiveness, avoidance tactics, person-
alizing, and sometimes deep despair, cynicism, grief, and hopelessness about ever getting anywhere—an accurate microcosm of the
woman-man relationship! The group also moves in and out of moments of breakthroughs into connection and creative, constructive dia-

logue and problem solving. An important breakthrough often comes when the men feel supported enough to follow up on their question to the women, "Why are you so angry?" In a recent workshop, this produced the following dialogue:

A WOMAN: I was really angry at what was going on in the group yesterday. When you asked us to visualize our images of the relationship in the group, I saw a wall of grey steel with the sound of fingernails going down it. You men don't really give a damn about us. (*Silence from the men; we ask what's going on*)

A MAN: If we respond, we'll take away her feelings.

THE WOMAN: No, if you're silent you will. We keep having to read your facial expressions, because you don't tell us the truth.

THE MAN: I guess I just have to let you be angry.

STEVE: Why not *ask* her what *she* wants?

THE MAN: What do you want?

THE WOMAN: I needed to express my anger—I need you to understand that.

A MAN: You want me to agree with you?

ANOTHER WOMAN: She wants a *response*, rather than a sheet of metal. (*The men try to respond, but it is difficult and awkward; the women respond to the men's difficulty—the focus is soon back on the men.*)

THE WOMAN: You men keep asking me what I want you to do, but again the *focus here isn't on you*, it's on me. I'm asking you to touch into my anger—to connect.

JANET: She wants you to "try on" her experience. She's asking for an empathic connection that feels like you're there with her, like you're interested.

THE MAN. It's hard for me to hear your anger, when I feel so responsible, but I'll try.

ANOTHER MAN: I hear you saying *not* to think about it in terms of myself, right? (*the woman nods*) You know something?—that's a *big* relief (*Much laughter from the group; a sense of real connection and movement*)

This shifted the quality of connection dramatically—and lastingly—towards what we call mutuality." Everyone sensed the shift. The men felt the relational space open up, and the opening up opened up more space—the negative spiral turned positive. No longer feeling dread, the men were able to listen to, be interested in, and respond to the women. Although there was intense conflict, there was relief in the sense of not being alone with it. Different participants offered different perspectives on how to break through the impasse, with various creative solutions being tried. There were several tries which led to disconnections, but *staying present* through the disconnection allowed a better connection to be made. As the men felt the relational space open, they could trust the women more and be more creative in what they said; as the women began to sense this mutual empathy, they began to trust the men more and take greater risks as well. Suddenly we all found ourselves engaged in the process of growth through and towards connection.

As groups begin to work on the impasses together, there develops a sense of shared responsibility and creativity. There follows a distinct moment when it is clear to everyone present that a shift has occurred, the group feels different. In fact *something has happened.* This we have called the "shift into mutuality." We have a sense, so far, that this shift occurs in our workshops, to a greater or lesser extent, depending on how much time we have for the process of mutual empathy to work. It isn't always clear how we got there, yet everyone can recognize the difference: there is an intense *sense of relational presence—people are really there.* In one-group, we asked the participants, at the end, to look back and describe the feeling after the shift had occurred. These were some of the words they used: "release, comfort, caring, safety, sharing, peaceful, easy, enjoyment of different styles, it's hopefulness, mutual nurturance, energizing, movement, insight, softening, appropriate confrontation, dynamic process, clearer recognition of others' experience."

In Stone Center language, we have described mutuality as a *way* of being in relationship—a dialogical, open, changing movement in relationship, where each person can increasingly represent her or his own experience, feelings, and perceptions, and each can move and be moved by the other and by the relationship. This sense of mutually-empathic joining is the basis for new power and new action. When men and women get to this place, something truly hopeful has happened. We don't yet know what is possible or what power this *shift to mutuality* between women and men can truly generate!

In the workshops, only after this shift and movement occur can the most difficult subjects be worked on. The issues brought up previously that led to the impasses are often the ones with the group really attending, responding, ruthlessly encountering the psychological "facts" without the burden of judgment, without a need to "agree," "disagree," or even "agree to disagree," and with an authentic desire to understand. It's amazing to us how the same questions which had brought hostile silence now bring animated discussion, how dread and anger—in one workshop nicknamed "the Big D" and "the Big A"—can be addressed unflinchingly. Humor is much in evidence, humor not in the service of sublimated aggression, but in the service of connection. Real information begins to be exchanged with real feeling. Real understanding occurs. For example, the men in one group said that one reason they fall silent when they sense a problem in relationship is that they've been taught they have to *fix* problems, and if they can't fix it, they won't say anything at all, won't even acknowledge that the problem exists—"if you don't talk about it, there's no problem."

With the affirmation of shared experience with other men, and freed from a sense of dread about the women's reaction, the men could show their pain about their sense of relational incompetence, and the women could feel it. At the same time, the men could appreciate and feel how crazy-making this is for the women. Through this mutually empathic joining—holding both sets of feelings, simultaneously—a creative moment happens, and the relationship can move.

In that same "fingernail-on-steel" group, after the shift to mutuality had occurred, for the first time we heard men describe how it is only in groups with other men that they can begin to be open about the losses in their lives—the loss of relationships with wives, children, and especially fathers. The men talked about how they could *not* be open about grief and loss with women—and then started to do it! As the men spoke of this, the women were leaning forward with exquisite attentiveness.

> THE MAN: All you women are leaning forward, listening really hard, and it's really quiet, like you can't believe that men have grief, or are lonely.
>
> A WOMAN: Are men lonely?
>
> THE MAN: God, don't you know?
>
> ANOTHER WOMAN: I thought so, but we've been waiting a long time to hear it. About a *millenium*, in fact.
>
> ANOTHER WOMAN: I'm drawn towards you, but I'm pulling back too, because I just don't want to take care of you anymore.
>
> THE MAN: I can understand that. But we're not asking you to take care of us anymore. Just hear it, that's all.

When the groups are working together in this way, we have heard the most extraordinary, honest, sensitive, intelligent, and thoughtful discussions of questions raised by each group about the other. We have discussed sexual differences and impasses, parenting issues, power imbalances, and even sexual abuse by therapists—to name a few. These are the moments that build our faith in the as yet untapped power of mutuality between women and men. Usually, only at the very end of this male–female encounter part of the workshop, with time running out, do we get to Question 3—"What do you most want the other gender group to understand about you?" By the time we get to these answers, the shift to mutuality has occurred, and we ask the men and women just to read their answers through, without discussion. In the quiet, attentive atmosphere, the answers are always not only touching, but healing.

WOMEN'S ANSWERS TO QUESTION 3

"What do you most want men to understand about you?"
We are not the enemy; even if I'm not clear, I have a point; to know what my experience of disconnection feels like; that conflict is an invitation to engagement which can bring closeness and resolution; conflict does not mean the dissolution of the relationship; how frightening men's power for violence is in limiting women's actions; don't trivialize my experience—go with my female creative process; what it feels like to make 67 cents to the dollar; that my way is not wrong, just different; that we are angry because we are hurt; that my sexuality is far beyond the physical connection; that I just want you to be there; that I am a human being too; we want to share, not take over; that we're not experts at relationships either.

MEN'S ANSWERS TO QUESTION 3

"What do you most want women to understand about you?"
I am not your enemy; how many of my actions are acts of love; my difficulties communicating feelings; my need for solitude; my difficulties in admitting powerlessness and asking for help; that I need space; that I need time; I'm scared too; not to have to censor my maleness; I love competition and play; how I feel about responsibility; the heavy burden placed on men to be successful and not look foolish; that being a son is often difficult; my sense of intrusion that often comes with relationships and my sense of shame for feeling that; I want to change; we care about relationships as much as women do;

men are scared of other men too; men have different priorities; the complexity of masculinity; our relational yearnings; our grief over losses; that I will come back after I go away.

In a workshop with college students, where the group encounter had been particularly heated and fragmented, after the men had read what they wanted the women to understand about them, one of the women was so moved, she spoke for the group: "There's a glow now. You gave us the other half of the string, and now we can make a tie."

THE DOUBLE STANDARD ON THE ROAD TO MUTUALITY

How does this shift to mutuality occur? At the end of the group encounter, when we have asked participants what they think helped the shift to mutuality to occur, these are some of their answers:

We realized we weren't getting anywhere by staying angry.

We felt, somehow, as if we were seen, together. Like we'd deeply seen a truth of the way we were treating each other, together.

We got out of the "I" to the "We," out of the authority/submissive role. We got into a movement rather than an obsessing.

We saw the danger of going on like that.

I think when that young lady there said that we were getting nowhere, I felt kind of ashamed, and didn't want any more conflict, and I tried to listen. And then when you bugged us men to respond, eventually we did.

We have seen that there is a "double standard" on this road to mutuality, and that men and women have different work to do on this shared journey. We also recognize that although men deeply feel women's power in relationships, men's power and privilege in the world has the major impact on the search for mutuality. Most frequently, it is the less powerful person or group who is more aware of the lack of mutuality and who initiates the struggle. Members of the more powerful group have different work to do as they begin to take responsibility for change.

WOMEN'S PATH TO MUTUALITY

1. The importance of sequence. At this time in our history, many women are feeling angry, despairing, and "tired of taking care of men, of doing all the *work* in the relationship." In the workshops, we have seen over and over how the beginning point of dialogue is around women's anger. Women *want* to hear men's experience but often first need to feel men moving towards them, learning to connect empathically, listening and seeking to understand their experience, especially to understand the origins of their anger. Only after this happens (or even after a slight forward movement is felt) are women able to listen fully to men and appreciate the depth of honesty the men are often able to express in the workshops.

2. *Women working together.* The power that results from the women meeting together and building a sense of solidarity and support before the intergroup dialogue is striking. The women often talk together about how different it feels to be among women. When men are present, especially their own partners, they feel more focused on the men's reactions. They notice together how much energy goes into watching the men—one woman called this "ego-tending," another, "hovering," as she was constantly checking out her husband to make sure that he wasn't either getting hurt, or hurting someone else. Women can validate each other's experience with this monitoring *and* the desire to change.

When the intergroup dialogue begins then, the women are able to offer enormous support to each other. Feeling this support, individual women are more able to effectively represent their experience to the men and to *stay with* their anger and their needs until the men respond. Other women can then relate to the men's confusion and suggest ways they might respond. This work can be done in a group much more easily and effectively than in a dyad.

There are significant divisions that emerge among women, especially around anger at men. We have seen enormous controversy about anger and where it belongs. These differences can be used to create mutuality if they do not lead to a split among women, that functions to resist change and to support the status quo.

3. *The search for new models of relationship.* Women in the workshops are often seeking a new model of relating to men—struggling to let go of what feels like "compulsive caretaking." The men often respond anxiously when the old forms are challenged, fearing that women are moving away or abandoning them. It is essential for everyone to work together towards a new psychology of a woman-man relationship, where women can stay *with* their own experience *and* hold an empathic connection to the men without feeling they have to "take care of men or the relationship." One woman described this situation as follows:

> It's like on a football field (she was trying to use men's language). We've been way down on your side and now we're going back to our side. We're having a good time together here. But we're still holding the relationship with you and are waiting for you to move towards us so we can play the game over the whole field.

This is a very important growth step—envisioning the possibility of different configurations of connection and allowing for different patterns of movement, distance and initiation within connection.

In the workshops, we have seen women shift to an appreciation of men's intelligence and perceptivity once the dialogue really opens up; we have heard women sharing aspects of their own experience in interesting new ways—ways that emerge as women and men begin to create a *shared relational context*. Appreciating and sharing are beautiful examples of Jean Baker Miller's description (1986) of the five outcomes of connection: new energy, an ability to take new action, new knowledge of self and other, an enhanced sense of self-worth, and a desire for more connection. (However, as growth in connection is never linear, such a positive experience can make it even more painful when, in real life, things revert—as they inevitably will—to old ways.) As a next step, many women say they need to examine why they resist and fear really seeing men's emotional vulnerabilities. Women, at this point, also have to face their own limitations and fears in relationship.

As a white, heterosexual woman (and a psychotherapist), I (Janet) am aware that in some other situations I hold the power and privilege. One of the important learnings for me in doing these workshops has been to understand better the *responsibilities* of the more powerful group in the struggle for relational mutuality, and then to apply that to myself—recognizing in other situations my initial blindness, my resistance to doing the work, and that it is up to me to be responsible for listening to the others' experiences, and for initiating change in relationships where I am in the more powerful position.

MEN'S PATH TO MUTUALITY.

In our workshops, men "get to mutual" in several steps—steps which may apply to men "getting to mutual" in any relationship, including therapy:

1. *Men naming their relational experiences.* It's surprising how rarely men have had their experience named. To use words like "relational dread," "a desire for connection," and to talk about a paradigm shift to thinking of "the relationship" as a "thing" give men a language which rings true and makes the relational world more real. As one man put it, "You mean we can take 'the relationship' on vacation with us to the Grand Canyon?"

2. *Men connecting with other men.* In our all-male subgroup, a man listens to another man describe in detail what he had always thought of as his own "secret" experiences—for example, "dread." Hearing

similarities may wake both men up, making each sharper and clearer, building a base of understanding through an interchange around *similarity*. Men feel a heightened sense of male identity, and male vulnerability, grief, and loss are often themes. Most Robert Bly / "men's movement" gatherings end at this point (Bly, 1990). Yet we see all-male work as a beginning, as a necessary step for the next phase, when men, facing women, are asked to do the uncomfortable and dangerous work, on their creative edges, of opening to women and connecting through difference.

3. *Men holding differences in relationship with women.* In the arena of relationship, men often feel incompetent, criticized, and defensive. This may lead to men disparaging the idea of "learning from women," or the fear of becoming "soft males" or "feminized men." We have seen the profound differences between women and men, and one of the differences is that *men are often not as aware of the relational differences*. If men are to learn about mutual empathic relationship and the nurturing of relationship, this learning will most likely take place through engagement with differences with women.

But first, men have to *see the differences*. Often, relational events are invisible to men. (After four years of this work, I (Steve) can vouch for this myself.) Men are not as aware of "the relational context" as women, are not as aware of women's attending to men's egos and responding to men's feeling states in relationship, and are not as aware of power imbalances involving the disempowerment of the subordinate gender. (Often, neither men nor women are aware of the gender differences in *relational timing*—women are often quicker than men.) To make these invisible relational facts visible is an essential step in men's learning mutuality—and crucial in working with men in psychotherapy. When these facts are revealed in a supportive environment, with other men seeing them at the same time so that the facts can be felt not as *personal* blindness but as *gender* blindness, men feel a sense of amazement, relief, and curiosity. Women's *relational* power is often frightening to men. For men to hear women's experience of diminished *institutional* power, and, further, to see that a shift from a power-over to a power-with model would mean not loss of men's power but in fact a further empowerment of all, has enormous implications for the culture and for the society.

Men often translate difference into conflict, and conflict with women can be intense. Men need to learn that they can encounter and hold conflict without something bad happening. Often, at the first sign of difference and conflict, a man may make a "flyswatter" response—trying to crush it. The fear of becoming violent is a prime element of male relational dread.

Men can get stuck in the paralysis of the dread of connection on the one hand, and, on the other, if they are in connection, in the fear of disconnection, of loss. This stuck stance can feel so precarious that men may do everything in their power not to change anything. If, as one man said, "the feeling of peace is when nothing happens," doing and saying nothing can protect a man from the anxious feeling that "something might happen." In relationship, men may be more at home with stasis, with a finished product, and fear process and relational movement. To get to mutual in relationship with women, it is essential that men be supported through conflict, dread, and fear long enough to have the experience of "something good happening."

4. *Men learning empathy in relationship with women.* Faced with women's anger, a crucial step for men to take is to *watch other men respond to women,* and *women respond to women, to see how* the process of attending and responding takes place. Men can learn to allow themselves to be moved by the feelings of the other as a way of becoming connected, and to know that it is possible to move in connection without endangering the sense of self.

At an early age men learn that self-worth means being competent at doing things well. In our workshops, men learn more about "doing empathy well." Empathy is "broken down" into its components, and becomes something real, unmysterious, even fascinating. Each component—"attending," "responding," "not being a blank screen," "trying on feelings"—becomes known, and then reassembled. Men learn what it is and how to do it, and then find that they can get better at it and feel valued for it.

Often in our workshops men will say, "But I *have* good relationships with men—me and my buddy can be out fishing for a whole day, and not talk much, but it's a good relationship." And yet men, when asked, will admit that "with my wife, it's different—both of us can really open up and talk. I feel she really understands me." When this happens–and it is almost always with a woman–men recognize how good it feels to be in mutual empathic relationship. This desire for mutuality may be hard to "get to" in men's awareness and may come out directly only at times when it is unalterably lost, or when men, almost despite themselves, find themselves experiencing it, or when they see women having it with their women friends, see that it is missing in their own lives and sense a deep lonely yearning, for connection.

Finally, the question that women often ask is *How do you get men to listen and attend to these matters?* While men may have a deep yearning for connection, a lot stands in the way of starting to learn about it–for about five thousand years "real men" didn't do this. So why do some men open up?

Sometimes, men will be opened up by a *loving relationship* with a woman, or by being a father, or by caring for a sick or dying father or mother or other family member.

Men may also open up through the *pain and suffering in relationship*. As in our workshops, getting to a painful and creative edge of an impasse with a women is often a precursor to a shift to mutuality. Men may have a difficult time *anticipating* relational events, so that often it is only *after* men say or do something to affect someone—or even to hurt someone—that they wake up. Men may have to flee—or damage or destroy—a relationship with a woman in order to really *feel* what they have to lose, and to realize that they want exactly what they are fleeing, or what they have damaged or destroyed. Men's being stuck between dread of connection and fear of loss, and being afraid of engaging in the movement of relationship, may have much to do with men's difficulty in both anticipating *and* recollecting relational events. It is rare that a man will say to a woman, without prompting, "I was thinking about what we were talking about yesterday."

A final way that men may open up to mutuality is *through men's groups*. Men connecting with men may lead to a separatist mentality which merely and archaically makes men more "male" and doesn't propel men towards making mutual connection; or it may lead to the realization that other men are a resource in learning to form mutually empathic, mutually authentic, mutually empowering relationships, with both men and women. There is a tremendous power right now in these men's groups. If this power can be *brought into relationship with women and shifted to mutual connection*, we might just be seeing a beginning in the transformation of the millenial pain shared by women and men to shared creative energy. Our workshop with four-year-old girls and boys gives us much hope for these possibilities.

CLINICAL APPLICATIONS

There are a number of applications of this model for clinical work that particularly emphasize the value of psychoeducational-process groups for studying and working with gender differences. (Useful educational material may be found in the Stone Center Working Paper series, Gilligan's and her group's writings (1982, 1989), and in Tannen (1990).) An interesting strategy for group therapy would be to alternate meetings of same-gender groups with the larger mixed-gender group. The value of groups is especially important in breaking down "individual pathology" attribution models and breaking out of the terrible isolation many couples experience. Most heterosexual couples lack a community where open exchange and constructive dialogue around relational struggles can take place.

We have developed an application of this workshop specifically for couples. A small group of couples meets on a Friday night and all day Saturday, with a similar formal of intergroup dialogue. We also discuss particular strategies and exercises for building connection, and couples leave with commitments to do particular assignments or projects together. We meet again one month later to see how people are applying the principles and to hear the couples report back on their work together. Mutual relationship has great power not only in one individual with another or others, but in one *couple* with another couple or other couples. As one man said to the group of couples, at the end of one workshop, "Your holding your relationships helps us to hold ours." Coleadership is of great value when the work towards mutuality is a vital and ongoing aspect of the coleadership pair. For example, while we are working together as leaders, we "check-in" periodically on the status of our own relationship both privately and in the group.

In the workshops for clinicians and for couples, we suggest particular "relational principles" which help to break through impasses. These principles, derived from the workshops, include: shifting to a relational paradigm; recognition and naming of impasses; early intervention; using a language of "connectors," staying with difference and conflict; creativity in action; moving through disconnection; letting go and coming back; and appreciating small changes.

We urge couples to map out the dialogue of a particular impasse they experience together (these are usually quite repetitive and fairly easy to choreograph), actually charting out in each line of dialogue what is going on in the woman, what is going on in the man, and what is going on in the relationship. Then, using our relational principles, we ask them to brainstorm ways to alter the dialogue, as a way of preventing or making early interventions in these destructive spirals and creatively changing impasses to breakthroughs. Looking together at their interaction helps couples to move into a space of mutual responsibility for the relationship.

In workshops for clinicians we also suggest particular strategies for building connection that may help clients work on developing relational mutuality. I'll give a few examples.

First we try to *enhance relational awareness*. To help men and women move into a relational paradigm, the use of "we" language is explored. One useful exercise has been to ask both people to close their eyes and *visualize the relationship*, and then to describe to each other the qualities of the relationship. What is the color, texture, sound, of the relationship. How does this change? For one man the texture went from "velvet" to "gravel" in an instant. Another question is "What animal is the relationship like?" One woman described the relationship as "a lioness, with two huge paws around both of us," while her partner saw "a spirited horse with a lot of energy—but it can gallop and get away from you."

Other ways to enhance relational awareness are (1) to have couples do *a relational inventory, together*—an informal assessment of the strengths and weaknesses of their relationship—and (2) to have both people together write a *relational purpose statement*—what is the purpose of the relationship, what are the questions it holds, what are we together to do or to learn. For example, one couple wrote: "To create a refuge, a safe place for us and children to grow and thrive, to create a place of peace and thus to contribute to the possibility of global peace."

We have noticed striking gender differences in *relational time*—the tempo and rhythm at which women and men attend to and respond to each other. We suggest several ways of bringing awareness to these gender-specific ways of handling relational time, such as the *check-in*, a simple, powerful, and useful exercise. Either person can call for a check-in, which consists of each person giving a brief "I-statement"— "I feel" or "I think." Discussion is not encouraged. As one couple said, "We have to be careful not to let our check-ins degenerate into conversation." Either person can also call for a *check-out*, with the proviso that the one checking out takes responsibility for checking back in, and saying *when* she or he will do this. Another strategy (Bombadieri, 1990) is the *20-minute rule*, which ensures but also limits talking about a particularly troublesome subject to 20 minutes per day. This creates a structure where men feel they don't have to take responsibility for setting time limits, while women can feel confident that they can expect full attention and engagement around the issue at hand.

To deal with the process/product impasse, we suggest *choosing a project*—or, better, *two* projects, one from each person's area of interest or expertise—finding a way to create together, whether this is a garden, a song, or a piece of serious writing—and to grow in the process of facilitating and building on each other's strengths.

We also suggest *ground rules for waging good conflict*, including check-ins (each person stating where he or she is in respect to the process of conflict) and check-outs (either person calling for a time out, if the conflict feels stuck, destructive, or abusive). Some ground rules need to be set in advance.

Couples can find humorous phrases which give perspective to impasses or conflicts, such as one man saying, in the middle of a fierce stuck place, "It's time to throw the garbage," or to find a phrase which, when the relationship seems to be disappearing, will *evoke* it—one couple's was: "We do it *together*."

CONCLUSION

From our work together over the past few years, we have grown even more cautious and gravely aware of how far we have to go, yet we also feel some hope that there can be creative change, movement, and growth towards mutuality in the woman–man relationship. It is only when we find ways to work together, to find the community and support we need to *participate* in this work, that such movement can take place. Perhaps what is needed is a "Women-*and*-Men's Movement."

Learning to live together creatively, facing into difference—difference of race, class, sexual orientation, ethnicity, and nation—is of vital significance as we move into the twenty-first century. We believe that this work on woman–man relationships is a potential model for the crucial work we all need to undertake, in transforming human impasses to possibilities.

DISCUSSION SUMMARY

After each colloquium presentation a discussion was held. Selected portions are summarized here. At this session Drs. Cynthia García Coll, Judith Jordan, Jean Baker Miller, Robin Cook-Nobles, and Irene Stiver joined Stephen Bergman and Janet Surrey in leading the discussion.

García Coll: As a developmental psychologist I am interested in how we develop these patterns. Can you talk about your work in other cultures and with four-year-olds?

Bergman: With four-year-olds at a preschool, we used the same format, first asking the boys and girls separately to answer three questions, modified for their level of understanding. Next the boys and girls sat on the floor facing each other.

The boys' answers to Question 1, "What do you like about girls?" were:

"They like to play what I like to play."
"They always play with me and help me with things."

The girls' answers were:

"We like kissing and hugging boys."
"We like when they chase us and tie us up and they thought we

were dead and we faked it and then we like sneaking away
and getting away."

This is appalling. But then something started to happen. The boys
were fidgeting, not paying much attention to the girls, and the girls
began to tell a story, together, each adding lines. The story was about
how one girl had tricked a wicked baby sitter. Soon the boys were listening wide-eyed. The girls—we realized this later—had found a way
to connect. Then a rather peculiar thing happened. I asked, "When
you play a game with the boys, who goes first?" One girl said, "Boys
go first." She looked to the other girls, and then, giggling, started to
chant, "Boys go first. Boys go first." Soon all the girls were getting into
it, "Boys go first. Boys go first" But the hopeful side was that, after this
encounter, there was a free-play period in a field. Soon the teacher, astonished, said, "This is amazing! I've never seen this before! The boys
and girls are playing together. And there are no more hierarchical patterns among the boys." He pointed out that the girls and boys were
running around holding hands—sometimes a foursome would run
by—and that the "top boy," the one usually on top of the hierarchy of
play, was by himself. No one was really paying much attention to him.
It hadn't been at all clear to us what had been going on in the group,
but now we could see that something had shifted, and the shift was
being incorporated immediately in their more interconnected play.

Surrey: We were in Turkey, a very gender-segregated society, with
very few cross-gender interactions except sexual ones, and with very
prescribed and male-dominated ways of being. People in Turkey kept
on saying "We're very relational, we define ourselves in relation, what
we need is more 'self.'" In fact, they were in very patterned relationships—with rigid and specified male and female roles and identities—
they were not dynamic, growth-fostering relationships. We saw that
the women were beginning to initiate the struggle for change, but that
the men were much further behind the men we'd seen in America and
seemed much less sensitized to relational matters.

It's a culture where men spend an enormous amount of time together—there's a strong male role and identity in family and society
and a richness of male ritual—no "soft males." It's a power-over culture, and that hinders mutuality in relationships. These observations
brought to mind some of the issues of the men's movement in this
country, where men are trying to create ritual and identity. Perhaps
men here are trying to recreate something that could be at odds with
building connection.

Question: Can there be other models of healthy relationship besides mutuality, such as a relationship based on action or autonomy?

Do men have to "sell out" to women's model of relationship, to mutuality?

Surrey: To me, mutuality simply means always holding an awareness of the other. You can be very active, doing things together or working "independently," but if you are out of touch with the impact of your actions on others, I don't think that's a healthy mode. Mutuality doesn't mean sitting around and talking all the time, it simply means maintaining a sense of self, a sense of the other, and a sense of what's happening in the relationship. You can be halfway around the world from someone and hold that, or you can be in a room with someone and *not* hold it. You could go off for days and write a book, if you negotiated that, and it still could be done with an awareness of the other and of the relationship—these are not mutually exclusive at all. But I do believe that action without awareness of its impact is extraordinarily dangerous and can lead to violence, so I would never say that that's a positive model. It's the same problem with autonomy—independence, creativity, working on your own—all those things are terrific, but never should be done without the awareness of the other and the impact on the relationship.

Bergman: We are not talking about men adopting women's ways; we are talking about both men and women moving to more healthy, human ways. This is not the "feminization" of men, but rather the "relationalization" of men and women both, together.

Stiver: This relates to the effect that the relational model brings to individual work as well as couples work. Whether you're working with a man or a woman, you can always bring the relationship into the work. The focus is to become aware not only of your own experience but to broaden your experience of the important people in your life. Whether I'm working with a man or a woman, I feel the work is more successful when something really changes in their important relationships. It's a dynamic of experiencing a relationship, often for the first time, in a different way.

Miller: It's a good question because sometimes we tend to get caught in old polarities, like relationships versus action or relationships versus something like autonomy. Relationships are very active if they're moving. Also, people can find their greatest sense of themselves, their fullest use of themselves within the context of relationships. In fact, I think people find their fullest selves when they are in a relationship that's moving towards mutuality.

Jordan: If men have been in a position of power-over and that position has brought them benefits, of course they're going to resist any change that will move them out of that position. Men not wanting to do it the "women's way," or selling out to women, is a crucial question because a huge part of male socialization is towards not being like women. The question is: How to present mutuality as having something in it for men? Steve has suggested very clearly that in these workshops men begin to get the sense that mutuality in relationship offers them a way to relieve and deal with their aloneness, their isolation, and their sense of being so armored and cut off.

Question: I'm wondering how your model applies in situations of difference among races, or gays and straights—the issues that arise from prejudice?

Cook-Nobles: I have been thinking about the male–female relationship within the African American experience. In the groups you have described, one of the questions the men asked the women was "What is it like to be oppressed?" In the African American experience, because both men and women have experienced oppression, the fear of the loss of the relationship takes on a different meaning qualitatively. The ultimate fear is that the safety net will be taken away if the relationship or the group is broken up. That threat may get in the way of hearing the other person's experience. I think that is some of what has happened in the African American community's response to the Thomas hearings. In dealing with the dynamics between two people, you are forced to look at the possible effect on the whole community. Will we lose the whole community? Who will be there to take care of us as a group? So you have those within-group conflicts which complicate the process on another level.

Question: I was also thinking of *different* races. How do people of color get members of the dominant race to sit down and recognize that there is a degree of interdependence that makes it worth their while to engage in the kind of intergroup conflict that these workshops address?

Cook-Nobles: I think there's a shift going on in which the minority group is not necessarily trying to get the majority group to sit down, but a shift in which the majority group needs to see its *need* to sit down. I think that's the shift not only in racial minority groups but also in the lesbian and gay community. We have to own the problem together.

Surrey: That was my point about the double standard and the importance to me of learning about initiating and taking responsibility as a white heterosexual woman. Watching men have to learn has helped me enormously.

Question: What about the danger of stereotyping men and women, polarizing into opposites human characteristics which are probably on a continuum rather than dichotomous?

Surrey: What we see really clearly is that the greater the impasse, the more gender stereotypical the behavior; the greater the movement towards mutuality, the more both women and men show the whole range of human characteristics, and the more we see everyone showing more individual, or "personal" behavior—and I believe that that's a microcosm of the larger situation in the society and in the world.

REFERENCES

Bergman, S. (1991). *Men's psychological development: A relational perspective.* (Work in Progress No. 48.) Wellesley, MA: Stone Center Working Paper Series.

Bly, R. (1990). *Iron John.* Reading, MA: Addison-Wesley.

Bombadieri, M. (1990). Personal communication.

Eisler, R. (1987). *The chalice and the blade.* New York: William Morrow.

Gilligan, C. (1982). *In a different voice.* Cambridge, MA: Harvard University Press.

Gilligan, C., Lyons, N., & Hanmer, T. (Ed.). (1989). Making connections: *The relational worlds of adolescent girls at Emma Willard School.* Troy, New York: Emma Willard School.

Jordan, J., Kaplan, S., Miller, J., Stiver, I., & Surrey, J. (1991). *Women's growth in connection.* New York: Guilford.

Miller, J.B. (1976). Toward a new psychology of women. Boston: Beacon.

Miller, J.B. (1986). *What do we mean by relationships?* (Work in Progress No. 22.) Wellesley, MA: Stone Center Working Paper Series.

Stern, D. (1985). The interpersonal world of the infant. New York: Basic Books.

Surrey, J. (1985). The "self-in-relation": A theory of women's development. (Work in Progress No. 13.) Wellesley, MA: Stone Center Working Paper Series.

Tannen, D. (1990). *You just don't understand.* New York: William Morrow.

This chapter was presented at a Stone Center Colloquium on November 6, 1991. © 1991 Stephen J. Bergman and Janet L. Surrey.

14

A Relational Approach to Therapeutic Impasses

IRENE P. STIVER

More than ten years ago I was asked to be a discussant at a symposium entitled "Regression in Psychotherapy." I am embarrassed to say that the title of my discussion was Regression in Borderline Personalities"; but that's only the half of it. I never recognized what I now know was a history of sexual abuse in most of the patients whose "regression" I described, and I used language such as: "fixated," "symbiotic relationship," "fusion," "merger," "false self/true self," and "sadomasochistic interactions" (Stiver, 1981, 1988).

On the positive side of this venture, I arrived at several interventions which I thought might reverse the "regressive" process in patients who began an apparent downhill course over several years of psychotherapy. One of these interventions was the use of an extended consultative process which I hoped would offer support to both patient and therapist to help them move out of stuck positions and "negative therapeutic reactions."

As a consequence, I have had many requests over these years to do such consultations, sometimes initiated by a therapist, sometimes by a patient, sometimes by both therapist and patient together. I have had, therefore, the opportunity to witness and learn from a range of impasses in the course of psychotherapy, from the patients', therapists', and consultants' perspectives.

But more important, over the ten years since I first became interested in what I would now call therapeutic impasses, I have traveled a revolutionary path with my colleagues at the Stone Center. At that time, we had already begun meeting regularly, struggling to move ourselves out of traditional assumptions, techniques, and perspectives, when they did not seem to fit our clinical experience, that is, listening and learning from our women patients. We spent many hours examining the language of our profession, with much of its pejorative connotations, language that is often objectifying, hierarchical, and pathologizing, as well as elitist, sexist, and the like. And we continue to struggle to find new ways and new language to talk about how we understand psychological difficulties and how to treat them. The work of Carol Gilligan and her colleagues has further enlightened my understanding over these years (Gilligan, Ward, & Taylor, 1988; Gilligan, Lyons, & Hanmer, 1990; Gilligan, Rogers, & Tolman, 1991).

A CATEGORY OF PATIENTS

I would like now to return to those patients who captured my interest more than ten years ago. These patients appeared at the outset of therapy to be functioning fairly well in the world and seemed to engage quickly in the therapeutic process; yet after a significant period of time (typically, two or three years), during which they appeared to be progressing, the therapy began to go downhill. The patient became more distressed, often disorganized, sometimes seriously suicidal and violent, and episodically entertained "delusional" ideas, and often had to be hospitalized. Once the downward course began, matters continued to get worse, and the therapy clearly reached a dramatic impasse. The patient felt desperate about how attached she felt to the therapist; yet she would often become enraged and aggressive towards him. The therapist, in turn, felt at a loss about how to respond effectively to this turn of events.

I thought then, and now too, that these impasses developed out of an interactive, relational dynamic since they reflected the patient's style of presenting herself and the therapist's countertransference reactions to it. Initially, these patients, all women, seemed to be engaging in the therapy with considerable verbal facility and the capacity to communicate their experiences in rather colorful ways. They quickly developed idealized transferences towards their therapists, who were mostly men, although there were some women therapists in this group too. They responded insightfully to the therapists' interventions and seemed soothed and comforted by the therapy.

Early in the treatment they appeared compliant and somewhat childlike; yet they put high value on their needs for independence and autonomy. Thus an appealing quality of helplessness emerged, which aroused rescue fantasies in the therapists, but simultaneously the patients apparently reassured the therapists about their ability to be self-sufficient. All of these features contributed to the "specialness" of these patients to their therapists who clearly appreciated them, sometimes presenting the course of their therapy at conferences as intriguing case examples and dramatic illustrations for teaching.

It should be noted also that, despite how engaging and competent these patients appeared, there were indications in their family histories that they had endured serious past difficulties and that their past relationships were very problematic. Typically these patients had a very intense relationship with one parent, while the other parent was either absent, or rarely mentioned and often devalued.

FORMULATION OF IMPASSE

I would like to summarize briefly how I understand the pattern I have been describing, in the context of a relational perspective. How did it happen that these women, who presented so positively to the therapist at the outset and appeared so motivated and responsive, began to look more and more harmed than helped during the course of the therapeutic process?

I believe that these patients' style of interacting in the beginning of therapy was a form of role play, which reflected a strategy to protect themselves against being wounded and violated in this new relationship. These women were, in fact, highly vigilant to the expectations others might have of them and were quite adept at figuring out how to win other's approval and acceptance. They had developed excellent interpersonal skills that allowed them to give the impression of a higher level of adaptation than they experienced inside; they were very good at hiding their deep feelings of inadequacy, terror and profound distrust of all relationships. Their interpersonal skills concealed from the therapists the extent of their underlying distrust, ultimately leading the patient to feel misunderstood by the therapist and the therapist to feel misled by the patient's presentation.

Before the beginning of disillusionment with each other, however, the patient had begun to build up a degree of trust in the therapist—who was so able to listen and who clearly liked and valued her—and gradually became more in touch with strong yearnings for connection with her therapist and began to relax the facade she had learned to present to the world. However, without the armor of previous protective strategies, she felt at a loss about how to behave and express her feelings. She became more and more overwhelmed by the intensity of her yearnings and as she felt increasingly vulnerable, her vigilance over her therapist's response to her heightened.

At the same time, the therapist became more and more troubled when he saw that the patient who had seemed so amenable to psychotherapy was becoming more acutely distressed and instead of being self-sufficient was becoming more dependent and demanding. Another facet that I understand better now than before, which relates to learning about the history of sexual abuse, is that the patient's intense yearnings were often sexualized. The therapist either overresponded, terrifying the patient, or suddenly began to distance himself, confirming the patient's worst fears—that the exposure of her yearnings and vulnerabilities would result in her violation or abandonment.

The increased intensity of feelings these patients experienced towards their therapists, together with the increased terror of exploitation and rejection, stirred up strong love/hate feelings. The patient, confused and terrified by these powerfully ambivalent feelings, in some instances developed psychotic transference reactions, which both patient and therapist felt impossible to manage. One of these patients said, "I want him always inside of me and I want to murder him."

Thus the downward course of therapy developed out of an interactional dynamic in which both therapist and patient struggled with the expression of yearnings for connection and the fear of such—yearnings that led to various modes of distancing and disconnection.

THE PARADOX

This therapeutic impasse can best be recast in terms of the central paradox conceptualized by Jean Baker Miller in her paper on *Connections, Disconnections and Violations* (1988). When a person's yearnings for connection are met with sustained and chronic rejections, humiliations and other violations, then the yearnings become even more intensified. At the same time these yearnings are experienced as dangerous. The person then tries to connect in the only relationship available but does so by keeping more and more of herself out of relationship. She tries to protect against further woundings and rejections by not representing herself authentically; rather she alters herself to fit with what she believes are the wishes and expectations of others. These inauthentic expressions become ways of distancing from others, hiding her vulnerabilities and deep longings for connection.

We believe this paradox is a central feature of all relationships, but more profoundly of those characterized by power inequities, which impede the development of mutually empathic and mutually empowering connections. Thus women in general, and patients in particular, struggle with their yearnings for connection, on the one hand, and on the other, their need to hide these yearnings by various means, which keep them more or less out of relationship.

For the group of patients described here, a history of sustained and chronic disconnections in their family histories contributed to their desperate needs to establish strong ties to their therapists, but they could do so only through playing a role. This role play allowed them to accommodate to what they saw as their therapists' need for a responsive patient, amenable to the process of psychotherapy; at the same time it kept large parts of themselves out of relationship. These patients also felt deep frustration and anger because they did not feel safe enough to represent themselves more fully; they remained highly vigilant to any sign that their therapists, like family members in the past, would violate their trust.

The therapists, in turn, struggled with their own paradox of connections and disconnections. As the patient's yearnings for connection became more intense, the therapist saw her as more dependent than he had expected, and he distanced himself from what he considered her increasing demands. And, as the patient's anger and violent outbursts became more frequent, the therapist often felt frightened and angry at a patient whom he had apparently misunderstood.

Before addressing the kinds of interventions that can begin to reverse the downward course of therapy with this particular group of patients, we need to move to a broader delineation of the concept of therapeutic impasse. I would like to explore its prevalence and meanings in all therapeutic relationships, not only those with the particular group of patients described so far. Here it is important to clarify how I will be defining therapeutic impasse.

IMPASSE DEFINED

My understanding of the term "therapeutic impasse" is that it refers to relatively protracted periods in which both therapist and patient feel increasingly less connected, more alone and isolated; *and* neither can see how to move from these feelings of disconnection back into connection. The reasons for feeling disconnected and the forms that it takes are highly variable and unique to each relationship. For example, these periods of disconnection can be experienced by either or both therapist and patient as boredom, disappointment, hopelessness, helplessness, anger, frustration, or preoccupation with "external" issues and other relationships.

Holding in mind this conceptualization of therapeutic impasses, what I have discovered over these years is that they are hardly limited to the kinds of patients I have just described; nor are the formulations of the dynamics leading to the impasses limited to this group of patients. In fact, I believe that these impasses reflect the dynamics underlying the central paradox of connections/disconnections, which characterize all relationships.

Perhaps what is most surprising is how little has been written about the different kinds of stalemates which occur during therapy, those painful ruptures when the therapy ends abruptly as a consequence of a significant impasse, and/or therapy which clearly has been experienced by the patient as harmful. Nor is there sufficient recognition of how often patients are blamed and blame themselves for these impasses and ruptures and how often many therapists also feel guilty and like failures as a consequence.

HARMFUL THERAPY

A few studies dramatically highlight the extent and consequences of various forms of impasse and therapeutic ruptures. Grunebaum (1986) interviewed 47 therapists (psychiatrists, psychologists, and social workers); they ranged in age from under 25 to 50. Thirty-two were females, 15 males. Twenty-two percent reported that they had been moderately harmed by their own therapy, 14% felt severely harmed, and 2% rated themselves as "very severely harmed." Thus a total of 38% of this group of therapists had had a moderately to "very severely" harmful therapy experience.

In a study of Jungian therapists (Auger, 1986), 43% reported negative therapy experiences of their own. Buckley, Karasu, and Charles (1981) found that 21% of therapists in their sample felt they had had harmful therapy. Elkind (1992) recently completed a study of 330 therapists. Fifty-three percent reported ruptures in their therapy, and 19% had more than two such ruptures. In 72% of these ruptures, the therapists felt they had been very harmed by the therapy

She also asked the therapists in her sample how many had had patients leave therapy in a therapeutic impasse, and 87% stated that they had. The therapists also reported that as a result they felt they were failures, angry at their patients, and devastated by the experience. The most common response in the face of impasse was the patient's belief that it was her fault. One patient said, "Even if I had thought that he did something , I kept coming back to feeling I should- have handled the situation differently; something was the matter with me for being so very hurt and upset" (Elkind, 1992, Chapter 3, p. 1).

Although Strupp and other researchers on the outcome of psy- chotherapy report that 47 percent of experts in psychotherapy believe that negative effects of therapy present a significant problem (Strupp & Hadley, 1985), there are limited data on the reasons behind these ef- fects. Grunebaum's study (1986) did do a breakdown of those thera- pists who felt harmed by their own therapy; 33% reported that their therapists were "cold, rigid, and distant"; 16% thought their therapists were emotionally seductive, that is, they fostered an intense and inti- mate relationship, yet blamed their patients for expressing their feel- ings when they were finally able to do so. Other reasons included poor matches and explicit sexual abuse. Other than Grunebaum's study there are no comparable studies of patients' opinions about what they felt was harmful to them.

THEORETICAL PERSPECTIVES

Over the years when therapeutic impasses, or "negative therapeutic reactions" have been addressed, the focus has been mainly on the pa- tient's pathology, her resistance and guilt as the basis for these reac- tions. Although countertransference reactions have been identified for some time as contributing to therapeutic failures, the emphasis has certainly been on the patient's recalcitrance, "actings out," and the like. Rarely has the focus been on the relationship itself.

Recently there has been a growing interest in therapeutic impass- es in more traditional therapies. Maroda (1991) stresses the need for greater awareness and admission of possible therapeutic blind spots. Kantrowitz and her colleagues (1989) have been investigating the mis- matching of psychoanalysts and patients as a source of impasse. She believes that many analysts significantly overestimate the positive ef- fects and outcomes of their treatments; in particular, she suggests that the analyst may prove to be a potential hindrance to the analytic process when narcissistic issues are involved. This research yielded two types of mismatching, but in both types, the analyst was unaware of his own "dynamic or characterological issues" in relation to the pa- tient. One type of mismatch occurred when the analyst was unaware that his style or personal issues were similar to the patient's; the other occurred when the analyst was unaware that the issues the patient was expressing were those he needed to disown and defend against in himself.

Kantrowitz (1992) uses her own case example to illustrate a stalemate in therapy as a result of her style in working with the patient. She was not aware of a possible stalemate until she ended an hour ten minutes early, which she understood to be a "countertransference enactment." These enactments result from the patient tapping into and stimulating some unconscious aspect of the analyst's emotions. In this instance, Kantrowitz believes that it was the patient's attempt to get her to experience his feelings of helplessness that led to the stalemate. Through her use of consultation, Kantrowitz was able to recognize that her own unconscious need to be helpful was interfering with her patient's ability to assume more responsibility for his own affairs. Through the use of consultation, she modified her style by using more confrontative as well as empathic interventions with this patient.

Atwood, Stolorow, and Trop (1989) offer a different perspective and see the therapeutic impasse as an opportunity to help both therapist and patient develop in the process. In fact, they see the impasse as offering "a royal road to change" in both therapist and patient. In particular, they note that when the intersubjective themes which unconsciously organize the experiences of therapist and patient in an impasse can be looked at, there are new understandings for them both and the therapeutic process is advanced.

Despite this growing recognition of the interactive nature of therapeutic impasse, most of the analytic writers focus on the need for the therapist to learn more about his unconscious intrapsychic issues, and blind spots, which have led to various countertransference enactments, such as mistakes and empathic failures. It does move away from blaming the patient for these impasses. While their approach does include relational dynamics, it does not focus sufficiently on the inevitability of impasses in any relationship in which two people struggle with their yearnings for connection and their needs to protect themselves from the pain of rejection and abandonment.

There are, however, a number of therapists who have made important new contributions to our understanding of therapeutic impasse, therapists who focus on their own powerful active personal participation in psychotherapy. They see the potential value of therapeutic impasses in moving the therapy and the therapist and patient into new, more authentic, and more growth-promoting interactions.

Ehrenberg (1985, 1992), an analyst from the William Alanson White School, brings an interpersonal perspective to therapeutic impasse which is in many ways consistent with our relational approach. She sees the impasse as the opportunity for the therapist to use her countertransference reactions as a way of moving into a more interactive and productive relationship. In particular she believes that stalemates can be avoided by going more deeply into the nature of the interactive impasse. She sees these periods in therapy as the occasion for the therapist to become more disclosing and communicative about her experiences within the relationship, particularly when she feels her patient distancing from her or when she believes she has distanced from the patient.

Elkind (1992) has recently written a book on therapeutic impasse which brings a strong relational perspective to this important topic. Again, it is amazing that it is the first book of this kind on a subject that is so central, so pervasive, so inevitable in the kind of work we do. Elkind makes a point of depathologizing different kinds of stalemates, impasses, and ruptures in the therapeutic process, observing how painful these experiences are for both patient and therapist She notes how isolated and shamed both therapists and patients are when they experience their therapeutic work as a failure, and how little our profession respects these occurrences or provides legitimate avenues of support.

RESPONSE TO IMPASSE

Although I believe all therapy inevitably contains a series of impasses, they may become more seriously problematic for a number of reasons, which I'll discuss a little later. At such times more formal outside intervention, in the form of a consultation, can sometimes be very helpful. In fact, what I will be proposing is that broader relational opportunities be available for both patient and therapist in all therapeutic endeavors.

It is not surprising that impasses are inevitable in the normal course of therapy, when one considers how very complicated and powerful the therapeutic relationship is. We at the Stone Center believe that when the therapy is characterized by "good enough mutuality," and the therapist engages authentically with the patient, then the therapeutic process should continue to evolve gradually and effectively through the necessary impasses. I will not discuss here our relational reframing of therapy, presented in a number of our working papers (Jordan, Kaplan, Miller, Stiver, & Surrey, 1991; Heyward, Jordan, & Surrey, 1992; Miller & Stiver, 1991), other than to note again the importance of creating a safe relational context in which the ethic of mutuality can find consistent and full expression.

I would, however, like to return to the paradox of connections and disconnections as the central source of therapeutic impasse throughout the course of therapy. That is, both patient and therapist will be continuously struggling with their yearnings for connection, and their needs to defend against exposing their vulnerabilities in the face of potential hurt, violation, and rejection. In a previous paper, Miller and I noted that "the therapist cues her listening, her understanding of the material that emerges, and her emotional attunement in the context of how connected or disconnected she experiences both herself and her patient at various stages of the encounter, (Miller & Stiver, 1991, p. 3). It is the therapist's major responsibility and task to help move the relationship back into connection from periods of disconnection.

This process requires the therapist's active involvement and responsiveness to her sense of disconnection in the relationship. By active I mean her full participation in the interaction, and her serious consideration of the disconnection. Surrey (1992) describes it as a kind of "jumping further into" the process, and becoming more engaged in what is going on. This acknowledgment of disconnection may be conveyed nonverbally or by a simple statement validating that something has shifted in the relationship. As Ehrenberg noted (1992), in this process the therapist needs to become more forthright and to disclose her countertransference reactions. We believe then that what is required of the therapist in the face of impasse is an energetic response—she struggles to understand the nature of the disconnection and how to move back into connection.

When patient and the therapist can move with the rhythms of connection and come to understand together what triggers disconnection and how these problems can be resolved, the therapeutic alliance becomes strengthened. This kind of work requires enormous resilience, courage, and faith *in the relationship*, which can develop over time in settings characterized by mutual empathy and mutual empowerment and where power issues are acknowledged and processed (Jordan, 1992).

IMPASSE THEMES

In reviewing the consultations I have done through the years, which were initiated because either the patient or therapist or both experienced a significant impasse in the therapy, one major theme emerges— a theme that reflects the central paradox as the underlying dynamic of these impasses. In the course of therapy, when the patient begins to feel safe enough to talk about what really matters and feels listened to, she becomes increasingly vulnerable, slowly shedding some of the protective strategies used in the past to protect against hurt and disappointment. Here, the therapist's presence and engagement help move the process along, in spite of the inevitable disconnections, such as empathic derailments, and transference distortions. When, however, there is a sudden shift in the therapist's involvement, and the patient experiences him as distancing himself from her just when she is becoming more vulnerable, a major impasse may evolve.

Sometimes an external event and significant change in the therapist's life, such as a marriage, divorce, a pregnancy, a death in the family, a suicide of a patient, can decrease her availability to her patient. Already feeling vulnerable, the patient becomes more vigilant for any sign of rejection and abandonment. She may respond by withdrawing herself, leaving the therapist feeling more alone, or she may become very angry, usually around a displaced issue, since she is often not consciously aware that the therapist is preoccupied or more distant. The patient may also become increasingly demanding and hostile, which leaves the therapist feeling helpless and hopeless about making a difference.

Sometimes a significant change in the patient's life may precipitate a similar impasse. For instance, when the patient loses an important person in her life through death or divorce, she may become more desparate about her need for the therapist. Whether she adopts a "clinging dependency" or a counterdependent stance, the therapist may distance herself from the patient.

What I have been struck by in talking to patients during the consultation process is how exquisitely perceptive they are about their therapists' personalities, their foibles, and the possible cues about changes in their lives. They typically keep these observations to themselves and only self-consciously report them to the consultant after several sessions. They apparently feel very protective of their therapists, not wanting to "tell on them" or embarrass them. It should be noted that this keen sensitivity to the flaws and foibles of the the the therapist's personality, needs to be spoken out loud because of the way the patient may distort her understanding of these "astute" observations—typically blaming herself for his behavior.

One young woman told me that she noticed that her therapist's picture of his wife had disappeared from his desk, yet she did not connect this with her sense of his distancing from her. She wondered if he were perhaps lonely and unhappy. She also felt he had "too much on his mind" to attend to her "insignificant" problems.

Another woman I saw in consultation began to wonder if her therapist was working too hard since she had started developing another area of interest in her profession. As we pursued this line of thought, it became apparent that the patient had been worried for some months that her therapist might be leaving her private practice to engage more fully in this new interest. When, with my encouragement, she talked to her therapist about her concern, her therapist acknowledged that she had just recently begun to wonder about how she might best allocate her time and was considering cutting down on her practice. Both therapist and patient were impressed by how astute the patient was to be aware of the therapist's conflict about her plans even before the therapist was fully cognizant of it herself.

With this awareness, the nature of their therapeutic impasse became clear to them both. They saw how the patient's improvement, namely, her increasing ability to be in touch with intense and painful feelings, and her greater awareness of her affection for her therapist, all led to her feeling more vulnerable, which terrified her. The patient believed, at some level, that her therapist was turning more and more to this new endeavor because she was "fed up" with her and because she saw her as "getting worse," not better.

FRAME OF THERAPY

Other major impasses may be triggered by acts or events arising from what is sometimes called the "frame" of therapy. I was, of course, taught that time and money were ultimately the central issues of therapy. Thus, when patients were late, missed appointments, didn't pay their bills, the interpretation was that these were all expressions of unconscious resistance, acting out and the like. The therapist's personal and power investments in these issues never came up.

Yet these are often the very issues which lead to impasses, primarily when the patient feels disempowered and disenfranchised; she recognizes at some level that this issue reflects the therapist's needs more than his concerns with the therapeutic relationship and its process. When therapists insist on charging their patients for missing appointments, even though the patient may cancel because of an automobile accident, a miscarriage, or the birth of a baby, there is a powerful impact on the patient and the therapeutic relationship. The patient may feel that the events in her life are insignificant, that she is powerless to negotiate real life issues with her therapist, or that she must be foolish and rebellious to even question the therapist about his policy. Yet she remains furious, and her trust in the therapist is seriously eroded.

Other more distressing examples of therapeutic impasses are those which reflect unacknowledged power inequities, such as the therapist's own lack of timeliness, his use of the telephone during sessions, or evidence of glitches in maintaining confidentiality. It is more

common than one would wish to be told in consultation that the therapist regularly answers the phone during sessions—a practice which is
understandably very upsetting to the patient. Sometimes a patient
tells me that she doesn't feel comfortable bringing this up with her
therapist because he might be angry, or "he's so important and busy";
sometimes others report they have brought it up but the therapist
doesn't change his behavior. On at least several occasions I have been
told that the therapist has said to the patient, "I don't know why it
should bother you; none of my other patients mind it at all."

I hear too that therapists often come late to their appointments
and do not make up the time, end sessions early because of "emergen-
cies" and the like. All of us are guilty of some of these lapses at certain
times. The fact of the behavior is less relevant than the refusal to accept responsibility for what has happened, with the result that the patient feels, and often is, blamed for responding by feeling awful. It is
crucial that the therapist acknowledges the power inequities as they
emerge and negotiates with the patient towards some resolution that
is reasonable for them both.

I particularly want to stress that all these instances of major disconnections, which are a function of the therapeutic frame, have a significant impact on the course of therapy, often long before the problem
becomes apparent. Thus patients notice these power inequities and
put a lid on their feelings about them because they feel so unentitled to
their reactions and have such a need for the therapist; but at the same
time they continue to distance themselves from him. Ultimately a major impasse or rupture develops, which may, at the time, appear mysterious to both patient and therapist.

INTERVENTIONS

I would now like to address interventions for those impasses, which
for a variety of reasons, do not seem to move through the rhythms of
connection and disconnection, but instead leave both therapist and patient feeling stuck. At such times some patients leave therapy abruptly
and, in many such cases, both therapist and patient continue for some
time to feel very wounded by the experience; in other instances the
therapist acknowledges that the work has come to a standstill and offers to refer the patient to someone else. When the latter option is discussed candidly, it sometimes helps both therapist and patient come to
terms with their limitations in this relationship and move on.

Another good and viable option in these circumstances is to invite
another person into the relationship who can serve as a consultant to

both therapist and patient. Ideally both people join together "to ask for help." Many times, however, it is either the therapist or patient who requests the consultation, but there is usually some degree of collaboration among all the parties involved. When either the patient or therapist resists and/or will not participate in the process, the effectiveness of the consultation is to some extent undermined.

Let us now return to the original group of patients I described on page 288, those whose therapy took such a dramatic downward course after what appeared to be a positive therapeutic experience over a significant period of time. These patients became intensely attached to their therapists, often feeling they could not exist without them; but they also felt betrayed by them since the therapists had promised so much at the beginning and then had backed off from the relationship. As a result, these patients became enraged and, at times, violent towards their therapists; the therapists found it increasingly difficult to tolerate the patients' demands and anger; and the patients found themselves more and more trapped by their own love/hate feelings.

CONSULTATION

With this group the first step in an intervention was a consultation, which introduced another person into the picture with whom both patient and therapist could establish a relationship. Because the impasses seemed so entrenched, these consultations could not be limited to one or two sessions. Rather the consultation process required a longer-term intervention, a total of perhaps four to six interviews, covering a period of a month or six weeks.

The consultation process provided the opportunity to address the struggles both the patient and therapist were experiencing. The therapist could clarify the relationship for himself by ventilating some of his "unspeakable" feelings towards the patient. The patient could better understand her therapist by having another person to look to as a source of help. Helping the patient verbalize as much as possible all her grievances about the therapist allowed her over time to bring them back into the therapy. For some of these patients it was the first time they could begin to speak some truths about their experiences to their therapists. This process began the rebuilding of trust in the therapist and the development of the relational confidence that Jordan (1992) describes as part of the process of fostering relational resiliency.

It is crucial that the patient not see the consultant as someone who will take the therapist away from her, a frequent concern expressed in the initial consultation interview. In helping the patient talk about both the positive and negative aspects of her feelings towards the therapist, it is impressive how truly terrified she often is that the consultant might tell the therapist about her negative feelings and thus jeopardize a relationship that is so important to her. The extent to which these negative feelings are split off is also evident when one realizes how openly hostile these patients had often been to their therapists during this impasse stage. But certainly the "detoxification" of many of the thoughts and feelings about the therapist, once verbalized to the consultant, makes it possible for therapist and patient to talk more openly about what was hidden for so long.

I believe a major component of the consultant's task is to help the patient and therapist see the other person more in context and to become more aware of the nature of their relationship. This will help them to broaden their perspectives about each other and to appreciate more fully their different modes of struggling to stay in connection.

Of course the consultation is usually not enough to resolve the impasse, although in my experience the therapy does move more smoothly once the consultation has begun. The consultation is, however, just the beginning of the process of diluting the transference, as it gives the patient the experience of talking to someone other than the therapist, with some benefit. It also communicates to the patient that the therapist encourages and fosters other relationships, something not typically experienced in their own families.

The therapist, at the same time, feels less alone as she has someone to talk to, and less burdened since she knows that there is someone else who can also be helpful to the patient. Working with this group of patients, whom I would describe as seriously traumatized by sexual and other significant abuse, often requires other treaters and modalities to prevent further impasses and to counter the hopeless and helpless feelings often aroused in the treaters.

In some cases the consultation process may be sufficient to help therapist and patient move back on course and no other intervention is necessary. However, in those instances of protracted and serious impasses, introducing other therapeutic relational opportunities serves to prevent future serious impasses.

Thus at the end of the period of consultation, the consultant can recommend that the patient continue to see her therapist but also see another person who can function as a cotherapist; an alternative to this cotherapy model is to refer the patient to a group. The cotherapist may continue to work with the patient through the course of therapy or see her intermittently or on a more time limited basis, or even become over time the only therapist working with the patient. Which path to take is not always evident at the time of the consultation. The particular role of the cotherapist can be negotiated with the patient and her therapist (e.g., cognitive behavioral interventions, clinical administration, or other therapeutic tasks).

What this form of intervention does is to encourage both therapist and patient to ask for help, to value the enlargement of relational opportunities, and to acknowledge each other's vulnerabilities in this difficult relationship. By adding another person's perspective, both parties can move into a more mutually empathic relationship. This movement often requires that the consultant help the patient to consider other constructions (from those developed in the past) of the meanings of the therapist's empathic failures, such as lack of sensitivity to power differentials.

The therapist also needs another person's perspective to acknowledge the changes in the patient over the course of therapy. This is particularly true in those therapies which have lasted a long time. That is, the therapist often holds on to some earlier view of her patient, even when she, the patient, has demonstrated considerable movement in her own growth. Thus, the therapist may not sufficiently appreciate the patient's increased ability to tolerate painful affects and her newly acquired competencies. The patient, in turn, realizes at some level that the therapist does not see her as clearly as she once did. It is often very moving for both therapist and patient, when the consultant shares her view of the patient in the here and now. As caretakers, therapists may sometimes feel more comfortable with their patients' vulnerabilities than with their competencies; yet therapists are usually gratified when they can see the progress their patients have made.

EXPANDING RELATIONAL OPPORTUNITIES

In addressing therapeutic impasses all along the continuum from episodic to more entrenched stalemates, we need to move out of the blaming mode to the empowering mode for both patient and therapist. As we appreciate and respect the fact that impasses are inevitable in all therapeutic work, we need to foster models of support that, as Jordan believes, facilitate mutually empathic connections and strengthen relational resilience (Jordan, 1992). Such models avoid the intensely ambivalent attachments that patients and their therapists can develop.

As a consultant, I see that part of my task is to help both therapist and patient appreciate the different (as well as similar) kinds of vulnerabilities each brings to the therapeutic relationship. I try to encourage the patient to develop a stronger voice, through practicing with me, and to bring that voice back into the therapy by communicating more about how the impasse has affected her and how she perceives her therapist. If I have access to the therapist too, I do the same with her.

One woman I saw in consultation told me how enraged she became when her therapist misunderstood her. I wondered with her if she could imagine that her therapist might feel intimidated by her when she started her critical assaults. At first this felt like a completely foreign idea to her, since her therapist loomed so large and seemed so intimidating to her. When she next saw her therapist and quoted what I had said, the therapist was able to affirm this observation immediately, and the patient was able to start seeing her therapist as human and vulnerable too.

In the same way, I can convey to the therapist the extent to which his patient was devastated by certain reactions or lack of reactions to something that mattered very much to her. Very often the therapist is surprised to hear of these reactions because of some of his own issues and/or because the patient has been unable to speak more openly to him. In my experience, most therapists are responsive to this new information and are motivated to change their own attitudes and style.

In this discussion I am reminded of the analogous work that Steve Bergman and Janet Surrey do in their workshops with couples (1992). In the face of impasses in relationships between men and women, the workshops provide opportunities to talk more openly with others who are not caught in the impasse, namely either Janet or Steve, or other members of a same gender group. This opportunity legitimizes turning to others for help and, in the process, speaking in a stronger voice of one's own as well as gaining a broader perspective about the other. More importantly, this workshop, like the consultation, can help all those involved in impasses to learn more about each other and to respect the nature and quality of their relationships. In these settings mutually empathic negotiations can begin to move from impasse to mutual empowerment.

PATIENT AND THERAPIST VULNERABILITIES

I think it is very important for the consultant to help both therapist and patient appreciate what kinds of vunerabilities each brings to the therapeutic impasse. The patient's vulnerabilities are easier to identify, namely that she is intimidated and fearful of exposing those secret thoughts and feelings which she experiences as "bad" and "dangerous." She believes that if she revealed her true feelings and thoughts she would be criticized, wounded, and rejected. In the face of any sign of confirmation of these fears, such as the therapist's silence, noncommittal stance, misunderstandings, and personal preoccupations, these vulnerabilities are both intensified and more deeply hidden.

The therapist, in turn, is under enormous pressure, from the culture at large and the profession in particular, to be expert, to always know what to do, and to help his patient move out of her current pain and difficulties into a more adaptive place. When the patient is in acute distress and at a loss about how to resolve it, the therapist may attempt to reassure and rescue the patient, often promising more than he can reasonably deliver, considering the constraints and limitations in the relationship. As we have seen, this situation often results in the therapist withdrawing as the patient requests more involvement with her; simultaneously the therapist feels guilty and ashamed since he recognizes that he has made some errors in the process.

The profession does not encourage acknowledging such feelings, sharing them, or asking for help. As the patient feels more and more hopeless, the therapist feels hopeless too, as well as burdened, in the face of demands that he feels he cannot fill. These vulnerabilities, especially when hidden and disowned, contribute to the therapist's sense of failure and greater distancing from the patient. The consultant can meet with patient and therapist individually (and sometimes together) to help legitimize these vulnerabilities so that the therapist can accept them as understandable and sometimes inevitable. The consultant may also give permission for, as well as actively encourage, enlarged relational opportunities for both patient and therapist.

The main point of this chapter is that impasses are inevitable, and therefore we need to learn more about how to move through them. It is also of paramount importance to know when impasses cannot be resolved and when therapy has become harmful and sometimes clearly destructive to the patient.

We know that in abusive relationships in general, the person abused often holds on to the relationship because she may be too terrified to move out of it, thinking it is all she has. In the therapy relationship too, patients hold onto powerful attachments to their therapists, even in the face of deep disappointment, betrayal, and other violations. In such cases the consultant needs to respect the power of the relationship on the one hand, and to serve as an advocate for the patient in helping her move out of the destructive, harmful therapeutic relationship, on the other.

In less dramatic instances of harmful therapy, a gradual process of moving out of it into a new therapeutic relationship is the preferred mode of intervention. In other instances where the harmful effects are more extreme, the consultant can help the patient leave the therapist in a relatively short period of time. The unfinished business of grief and mourning obviously will need to be addressed with the new therapist.

CONCLUSION

In bringing a relational perspective to therapeutic impasses, we discover how inevitable they are in the course of therapy and how their resolution can lead to growth and change in both therapist and patient. I believe the paradox of connections/disconnections helps us understand the dynamics of these impasses and guides us in our efforts to move the therapy out of impasse and into more authentic relationship.

This perspective must necessarily move us out of the blaming mode and into the empowering mode. In not pathologizing therapeutic impasses, we give permission to both therapist and patient to ask for help without feeling like failures and blaming themselves. Most important is the need to value the enlarging of relational possibilities for both patient and therapist, so that in the face of episodes of disconnection between them, neither feels so at risk of being left alone and abandoned. The consultation is one model of support to both therapist and patient, but other models are the use of cotherapists as well as various kinds of groups for therapists and patients.

A relational reframing of therapy in general and impasse in particular stresses the need for an ethic of mutuality in the therapeutic encounter, with a profound appreciation of how much patient and therapist have in common. This conceptualization means rejecting the power-over model of therapy with its view of the therapist as expert and the patient as "the troubled one," "sicker" and "more disturbed."

I would like to close with Harry Stack Sullivan's definition of the therapeutic relationship: "Two people, both with problems in living, who agree to work together to study those problems, with the hope that the therapist has fewer problems than the patient" (Kasin, 1986, p. 455).

DISCUSSION SUMMARY

After each colloquim presentation, a discussion was held. Selected portions are summarized here. At this session, Drs. Jean Baker Miller, Robin Cook-

Nobles, Judith Jordan, Suzanne Slater, and Janet Surrey joined Irene Stiver in leading the discussion.

Slater: I think the ideas expressed in this chapter present a profound challenge to the therapist. As therapists we have to agree to do therapy on such an authentic, mutual basis, and we have to agree to do this in maybe fifteen to twenty-five relationships simultaneously. The temptation then to take those clients who are "entertaining," and don't appear to be demanding and needy, can be compelling. We need to be vigilant about this tendency as well as not to underestimate what it takes for us to do our work well.

Jordan: I think it's so important to look at the shame of the therapist when the therapy feels stuck; at such times both parties move into isolation, and they don't feel they can get out of feeling stuck. The first step is for the therapist to acknowledge her sense of distance and then try to make the connection happen again. It must be very relieving for the client to have that reality acknowledged by the therapist.

Surrey: I think one of the hardest things for the therapist to acknowledge is anger. This raises the big question of what kinds of feelings is it ok for the therapist to express. Therapists' feelings of anger are inevitable yet are very problematic. Therapists are often ashamed of their anger and disown it, yet patients are keenly aware of its being there. In another way, we therapists often encourage our clients to express their anger, but we don't always like it when they do.

Question: I was struck by your phrase, "paradox of connections/disconnections," and I think of my own experiences as a therapist. Recently a client said to me, "I haven't heard a thing you said in the last five years!" I was struck at that moment as I realized that she was finally allowing that part of herself to say "I can't hear you if you're too close or too real." Her simple acknowledgment of that was very powerful. It was at first very jarring since I thought we were connecting and what was happening is not what I thought it was.

Stiver: I think that's a very good example of what happens a lot in therapy, although not often verbalized. But I also don't take what she said too literally. That is, I think she was saying, "Now I can begin to hear you." But probably she heard some things you said all along the way and that both hearing you and not hearing you made it possible finally to hear you in a new way and to feel free to tell you more of the truth of her experience. This decreased the distance between you.

Jordan: I was thinking how much in situations of impasse clients push the therapist out of role playing. Therapists role play a lot and it's amazing how many of our clients put up with it; certain clients won't. I think the impasses you described force the therapist out of role play into real connection.

Stiver: I agree. The traditional model of therapy is indeed a form of role play—all the ways we have been taught to be, such as, not to show our feelings, present a blank screen, behave as if we have our lives in order and as if we understand the client at all levels and at all times. These are the therapist's ways of distancing, of being "out of relationship."

Question: You've been talking about psychological forms of connections, but what about the physical forms of connection, that is, touching, hugging, how do they fit into the paradox of connections/disconnections?

Stiver: I think as therapists we need always to be careful of the ways we can communicate our feelings, and I think it may be more precarious when we move into the physical realm with our clients. Physical connection can easily be misunderstood and frightening, and we know it has also been seriously misused. At the same time physical contact can also be a natural expression of affection, warmth and connection—like touching a hand or helping ground a person who is terrified. However, we need always to be alert to the dangers inherent in physical contact for our many clients who have histories of physical and sexual violations.

Cook-Nobles: We need also to take a cross-cultural perspective. In certain cultures if you don't respond physically it may be experienced as distancing and rejecting. In cultures where nonverbal expressions of connection are familiar, the therapist who does not respond may be experienced as disconnecting.

Question: As you talk of therapist and client moving closer by being mutually empathic and struggling together, how do you see the future? How will we determine who qualifies to be a therapist, who is strong enough to do this work? In the therapy you're describing, the lines are often crossed in the mutuality of the relationship. You're sort of saying to the client that she has to be empathic with the therapist. The therapist is no longer functioning as a leader. How do we know if the therapist is the stronger partner?

Stiver: The therapist has certain responsibilities and tasks. The same person can be a client in one situation and a therapist in another, and her tasks and responsibilities shift accordingly. Our hope is that the therapist is experienced and trained. I believe the model of therapy we are talking about requires a different kind of training from what most of us have had.

Slater: I think what we are asked to do as therapists is extremely complex. We are talking about a relationship being mutual without equal focus on each person's needs; yet, when the therapist is emotionally present and authentic, some of her needs have to come in. But certain lines, such as expecting clients to take care of the therapist, cannot be crossed. Our training falls short of addressing these issues. People can also misunderstand the relational approach as giving permission to the therapist to express her personal needs, or that it's a fifty-fifty relationship. That is not what we mean.

Miller: I think the therapist has a great deal of responsibility. Her purpose is to try to advance the relationship so that it becomes more mutually empowering but that can never be in the direction of exploiting another person. I certainly agree with all the things that have been said, including helping therapists become less isolated in their own lives. I think that is our best hope and protection. But I think all therapists need a great deal of training and help, certainly initially, but also all through their lives. Therapists have the responsibility to see that they get that training and the fact that their responsibility is very different from the client's can't ever be forgotten.

REFERENCES

Atwood, C., Stolorow, R., & Trop, J. (1989). Impasses in psychoanalytic therapy: A royal road, *Contemporary Psychoanalysis, 25*(4), 554–573.

Auger, L. (1986). The patient's experience of the analyst's subjectivity. *Psychoanalytic Diologues: A Journal of Relational Perspectives, l*(1), 29–51.

Bergman, S. & Surrey, J. (1992). The woman–man relationship: Impasses and possibilities. (Work in Progress No. 55.) Wellesley, MA: Stone Center Working Paper Series. (Reprinted as Chapter 13, this volume)

Buckley, P, Karasu, T., & Charles, E. (1981). Psychotherapists view their personal therapy. *Psychother. Theory, Res. Pract, 18*, 299–305.

Ehrenberg, D. B (1985). Countertransference resistance. *Contemporary Psychoanalysis, 21*(4), 563–576.

Ehrenberg, D. B.(1992). On the Question of analyzability. *Contemporary Psychoanalysis, 28*(l),16–31.

Elkind, S. (1992). *Resolving impasses in therapeutic relationships.* New York: Guilford.

Gilligan, C, Ward, J. V., & Taylor, J. M. (Eds.) (1988). *Mapping the moral domain.* Cambridge, MA: Harvard University Press.

Gilligan, G, Lyons, N., & Hamner, T. (Eds.) (1990). *Making connections: The relational worlds of adolescent girls at Emma Willard School.* Cambridge, MA: Harvard University Press.

Gilligan, C., Rogers, A. G., & Tolman, D. L. (Eds.) (1991). *Women, girls and psychotherap:, Reframing resistance.* New York: Haworth Press.

Grunebaum, H. (1986). Harmful psychotherrapy experience. *American Journal of Psychotherapy, XL*(2) 165–176.

Heyward, C., Jordan, J., & Surrey, J. (1992). *Mutuality in therapy. Ethics, power and psychology.* (Work in Progress No. 60.) Wellesley, MA: Stone Center Working Paper Series.

Jordan, J. (1992). Relational resilience. (Work in Progress No. 57.) Wellesley, MA: Stone Center Working Paper Series.

Jordan, J. V., Kaplan, A., Miller, J. B, Stiver, I. P., & Surrey, J. (1991). *Women's growth in connection: Writings from the Stone Center.* New York. Guilford Press.

Kantrowitz, J., Katz, A., Greenman, D., Morris, H., Paolitto, F., Sashin, J., & Solomon, L. (1989). The patient-analyst match and the outcome of psychoanalysis: A pilot study. *Journal of the American Psychonalytic Association,* 37(4) 893–919.

Kantrowitz, J. (1992). The analyst's style and its impact on the analytic process: Overcoming a patient-analyst stalemate. *Journal of the American Psychoanalytic Association,* 40(7), 167–191.

Kasin, E. (1986). Roots and branches. *Contemporary Psychoanalysis, 22,* 452–458.

Maroda, K. J. (1991). *The power of countertransference: Innovations in analytic technique.* New York: Wiley.

Miller, J. B. (1988). *Connections, disconnections and violations.* (Work in Progress No. 33.) Wellesley, MA: Stone Center Working Paper Series.

Miller, J. B. & Stiver, I. P. (1991). *A relational reframing of therapy.* (Work in Progress No. 52.) Wellesley, MA: Stone Center Working Paper Series.

Stiver, I. P. (1981, April 3). Regression in psychotherapy: Conceptual and clinical considerations. The Paul C. Myerson Symposium on Psychotherapy, Annual Tufts Symposium.

Stiver, I. P. (1988). Developmental dimensions of regression: Introducing a consultant in the treatment of borderline patients. *Mclean Hospital Journal,* XIII, 89–113.

Strupp, H. H. & Hadley, S. W. (1985). Negative effects and their determinants. In D. T. Mays & C. Franks (Eds.) *Negative outcome in psycotherapy and what to do about it,* pp. 20–55. New York: Springer.

Surrey, J. (1992). Personal Communication.

This chapter was presented at a Stone Center Colloquium on May 6, 1992. © 1992 Irene Stiver.

15

Intimacy in Lesbian Relationships: A Critical Reexamination of Fusion

JULIE MENCHER

I appreciate the opportunity to be here tonight to share with you my work on intimacy patterns in lesbian relationships. The work of Surrey, Stiver, Miller, Kaplan, and Jordan has been crucial to my understanding of women's development and has greatly informed my analysis of lesbian psychology. I congratulate and thank these women for their growing acknowledgment that the relational experience of lesbians is a critical topic of inquiry for any students of women's development. My presence here tonight reflects the recognition that diversity exists among women, that the experience of some women can inform our understanding of all women, and that women must speak for ourselves—while there are many commonalities among us, we must enrich our understanding of women through work by lesbians about lesbians, by women of color about women of color.

Underlying the relational perspective is the notion that context is fundamental, that the social and psychic context of gender decisively shapes the female experience. In that vein, I would like to make clear that my personal and professional context consists primarily of white women, of varying ages, classes, educational backgrounds, and physical abilities. In our discussion tonight, I would welcome the input of women of other contexts to add to our collective understanding.

Recent endeavors in feminist psychology have questioned the

male bias of traditional theoretical frameworks which emphasize separation and autonomy as the hallmarks of healthy human development. Instead, some feminist theorists propose that women grow
through connection, that women's development relies on participation
in mutual, authentic relationships. However, attempts to study the relational nature of women have been colored by a predominant focus
on women in heterosexual relationships. In these relationships, the
woman's authentic expression of self may be hindered by the need to
adjust to the different developmental pathway of her male partner,
which may produce distinct behavior in relationships. An examination
of women's behavior, emotional dynamics, and patterns of intimacy in
lesbian relationships may offer a unique window through which to
view women's psychological development.

Several researchers have measured patterns of intimacy in lesbian
relationships by a male standard of separation and autonomy and
have pathologized as "fusion" the intimacy they observe. This chapter
will explore lesbian relationships within the context of women's relational development and will critique traditional notions of healthy
and unhealthy relational dynamics, particularly the notions of fusion
and intimacy.

Tonight I will be weaving together an examination of several different questions:

- What are the sources of fusion in lesbian relationships, i.e., why is
  fusion a predominant relational pattern for lesbians?
- Is fusion in lesbian relationships inherently maladaptive or pathological?
- How are traditional notions about fusion altered by new understandings of women's development?
- How does an understanding of lesbian relational patterns of fusion contribute to a more generic understanding of female patterns of intimacy?

"Fusion in lesbian relationships" is a topic which has received
much air time in settings as diverse as lesbian dinner party conversations and articles in the psychological literature. In the relatively small
body of literature on lesbian couples, at least fourteen articles have appeared in the last ten years which feature fusion as the prominent issue; it is rare to find an analysis of lesbian couples which does not address fusion (Burch, 1982, 1985, 1986, 1987; Decker, 1983-84; Elise,
1986; Kaufman, Harrison, & Hyde, 1984; Krestan & Bepko, 1980, Lindenbaum, 1985; Lowenstein, 1980; Pearlman, 1988; Roth, 1985; Schneider, 1986; Smalley, 1987). The topic of fusion has found its way into

colloquial settings as well. In a recently overheard conversation on a predominantly lesbian beach, three lesbians debated whether a lesbian couple is "fused" if they trade underwear back and forth.

So, what is all this fuss about fusion? Fusion, merger, and enmeshment are terms that have been used interchangeably in the literature to describe a common relational dynamic for lesbian couples. Fusion is variously defined in the psychological literature, but several features are common to most definitions: Fusion is a state of "psychic unity" in which individual ego boundaries are crossed and two individuals experience a sense of oneness (Burch, 1986). In the state of fusion, the self is embedded within a relational context, and boundaries between self and other are unclear (Karpel, 1976). Intense intimacy, a lack of separation, and overidentification are defined as characteristics of fusion.

We may argue about whether what is being defined as fusion is in fact fusion. However, for purposes of semantic simplicity, I will use the word fusion as it is used in both the traditional literature and the literature on lesbian fusion—and I will return later to explore the semantic problems with how fusion is used to describe particularly intense states of intimacy.

FUSION IN LESBIAN RELATIONSHIPS

Based on these definitions, several commentators have observed certain relational patterns in lesbian couples, have labeled these patterns fusion, and have marked fusion as a prominent problem in lesbian relationships. These patterns include both interpersonal dynamics and behavioral indicators.

The literature depicts these problematic dynamics in the following manner: It notes that lesbian women place a high premium on being intimately involved and experience difficulties when they are without an intimate relationship, frequently resulting in excessive tenacity to unsatisfying partnerships. The literature depicts the lesbian couple locked in an embrace of intimacy which values identification; mutual understanding and acceptance; and shared beliefs, behaviors, goals, and wishes. Differences between partners are feared, often to the extent that denial of differences is readily employed. Conflict is either avoided or constantly remains unresolved. The individual develops an acute sensitivity to her partner's needs and feelings, often at the expense of fulfilling her own needs. Individual identities become "merged" or "blurred," and partners have difficulty articulating, "I feel." Relative to the heterosexual pattern of ostensibly asymmetrical dependency needs, the lesbian couple is viewed as mutually dependent, with both partners highly dependent on each other. The women often describe a sense of being able to share "everything" with their partners, and the ability to self-disclose is often seen as nearly total. Growth and the continued development of individual identity is seen as dependent on continued involvement in the relationship.

Other features identified in the literature as indicators of fusion are more behavioral: The couple attempts to spend all or most of its leisure time together; social contacts are limited primarily to mutual friends, with few individual ones. They share professional services, e.g., doctors, lawyers, therapists, financial planners. Monies are pooled. Clothing and other possessions are shared, and the couple is in frequent telephone contact when apart, even if apart only during the work day (Kaufman, Harrison, & Hyde, 1984). These are the dynamic and behavioral characteristics which have been called fusion and which I am describing for the moment when I use the word fusion. Taken together, these characteristics form the aggregate picture of a typical lesbian relationship, as depicted in the literature. While some of these features are also shared by heterosexual couples and some are undeniably problematic, in the literature it is all of these characteristics together that are viewed as pathological.

Speculation about why lesbian relationships show greater fusion than heterosexual or gay male relationships generally describes two factors. Krestan and Bepko (1980) view lesbian fusion as the couple's response to the situating of a lesbian relationship in a homophobic culture. In constant contact with a culture which ignores, denies, invalidates, pathologizes, and attempts to destroy lesbian relationships, the partners bond together in a "two-against-the-world" posture. In Krestan and Bepko's view, fusion is an attempt—though misguided and ultimately self-destructive, they believe—to respond to the culture's diluting of the relationship externally by concentrating and reconstituting togetherness internally. Fusion may help the partners to develop the sense of "relationship constancy" that society usually bolsters for heterosexual couples, but badly batters for lesbian couples (Pearlman, 1988).

Others locate the source of lesbian fusion in the gender differences of pre-Oedipal relational life (Burch, 1982, 1985, 1986, 1987; Lindenbaum, 1985; Lowenstein, 1980). They argue that fusion is a consequence of the presence of two women in the lesbian dyad. Leaning heavily on the work of Chodorow (1978), they assert that while all erotic relationships involve a yearning for replication of the unity of the mother-infant dyad, only heterosexual men and lesbian women can hope to recall that primary connection in their adult romantic rela-

tionships because only heterosexual men and lesbian women are involved with women. In order to develop with a sense of maleness,
boys must develop defenses which enable them "to individuate" and
to separate from the mother–child connection. On the other hand, girls
can develop while remaining attached to their "primary love objects."
Ultimately, adult males end up with greater skills in separating and
distancing, while adult females end up with greater skills in connecting and empathizing.

According to these authors, a man in a heterosexual relationship
may begin to re-experience the merger of the mother–infant relationship, but he can readily employ the familiar defenses against merger
which are quickly aroused in him. (Parenthetically, men's defenses
against merger with mother may significantly contribute to male
misogyny and male avoidance of intense intimacy.) In contrast, a
woman brings to her relationship with another woman a set of skills
in connection without the man's highly developed defenses against
the recollection of mother-infant merger. Because both partners are
women, there is an unstymied regressive pull, according to this argument, toward fusion.

Framing the sources of fusion in these particular ways contributes
to these authors' assumptions that fusion is inherently pathological,
maladaptive, or dysfunctional. Fusion as a response to oppression is
then seen as a necessary evil, a consequence of homophobia from
which lesbians must free themselves. The long-standing psychoanalytic tradition that views sustained regression as inimical to healthy
development enables the psychodynamic explanation of lesbian fusion to serve as sufficient justification for the inherent harm of fusion.
These observers of lesbian relationships point to the isolation of the
couple, rigidity of relational patterns and roles, diminished tolerance
for individual differences, and the lack of opportunity for the development of individual identity as the inevitable and dangerous consequences of fusion.

There is ample evidence in the literature of lesbian psychology to
suggest that the patterns of intimacy of lesbian couples are different
from those of heterosexual and gay male relationships, and that many
of these distinctive features have been pathologized by labeling them
as fusion. However, as the literature stacks up to argue that what is
called fusion is inherently pathological, I believe that we see these
commentators doing to lesbians what we so often (and so accurately)
accuse traditional theorists and clinicians of doing to women: Similar
to the ways in which traditional psychology has failed to examine
what is normative for women and consequently has found pathology
in women when measured by male norms, so the literature on fusion

fails to examine what is normative for lesbians and finds pathology in lesbians when measured by male and heterosexual norms. It is erroneous to assume that lesbian relationships will follow heterosexual patterns, especially when we are confronted with the evidence—i.e., that fusion is so prevalent—that they do not. These authors may be putting the cart before the horse, highlighting the pathological before we have adequately determined what is normative for lesbians.

In fact, empirical data suggests that the prevalence of the relational dynamics that have been called fusion do not necessarily create pathology or dysfunction in lesbian relationships. Several studies have found that lesbians express a high degree of satisfaction in their relationships, and account for this satisfaction by crediting the by-products of intense intimacy—equality, companionship, the connection between friendship and love, and the valuing, by both partners, of communication and emotional support, many of the features which have been interpreted as fusion (McCandlish, 1982; Moses, 1978; Vetere, 1982).

In 1984, I examined lesbian relationship patterns in a small, qualitative study of well-functioning, stable lesbian couples (Mencher, 1984). Based on a series of individual and couple interviews with six women in relationships of six to eight years, my study differed from existing work on fusion by taking a detailed look at a nonclinical sample. A critical finding was that these satisfying, enduring lesbian relationships were characterized by fusion—but that these patterns did not cause the couples particular disturbance. In fact, the women interviewed accounted for the success of their relationships by naming as relational advantages the very same traits which often are labeled fusion. The intense closeness of the partners and the placement of the relationship as an axis around which their lives turned were cited as significant advantages of these relationships. Contrary to the idea that fusion limits the growth of individual identity, these women conveyed that the intense intimacy creates the trust and safety which foster self-actualization and risk-taking. For these women, the intimacy patterns that some would call fusion promoted a sense of security and faith in the relationship, and assurance that the women would be accompanied along life's journeys.

In an interesting study of eighteen heterosexual women's valued female friendships, Berzoff (1990) found that the four women who described an experience of fused self-other boundaries with a close female friend are the same four women who tested at the highest levels of ego development in the sample—that the healthiest women were those who described experiences of fusion.

These studies suggest that what has been identified as fusion may not be inherently disturbing to women and may indeed be both normative and growth-enhancing for lesbian couples. Confusion about both the function of fusion and the malignancy of fusion has resulted in a spate of articles which direct clinicians to prescribe separation and differentiation to their lesbian clients. In doing so, these authors ignore the vital use of fusion as a strategy to cope with homophobia, and fail to consider the syntonicity of fusion and women's preference for certain relational structures.

At times, fusion has been a creative and useful strategy employed by lesbians to strengthen a sense of couplehood and to fight active and passive cultural resistance to the lesbian relationship. Slater (1989) notes that it is the lesbian couples who fail to create this compensatory fusion whose relationships are at risk. She argues that if the outside pressure for the couple to act as separate, disconnected individuals is supplemented by one of the women fearing this level of connectedness, the couple will fail to generate sufficient cohesiveness and will separate. The existence of the couple within the context of a homophobic society is one source of fusion in lesbian relationships, and provides one way to understand how fusion is functional for lesbian women.

In the remainder of this chapter, I will focus on the question of why fusion is a relational pattern which particularly characterizes an intimate dyad composed of two women. I believe that women's development is the principal source of lesbians' tendency towards fusion, and that fusion may function constructively as a relational pattern which allows women to express their relational strengths. Before we begin to rework the notion of fusion, it is necessary first to understand its underpinnings in classical psychoanalytic theory, and how fusion came to acquire a pathological reputation. At that point, we can utilize new understandings of women's development to rework our understanding of the malignant nature of fusion. Finally, we will discuss how this examination of lesbian fusion informs our understanding of more generically female patterns of intimacy.

TRADITIONAL VIEWS OF FUSION

Traditional psychodynamic theory, particularly object relations theory, depicts psychic life as beginning in fusion and proceeding as a struggle against an intense desire to return to this state of blissful merger. The individual throughout life longs for and searches for a union with a "symbiotic love object" that will recall the primary relationship with mother. This longing continually alternates with the "fear of re-engulfment which threatens the personal identity and entity of the individual. The longing for union and fear of re-engulfment is the basic conflict of human existence" (Pacella, 1980, p. 117).

This merger (momentary as it is before a fear of engulfment sets in) is the primal relational configuration from which further object relations develop. According to theorists such as Fairbairn (1952), Guntrip (1969), and Mahler (1975), the merged relational matrix of mother and infant is the vital prerequisite for the healthy development which ensues (we might say, paradoxically) from the child's separation from this matrix.

Mahler goes on to describe a series of stages in the child's separation and individuation from this primary relational matrix, from union with the mother (1975). In this scheme, the goal of development is separation from the fused state of infancy. Although the object relations theorists focus on pre-Oedipal relationships, the Oedipal crisis, as articulated in the psychoanalytic literature, is viewed as a further developmental push towards separation, away from intense intimacy with mother. Development proceeds as a series of successive disengagements from the primary, merged attachment with mother and progressive delineations of individual boundaries and personal autonomy.

According to this theory, erotic adult relationships involve transitory but precious moments of fusion, moments which recapitulate—however briefly—the early fused relationship with mother. The essence of what is called "mature love" consists of the ability to experience fusion in these moments, and only momentarily. Fusion as a sustained relational pattern is seen as taboo. Erikson (1963, 1968) insists that the experience of true intimacy requires that the individual has successfully negotiated an adolescent process of building a firmly delineated identity with strong individual boundaries. These strong boundaries and firm identity will enable the individual to withstand the momentary fusion experiences that characterize intimacy, without threat of ego loss. In contrast, Erikson describes adolescent love as "an attempt to arrive at a definition of one's identity by projecting one's diffused self-image on another and by seeing it thus reflected and gradually clarified" (Erikson, 1968, p. 132).

Likewise, Kernberg (1976, 1980) believes that mature love involves the ability to re-experience fusion without loss of self. For Kernberg, individual identity consolidation and increasing individuation of self from "object" are the goals of development. When successfully accomplished, the individual can experience without harm the crossing of the of boundaries of the self that characterize what Kernberg calls "mature love."

The psychoanalytic literature views infancy as the sole province of the fulfillment of yearnings for fusion. These theorists depict the momentary recapitulations of fusion in adult erotic relationships as the pay-off for the individual's successful repudiation of infantile merger and successful disengagement from the mother–child dyad.

However, both Erikson and Kernberg are clear that their descriptions of the pathways of healthy development have only limited applications. After constructing a developmental theory without reference to gender and thus with implied universal application, Erikson (1968) parenthetically adds that for women development may proceed differently. He states that the determination of female identity remains incomplete until a woman engages in an intimate relationship, that she evolves identity within a relational context (based on the man she marries). Lest we begin to build enthusiasm for Erikson as the precursor of the self-in-relation perspective, it is important to remember that Erikson's parenthetical observations of the confluence of female identity and involvement in intimate relationships did not motivate him to alter his developmental scheme nor to make significant gender distinctions about what constitutes healthy development. For our purposes, the extreme similarity between Erikson's definition of "adolescent love" and his description of female patterns of intimacy and identity is eloquent.

The juxtaposition of Erikson's comments on love and those on female development suggests that he believes young women to be incapable of mature love, since they do not bring a firmly established identity to intimate relationships, but instead rely upon intimate relationships to shape their identities. Thus, for Erikson, female development may be necessarily delayed or impaired.

Kernberg's explanation of how two individuals in a mature love relationship can experience fusion without ego loss also illustrates the limited application of this theoretical perspective. Discussing heterosexual relationships only, Kernberg contends that the couple maintains individual boundaries in the midst of moments of crossing boundaries by creating individually, "elements of secrecy and mystery" (Kernberg, 1980). The secrecy and mystery derive from the recollection of the Oedipal constellation in the adult relationship, a recollection made possible by virtue of the fact that it is a man and woman who are joining in an intimate dyad. It is probable that the Oedipal constellation would not be recalled in the same way in an intimate dyad of two women; thus, the elements of secrecy and mystery would not be present to protect the couple from (what Kernberg calls) "uncontrolled intimacy," what we might call sustained fusion.

Indeed, it can be postulated that, in traditional psychoanalytic terms, a pre-Oedipal constellation would be more likely to be recalled in an intimate relationship between two women. While, according to psychoanalytic theory, the re-enacted Oedipal constellation for a female may recall issues of separateness and differentness from a male which prevents patterns of sustained fusion in normative heterosexual relationships, the pre-Oedipal constellation may recall issues of primary oneness and female identification which promotes sustained fusion in normative lesbian relationships. Whatever the explanation, it is clear that Oedipal regression has been viewed as desirable, while pre-Oedipal regression has been seen as dangerous.

From this brief review, we can see that the psychoanalytic literature views adult fusion as pathological because it illustrates impaired development of the self and immature or regressed object relations. This summary, however, also raises the likelihood—indeed, the normative expectation—that women will evolve identity within a relational matrix and that intimate dyads of two women will normatively be characterized by fusion. In order to move on from the traditional literature's pathologizing of these normative female relational patterns, we must examine more recent, female-centered theories of women's development.

FUSION AND WOMEN'S DEVELOPMENT

The fusion-as-pathology arguments rest on three basic assertions: First, life begins in a state of symbiotic merger with mother. Second, development consists of a series of progressive disengagements from this (and subsequent) relationships; ". . . we start in a state of dual oneness and wind up in a state of singular oneness" (Benjamin, 1988, p. 18). Third, fusion in adulthood represents regression to an infantile state of merger and must therefore be held at bay. Recent revisions in developmental theory, revisions which attempt to correct the male and (male-based) separation bias of traditional theory, resoundingly critique these three assertions.

Infant research in the past decade, particularly the work of Stern (1985), has substantially refuted the notion that infancy is a state of unity with mother. Contrary to the notion of mother–infant symbiosis, Stern presents evidence to suggest that even the newborn is "primed" to be interested in others and to experience itself as distinct from others.

We have only begun to understand how Stern's and others' findings about the absence of mother–infant merger alter psychoanalytic notions of development, separation, dependency, regression, health, intimacy, and fusion. In her provocative book, *The Bonds of Love*, Benjamin (1988) begins to articulate a theory of "intersubjectivity" which is partially based on Stern's findings:

> Once we accept the idea that infants do not begin life as part of an undifferentiated unity, the issue is not only how we separate from oneness, but also how we connect to and recognize others; the issue is not how we become free of the other, but how we actively engage and make ourselves known in relationship to the other. (p. 18)

Stern (1985), Surrey (1985), Jordan (1986), and Benjamin (1988) all question the very telling language of psychoanalytic thought, the language of subject and object, of the doer and the done-to, in which the child is subject and the mother is object, which has grown out of an "infantocentric" view of mother-infant merger. Instead, as Benjamin asserts, the dyad of the mother and the social infant who can respond to and distinguish others represents not a oneness which is destined to be separated into subject and object; but that of subject and subject. The intersubjective view is different from the intrapsychic view in that it "reorients the conception of the psychic world from a subject's relations to its object towards a subject meeting another subject" (Benjamin, 1988, p. 20). It emphasizes what happens "in the field of self and other," in the connective space between two individuals, rather than emphasizing the internal, intrapsychic field of internalizations.

If we view the mother–infant relationship within an intersubjective frame, we remove it from the symbiotic matrix of oneness, total dependency, and total selflessness (of both infant and mother); it is no longer a relationship to be forsaken, either through separation or through internalization.

The contributions of Stern and Benjamin to refute the notion of the blissful merger of infancy have profound implications for the psychoanalytic view of development. If development consists of a series of separations from the primary fused relational matrix of infancy, if all subsequent relationships involve the negotiation of the essential life dilemma between the yearning for fusion and the terror of engulfment, then what happens to our view of development if we radically alter our ideas of that primary relationship? If we pull the main thread, does the whole fabric unravel? How does a different understanding of how we begin life alter our understanding of how development proceeds? In examining the second assertion on which the fusion-as-pathology argument is based—that development consists of a series of separations—it is helpful to turn to the relational perspective of the Stone Center (Jordan, 1984, 1986; Kaplan, 1984; Miller, 1984, 1986, 1988; Stiver, 1984; Surrey, 1985, 1987). In proposing new models of female development, the theory group of the Stone Center begins to offer clues as to why the intimacy patterns of lesbians differ, and why they differ particularly in the direction of fusion.

In shifting the emphasis from *separation* to *relationship* as the basis for women's self-experience and development, the relational perspective complements Stern's assertion that life begins in a relational template. According to this perspective, for women, "The primary experience of the self is relational; the self is organized and developed in the context of important relationships" (Surrey, 1985). The primary emotional motive for women is to seek a relational process. The goal of development is the increasing ability to build and to enlarge mutually enhancing relationships. The pathway toward this goal involves what Surrey (1985) has termed *relationship differentiation,* a process of differentiation in the embryological sense—in which the individual articulates increasing levels of complexity, fluidity, choice, and satisfaction in her constellation of relationships. Women's development, in this scheme, hinges neither on the assertion of difference of self from other, nor on a lessening degree of need for or connection to the other. The ongoing actual relational process between self and other, between subject and subject, is critical, along with the internalization of intrapyschic relational images.

Based on these notions of the goals of women's development, the relational perspective redefines what constitutes a healthy adult relationship. Unlike Kernberg and Erikson, who measure healthy adult relationships by the "individual-ness" of the two selves, the Stone Center theorists mark healthy relationships by the quality of the relational processes. They view mutual engagement, mutual empathy, and mutual empowerment as the fundamental processes of a healthy relationship. A key feature is relational authenticity.

Mutual engagement—the capacity, in both people, for attention and interest—is illustrated by a comment from Adrienne, one of the subjects in my 1984 study of lesbian couples:

> [I get] so many things from the relationship]. I can validate myself as a caring, giving, loving person through her. And I certainly receive all those things when I need to receive them. I get companionship, the sharing of experiences together, the freedom of being able to express anything I need to—there doesn't have to be a filtering system there. (Mencher, 1984, p. 118)

Mutual empathy refers to being attuned to and responsive to the subjective, inner experience of the other, and the capacity to share in and comprehend the momentary psychological state of the other person. Mutual empathy requires neither sameness nor differentness, but can exist in either case.

JESSE: "I would say that the effects of homophobia and having to be closeted are that they just bring us closer. It's the subtle homophobia—assumptions of heterosexuality. [Laurie] and I understand that immediately and share without any questions at all." (Mencher, 1984, p. 107)

KATHLEEN: "She lets me be who I am even if it's not her. And if she doesn't understand it, she lets me be in those ways. She encourages me to go with those places that are different from her." (Mencher, p. 98)

ADRIENNE: "She's never not understood me. We're usually able to talk and talk." (Mencher, p. 103)

Mutual empowerment consists of the mutual capacity to be moved by, respond to, and move the other. Even when interviewed separately, Kathleen and Cory described with remarkable similarity how the intimacy of their couple relationship has moved them each towards growth.

KATHLEEN: "I think that lesbian relationships allow for a lot more expansion. My relationship is what has allowed me to change so much in this period of time and to allow [Cory] to change and grow." (Mencher, 1984, p. 105)

CORY: "This relationship provides me with a safety and sustenance. When people feel safe, they learn, grow, and change. Since the relationship is so safe, I've been able to change. I've allowed myself to be more inward, to feel painful feelings, and to show them in ways that I couldn't before. . . . When I'm loved, I know I can love myself better. . . . It's a very life-affirming relationship." (Mencher, pp. 105–106)

Relational authenticity is the ongoing challenge to feel emotionally real, connected, vital, clear, and purposeful in relationship.

JOAN: "I would be who I am without her, but I am certainly more complete with her." (Mencher, 1984, p. 101)

JESSE: "In being together, both of us have been able to become who we really were all along. . . . We've really helped each other become something that we're comfortable with. (Mencher, p. 105)

These are the comments of women in lesbian relationships which exhibited marked patterns of what is traditionally viewed as fusion. I present these comments within a discussion of the relational perspective's definitions of the features of a healthy relationship in order to suggest the following: If we identify norms for relational structures which are based on women's developmental experience, then some of the features of lesbian relationships that have been described as fusion—e.g., intense intimacy, acute sensitivity to the inner emotional world of the other, and the embeddedness of individual identity within the relationship—these features lose their pejorative connotation. Instead, these intimacy patterns in lesbian relationships appear to be the likely result of two women—both of whom have travelled developmental pathways marked by movement toward connection—coming together in an intimate erotic pairing. Contrary to the notion that these relational patterns indicate something gone awry, these patterns may indicate movement toward the fulfillment of women's preferences for relational structures which feature mutual engagement, mutual empathy, mutual empowerment, and relational authenticity.

In discussing fusion as pathology in lesbian relationships without first identifying the normative patterns of intimacy, researchers and clinicians may have unwittingly pathologized women's ways of being and loving. An examination of intimacy patterns in lesbian couples may allow us to understand a bit more about how women experience themselves and their relationships when that experience is unfettered by the different intimacy patterns of men and by patriarchal assumptions about how women should love. Whereas the presence of men may, as Erikson and Kernberg describe, bring to heterosexual pairings a movement toward individuation and away from intense sustained intimacy, a similar pushing-against women's preference for connection does not exist in a lesbian dyad.

Certainly, this does not indicate that either the heterosexual pattern or the lesbian pattern is better or worse than the other; they each have their possibilities and problems, to be sure. I am suggesting, simply, that the lesbian pattern—a more fused pattern—is not inherently disturbed and that the lesbian pattern may further explicate women's relational patterns in general. In a relationship in which both partners, as women, are consistently directed toward connection, there can exist a full range of possibility for mutuality, empathy, and authenticity.

CONCLUSION

In closing, I'd like to refer again to Benjamin for her comments on how psychoanalytic thought may have distorted our understandings of intimacy:

> The classic psychoanalytic viewpoint did not see differentiation as a balance, but as a process of disentanglement. Thus it cast experiences of

union, merger, and self-other harmony as regressive opposites to differentiation and self-other distinction. Merging was a dangerous form of
undifferentiation, a sinking back into the sea of oneness—the "oceanic
feeling" that Freud told Romain Rolland he frankly couldn't relate to.
The original sense of oneness was seen as absolute, as "limitless narcissism," and, therefore, regression to it would impede development and
prevent separation. In its most extreme version, this view of differentiation pathologized the sensation of love: relaxing the boundaries of the
self in communion with others threatened the identity of the isolate self.
(Benjamin, 1988, pp. 46–47)

The actualization of the self and the intense intimacy of a relationship need not be mutually exclusive. As Jordan (1984) suggests, there
may exist a paradox of empathy: by joining in an intimate connection,
self and other may become more accurately articulated. As a woman,
the more I feel connected, the more I feel myself.

The dichotomizing of "oneness" and "separation" offers a distorted vision of relational life—which Miller (1990) suggests arises from
male theorists' difficulties in conceptualizing true relatedness. Within
this dichotomous vision, oneness is associated as mother and as female, while separation is associated as father and as male. If men control the world, it's not difficult to guess which part of the dichotomy
will be idealized and which will be pathologized.

In this chapter, I have attempted to re-examine traditional notions
of fusion. I have tried to understand how the pathologizing of what
have been viewed as more fused patterns of intimacy represents a
pathologizing of lesbians' ways of loving in particular and of women's
ways of loving in general. I have used the word *fusion* tonight within
an attempt to de-pathologize some of the behaviors and dynamics it
describes and to assert that fusion may represent a relational pattern
which allows women to express our relational strengths. However, in
the state of distortion and bias which surrounds fusion in the literature, it may be impossible to de-toxify the term and to relieve it of malignant connotations.

Instead, we might substitute a nonpejorative word, such as *embeddedness*, to describe the situating of women's identity within relationships. According to the *Oxford English Dictionary, to embed* means "to
fix firmly in a surrounding mass of some solid material" (Murray et
al., 1933, p. 106). For women, the relational world is made of solid material. The use of embeddedness bypasses the confusion and inaccura-
cy of the word fusion. Embeddedness as a description of healthy relational involvement acknowledges the normative developmental needs
and intimacy patterns of women and revises the traditional standards
of autonomy and separation which are so male-derived. The use of a

nonpejorative term, such as embeddedness, may enable us to view relational patterns which differ from the prescribed heterosexual norm without foregone conclusions about the pathology.

It is critical to examine our fundamental assumptions about love before we move to a critique of certain patterns of intimacy. These assumptions have arisen from the male experience of separation and the heterosexual experience of difference and distance within relationship. We must re-assess whether these notions resonate with the experience of women. In critiquing how lesbians tend to love, I am afraid that some have depreciated how most women would prefer to love—with mutuality, with trust, with passion, with empathy—with abandon.

DISCUSSION SUMMARY

A discussion was held after each colloquium presentation. Selected portions of the discussion are summarized here. At this session Carolyn Dillon (Clinical Professor, Boston University School of Social Work), Alexandra Kaplan, Jean Baker Miller, Lourdes Rodriguez (Counseling Psychologist, Simmons College), and Irene Stiver joined Julie Mencher in leading the discussion.

Question: Is fusion related to decreased sexual activity in long-term lesbian relationships? Did you find that in your 1984 study?

Mencher: I did not measure my subjects' levels of sexual activity, but I do have some ideas about decreased sexual activity in long-term lesbian relationships. First, we have to remember that as lesbians we have not been taught how to be sexual with our partners. Heterosexual women are taught from an early age, implicitly and explicity, how to carry on sexual relationships with men. But as lesbians, no one taught us how to date, how to be sexually aggressive, how to initiate sex, etc. So, I think that may have something to do with many lesbians not being able to sustain eroticism past that initial period of wild passion. Secondly, since such a high percentage of women have been sexually abused as children, and since the consequences of child sexual abuse are often reflected in adult sexual activity, there is an increased likelihood that two women coming together in an intimate dyad will reflect those difficulties.

Rodriguez: It occurs to me that lesbian relationships reflect the psychology of an oppressed people. Sometimes internalized homophobia and internalized self-hate are played out in the sexual context.

Comment: We need to look at the definition of sexuality, just as we have to look at the definitions of fusion and intimacy.

Kaplan: We need to think about lesbian relationships in relation to what? In relation to heterosexual relationships? One way to turn it around is to say that in the heterosexual culture, the level of sexual activity (who knows what it is?) is heavily determined by the men. Maybe that's the aberration. Maybe lesbians have found the level of sexual activity that is comfortable. We shouldn't think of that level as something that we have to excuse, vis-à-vis the other.

Dillon: There's so much homophobia in the culture. It's very hard to come home to the couple and feel sexy when what you really want to do first is to discharge the conflicts, tensions, disempowerments, devaluations, slight remarks, avoidances of the day.

Mencher: Many lesbian women spend their days pretending that they are not lesbian women, confronting homophobia with that kind of silence. The cumulative effect of this may, as Carolyn and Lourdes have stated, affect lesbians' interest in making love.

Stiver: The notion of reframing sexuality, just as Julie has reframed fusion, is not a small matter. Women don't want to talk about it. We are often obliged to accept a male understanding of sexuality. Women have had male sexuality imposed upon them so much, that they believe they have to accept this view or they will reveal themselves as defective or inadequate in some powerful, central way. This makes it difficult to develop and explore one's sexuality in a free kind of way—for all women, but particularly for lesbians. We have had a sexuality imposed on us that doesn't feel congenial. We haven't felt the freedom to explore our sexuality.

Also, I want to comment on what you have implied about fusion: that men are so cut off from the opportunity to experience connection with their mothers that they "romanticize" the yearned-for state of symbiosis (that has nothing to do with what was). Thus, they see it as a paradise that they long to return to but are terrified of. Then, the male theorists develop and present a theory which devalues and makes one horrified of the longing and fantasy that men carry into adulthood.

Miller: The basic theory is a male-made-up notion, about the life of mothers and babies that never existed. It has to do with this culture's lack of understanding of relationship. There's this notion of this so-called paradise of people sort of glommed together into a "oneness" or of separation—not a conception of the interplay, flow, and interaction that is relatedness.

Question: Can you comment on the experience of being multicultural from a lesbian perspective?

Rodriguez: There is a difference. As a Hispanic woman, I found validation for being Hispanic within my family, growing up. That's very different for lesbians and gay men, where identity formation and validation does not happen inside the family. That's why going inside ourselves, within the couple, and the community for that validation is so important.

Question: Is fusion another word for codependency?

Mencher: That is a really interesting question. I'd like that topic to be my next paper. I think that the feminist critique on codependency has yet to be written. We need a gender-based analysis of codependency to really understand if what is being called codependency is pathology or caring.

Question: I wonder if you can comment on what would be a more accurate understanding of women's sexuality.

Mencher: I can't possibly. The point that several panelists have made tonight is that because men have always been in control of women's sexuality, we don't know what women would want sexually if we weren't schooled in those male-derived norms.

I hope that we all can collectively define what women's sexuality is, both for heterosexual and lesbian women.

REFERENCES

Benjamin, J. (1988). *The bonds of love: Psychoanalysis, feminism, and the problem of domination.* New York: Pantheon.

Berzoff, J. (1990). Fusion and women's friendships: Implications for expanding our adult developmental theories. *Women and Therapy, 8,* 93–107.

Burch, B. (1982). Psychological merger in lesbian couples: A joint ego psychological and systems approach. *Family Therapy, 9,* 201–208.

Burch, B. (1985). Another perspective on merger in lesbian relationships. In L. B. Rosewater & L. E. A. Walker (Eds.), *Handbook of feminist therapy: women's issues in psychotherapy.* New York: Springer.

Burch, B. (1986). Psychotherapy and the dynamics of merger in lesbian couples. In T. S. Stein & C. J. Cohen (Eds.), *Contemporary perspectives on psychotherapy with lesbians and gay men.* New York: Plenum.

Burch, B. (1987). Barriers to intimacy: Conflicts over power, dependency, and nurturing in lesbian relationships. In Boston Lesbian Psychologies Collective (Eds.), *Lesbian psychologies.* Urbana: University of Illinois.

Chodorow, N. (1978). *The reproduction of mothering: Psychoanalysis and the sociology of gender.* Berkeley: University of California.

Decker, B. (1983–1984). Counseling gay and lesbian couples. *Journal of Social Work and Human Sexuality, 2,* 39–52.

Elise, D. (1986). Lesbian couples: The implications of sex differences in separation-individuation. *Psychotherapy, 23,* 305–310.

Erikson, E. (1963). *Childhood and society.* New York: Norton.

Erikson, E. (1968). *Identity: Youth and crisis.* New York: Norton.

Fairbairn, W. R. D. (1952). *Object relations theory of personality.* London: Tavistock.

Guntrip, H. (1969). *Schizoid phenomenon, object relations and the self.* New York: International University.

Jordan, J. (1984). *Empathy and self-boundaries.* (Work in Progress No. 16.) Wellesley, MA: Stone Center Working Paper Series.

Jordan, J. (1986). *The meaning of mutuality.* (Work in Progress No. 23.) Wellesley, MA: Stone Center Working Paper Series.

Kaplan, A. (1984). *The "self-in-relation": Implications for depression in women.* (Work in Progress No. 14.) Wellesley, MA: Stone Center Working Paper Series.

Karpel, M. (1976). Individuation: From fusion to dialogue. *Family Process, 15*(1), 65–82.

Kaufman, P. A., Harrison, E. H., & Hyde, M. L. (1984). Distancing for intimacy in lesbian relationships. *American Journal of Psychiatry, 141,* 530–533.

Kernberg, O. (1976). *Object-relations theory and clinical psychoanalysis.* New York: Jason Aronson.

Kernberg, O. (1980). *Internal world and external reality: Object relations theory applied.* New York: Jason Aronson.

Krestan, J., & Bepko, C. S. (1980). The problem of fusion in the lesbian relationship. *Family Process, 19,* 277–289.

Lindenbaum, J. (1985). The shattering of an illusion: The problem of competition in lesbian relationships. *Feminist Studies, 11*(1), 85–103.

Lowenstein, S. F. (1980). Understanding lesbian women. *Social Casework, 61*(1), 29–38.

Mahler M. (1975). *The psychological birth of the human infant: Symbiosis and individuation.* New York: Basic Books.

McCandlish, B. M. (1982). Therapeutic issues with lesbian couples. *Journal of homosexuality, 7*(2/3), 71–78.

Mencher, J. (1984). Changing the lens on female personality development: A challenge to the notion of fusion in lesbian relationships. Unpublished master's thesis, Smith College School for Social Work, Northampton, MA.

Miller, J. B. (1984). *The development of women's sense of self.* (Work in Progress No. 12.) Wellesley, MA: Stone Center Working Papers Series.

Miller, J. B. (1986). *What do we mean by relationships?* (Work in Progress No. 22.) Wellesley, MA: Stone Center Working Papers Series.

Miller, J. B. (1988). *Connections, disconnections, and violations.* (Work in Progress No. 33.) Wellesley, MA: Stone Center Working Papers Series.

Miller, J. B. Personal communication. January, 1990.

Moses, A. E. (1978). *Identity management in lesbian women.* New York: Praeger.

Murray, J. A. H., Bradley, H., Craigie, W. A., & Onions, C. T. (Eds.). (1933). *Oxford English Dictionary* (Vols. III–IV). Oxford: Clarendon.

Pacella, B. L. (1980). The primal matrix configuration. In R. F. Lax, S. Bach, & J. A. Burland (Eds.), *Rapprochement: The critical subphase of separation-individuation* (pp. 117–131). New York: Jason Aronson.

Pearlman, S. F. (1988). Distancing and connectedness: Impact on couple forma-
    tion in lesbian relationships. *Women & Therapy, 8(1/2),* 77-88.

Roth, S. (1985). Psychotherapy with lesbian couples: Individual issues, female
    socialization, and the social context. *Journal of Marital and Family Therapy,*
    11, 273–286.

Schneider, M. S. (1986). The relationships of cohabiting lesbian and heterosex-
    ual couples: A comparison. *Psychology of Women Quarterly, 10,* 234-239.

Slater, S. Personal communication. August, 1989.

Smalley, S. (1987). Dependency issues in lesbian relationships. *Journal of homo-*
    sexuality, 14, 125–135.

Stern, D. (1985). *The interpersonal world of the infant: A view from psychoanalysis*
    and developmental psychology. New York: Basic Books.

Stiver, I. (1984). *The meaning of "dependency" in female-male relationships.* (Work
    in Progress No. 11.) Wellesley, MA: Stone Center Working Paper Series.

Surrey, J. (1985). *Self-in-relation: A theory of women's development.* (Work in
    Progress No. 13.) Wellesley, MA: Stone Center Working Paper Series.

Surrey, J. (1987). *Relationship and empowerment.* (Work in Progress No. 30.)
    Wellesley, MA: Stone Center Working Paper Series.

Vetere, V. A. (1982). The role of friendship in the development and mainte-
    nance of lesbian love relationships. *Journal of Homosexuality, 8(2),* 51–65.

This chapter was presented at a Stone Center Colloquium on February 7, 1990.
© 1990 Julie Mencher.

Index